Occupational Therapy and Women's Health

This innovative and comprehensive textbook provides a detailed exploration of the role of occupational therapy in addressing the unique needs of women across the lifespan.

Structured into 14 parts, the book begins with the foundations of women's health, delving into its historical evolution, the significance of gender equality in medical research, the implications of employment on women's well-being, intricate sociocultural influences, and the intersection of women and occupation from an occupational therapy perspective. Following this foundational context, the book journeys through diverse areas such as gynecological and obstetric health management, endocrine health, autoimmune conditions, non-cisgender health in the context of women's health, mental health and biopsychosocial aspects, cardiovascular health, sleep, weight, and lifestyle factors, oncology, neurological health, women's health across the lifespan, inter-partner violence and trauma-informed care, and special topics in women's health.

Women's health is a universal concern that transcends geographical boundaries, cultural differences, and socioeconomic disparities, and this important book will be key reading for both students and practitioners of occupational therapy.

Sabina Khan is a women's health specialist, occupational therapist, educator, researcher, leader, and advocate. Her research expertise spans the areas of women's health, neurological rehabilitation, trauma-informed care, and promoting diversity, equity, and inclusion in healthcare. She has published extensively on topics related to women's health and occupational therapy.

Occupational Therapy and Women's Health
A Practitioner Guide

Sabina Khan

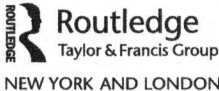

NEW YORK AND LONDON

Designed cover image: Shutterstock

First published 2025
by Routledge
605 Third Avenue, New York, NY 10158

and by Routledge
4 Park Square, Milton Park, Abingdon, Oxon, OX14 4RN

Routledge is an imprint of the Taylor & Francis Group, an informa business

© 2025 Sabina Khan

The right of Sabina Khan to be identified as author of this work has been asserted in accordance with sections 77 and 78 of the Copyright, Designs and Patents Act 1988.

All rights reserved. No part of this book may be reprinted or reproduced or utilised in any form or by any electronic, mechanical, or other means, now known or hereafter invented, including photocopying and recording, or in any information storage or retrieval system, without permission in writing from the publishers.

Trademark notice: Product or corporate names may be trademarks or registered trademarks, and are used only for identification and explanation without intent to infringe.

Library of Congress Cataloging-in-Publication Data
Names: Khan, Sabina (Occupational therapist), author.
Title: Occupational therapy and women's health : a practitioner guide / Sabina Khan.
Description: Abingdon, Oxon ; New York, NY : Routledge, 2025. | Includes bibliographical references and index. |
Identifiers: LCCN 2024040192 | ISBN 9781032934457 (hardback) | ISBN 9781032872520 (paperback) | ISBN 9781003531678 (ebook)
Subjects: MESH: Occupational Therapy | Women's Health
Classification: LCC RM735.3 | NLM WB 555 | DDC 615.8/515082--dc23/eng/20241122
LC record available at https://lccn.loc.gov/2024040192

ISBN: 978-1-032-93445-7 (hbk)
ISBN: 978-1-032-87252-0 (pbk)
ISBN: 978-1-003-53167-8 (ebk)

DOI: 10.4324/9781003531678

Typeset in Optima
by SPi Technologies India Pvt Ltd (Straive)

To my husband, Sattar; my daughters, Leila and Yasmin; my son, Adam. To my parents, Rana and Mohammad. To my clients, colleagues, and students over the years, and to the practitioners who strive to provide the best possible care in all settings.

Contents

List of Figures   *viii*
List of Tables   *ix*

1 Foundations of Women's Health in Occupational Therapy   1

2 Occupational Therapy in Gynecological Health Management   39

3 Occupational Therapy in Obstetric Health Management   87

4 Endocrine Health   155

5 Autoimmune Conditions   177

6 Non-Cisgender Health in the Context of Women's Health   203

7 Mental Health and Biopsychosocial Aspects   224

8 Cardiovascular Health   246

9 Sleep, Weight, and Lifestyle Factors in Women's Health   263

10 Oncology in Women's Health   290

11 Neurological Health in Women   317

12 Women's Health Across the Lifespan   339

13 Inter-Partner Violence and Trauma-Informed Care   370

14 Special Topics   388

Index   *421*

Figures

2.1	The bony pelvis	40
2.2	The male pelvis (left) compared to female (right) pelvis	41
2.3	The female external genitalia	44
2.4	The female internal reproductive organs	45
2.5	Female pelvic floor muscles	48
2.6	Pelvic floor strengthening exercises: (a) Glute bridge; (b) Squat; (c) Squat graded up with resistance band for adductor activation; (d) Plank; (e) Plank graded up with single leg raise	54
2.7	Pelvic floor relaxation exercises: (a) Seated adductor stretch; (b) Hip opening and pelvic alignment stretch; (c) Pregnant pelvic stretch and breathing exercise	55
3.1	Fluctuating hormone levels throughout pregnancy	89
3.2	Embryo developmental stages	92
3.3	Postural changes in pregnancy	94
3.4	Gender differences in neuroanatomy	94
3.5	Lobes of brain	95
3.6	Child carrying techniques: (a) Proper spinal alignment; (b) Hip carrying position: spinal misalignment	120
3.7	Stages of grief	139
5.1	Stages of rheumatoid arthritis	179
5.2	Symptoms of lupus	183
5.3	Symptoms of Hashimoto's	186
5.4	Normal villi and villi atrophy in celiac disease	191
7.1	Body changes during menopause	239
8.1	Cholesterol is a waxy substance in the blood	247
8.2	Reduced level of cholesterol plaque in blood vessels	252
9.1	Melatonin and cortisol fluctuations along circadian rhythm	265
10.1	Anatomy of the breast	292
10.2	Stages of breast cancer	294
10.3	Manual lymph drainage being performed on lower extremity (LE)	310
10.4	Compression bandaging on LE	311
12.1	Stages of menstrual cycle	340
13.1	Trauma response	373

Tables

1.1	Strategies for promoting gender equity in rehabilitation research	15
1.2	Gender disparities in the workplace	16
1.3	Role of the OTP in promoting women's health and well-being at work	18
1.4	Strategies for empowering women's professional development	19
1.5	Strategies for the OTP to build cultural competence	23
1.6	Considerations for addressing cultural factors in women's health interventions	24
1.7	Complexity levels in women's health occupational therapy evaluation, including CPT codes, descriptions, and examples	30
1.8	Comprehensive initial consultation checklist for women's health in occupational therapy	31
1.9	Common billing mistakes and mitigation strategies	37
2.1	The muscles of the pelvis	46
2.2	Pelvic floor muscle functions by gender assigned at birth	48
2.3	Do's and don'ts of an effective pelvic floor muscle exercise program	53
2.4	Types of pelvic pain and corresponding occupational therapy strategies	58
2.5	Pelvic floor pain assessments and contraindications	60
2.6	Functional assessment of the muscles of the pelvis	65
2.7	Manual muscle testing grading scale	66
2.8	Overview of occupational therapy considerations for key signs and symptoms in women's health	67
2.9	Common gynecological conditions and occupational therapy interventions	70
2.10	Postoperative rehabilitation and recovery considerations for gynecological surgeries	75
3.1	Key pregnancy hormones, their functions, and impact on daily activities	88
3.2	Fetal development stages and occupational therapy considerations	90
3.3	Physiological changes during pregnancy and their impact on body functions and occupational functioning	93
3.4	Comprehensive prenatal interventions by occupational therapy practitioners	98
3.5	First trimester exercises to enhance maternal comfort and prepare for labor	99
3.6	Second trimester strengthening and stability exercises	100
3.7	Third trimester preparatory exercises	101
3.8	Key areas of support by OTPs during the prenatal phase and their impact on occupational functioning	101
3.9	Key additional questions in OT evaluation for pregnant clients	104
3.10	Common musculoskeletal issues in pregnancy	107

3.11	Occupational therapy assessment tools for pregnant patients	110
3.12	Mental health and psychosocial assessment tools for pregnant patients	111
3.13	Assessment tools for pelvic floor health in occupational therapy	112
3.14	OT Interventions for common musculoskeletal issues in pregnancy	113
3.15	Trauma-informed assessment tools for OTPs	117
3.16	Adaptations for safe and comfortable playtime, childcare, and daily activities during pregnancy	119
3.17	Comprehensive occupational therapy interventions for labor and delivery	124
3.18	Labor positions and their adaptations for women with disabilities	125
3.19	Comparison of postpartum OT considerations for C-section and vaginal deliveries	126
3.20	Common pelvic floor rehabilitation interventions used by OTPs	130
3.21	Occupational therapy considerations for high-risk pregnancies	135
3.22	Strategies for high-risk pregnancies and specific occupational therapy interventions	138
4.1	Hormonal changes and symptoms across a woman's life	156
4.2	Key hormones in women's health, their primary functions, and considerations during occupational activities	157
4.3	Common endocrine conditions and associated hormonal imbalances, including associated symptoms that can affect daily functioning	158
4.4	Occupational therapy interventions in contraception and family planning	166
4.5	Comparative overview of perimenopause and menopause symptoms and their impact on daily living	168
5.1	Occupational therapy interventions for women with rheumatoid arthritis—Factors, interventions, descriptions, and considerations	180
5.2	Occupational therapy interventions for women with systemic lupus erythematosus (SLE)—Factors, interventions, descriptions, and considerations	184
5.3	Occupational therapy interventions for women with Hashimoto's thyroiditis—Factors, interventions, descriptions, and considerations	187
5.4	Occupational therapy interventions for women with celiac disease—Factors, interventions, descriptions, and considerations	192
6.1	Key terminology related to gender diversity	204
6.2	Effects and potential risks of hormone replacement therapy for transgender individuals	211
6.3	Strategies for creating safe and inclusive environments in rehabilitation for non-cisgender clients	213
6.4	Mental health and well-being interventions for non-cisgender clients	216
6.5	Gender affirming care examples	218
6.6	Gender-affirming care interventions for non-cisgender clients	219
7.1	Scenarios in sexual counseling for women's health, OT interventions, and their impact on mental health and biopsychosocial aspects	226
7.2	Strategies for empowering women in childbearing: Interventions and their impact on women's psychosocial health	231
7.3	Occupational therapy interventions for managing psychiatric symptoms during pregnancy and their impact on mental health and occupational participation	232
7.4	Infant cues indicating hunger and fullness	236

8.1	Key differences in heart disease between men and women and their implications for OT interventions	249
8.2	Common MET levels in cardiac rehabilitation and variations for women vs. men	250
8.3	Overview and considerations of high-risk populations for heart disease in women	256
9.1	Common sleep disorders in women	266
9.2	Assessments and interventions for sleep disorders in women	267
9.3	Common eating-related disorders in women	270
9.4	Factors contributing to obesity in women	272
9.5	Assessments and interventions for eating-related disorders and obesity	273
9.6	Assessments and interventions for promoting physical activity and healthy lifestyle choices	276
9.7	Assessments and interventions for substance use in women	280
10.1	TNM Staging of breast cancer	293
10.2	OT interventions for women with breast cancer	297
10.3	Staging of lung cancer using the TNM System	299
10.4	OT Interventions for women with lung cancer pre- and post-surgery	302
10.5	Staging of gynecological cancers	304
10.6	Pre-surgery and post-surgery interventions	306
11.1	Types of migraines	317
11.2	Phases of migraines, symptoms, and impacted occupations	318
11.3	Occupational therapy interventions for women with migraines	320
11.4	Types of stroke and relevance in women's health	320
11.5	Phases of stroke, symptoms, and changes in occupational performance	321
11.6	Occupational therapy interventions by phase	322
11.7	Types of multiple sclerosis and relevance in women's health	325
11.8	Phases of MS, symptoms, and changes in occupational performance	326
11.9	Occupational therapy interventions by phase	327
11.10	Types of Alzheimer's disease and relevance in women's health	330
11.11	Stages of Alzheimer's disease, symptoms, and changes in occupational performance	331
11.12	Occupational therapy interventions for women with Alzheimer's disease by stage	332
13.1	Common non-verbal cues indicative of trauma during an interview	374
13.2	Implementing trauma-informed practices in various OT settings	381
13.3	Actionable steps for OTPs to enhance cultural competence	384
14.1	OT techniques and assistive devices for performing breast self-examination (BSE) with limited mobility	389
14.2	Physiological differences impacting sports performance between women and men	394
14.3	Comparison of women with disabilities from birth vs. acquired disabilities	398
14.4	Nutritional needs and considerations across different life stages and conditions for women compared to men	401
14.5	Nutritional needs and considerations across different life stages and conditions for women compared to men	404
14.6	Contraindications for common alternative medicine practices	408

1 Foundations of Women's Health in Occupational Therapy

Chapter Objectives

Upon completion of this chapter, the reader will be able to:

1. Explain the importance of considering cultural, social, and economic factors in women's health and occupational therapy practice.
2. Identify key global regions with distinct healthcare challenges affecting women, and describe these challenges and their implications on women's health.
3. Discuss the historical development of women's healthcare and the evolution of occupational therapy's role in this field.
4. Evaluate the impact of employment and gender inequities on women's health and describe occupational therapy interventions that can mitigate these effects.
5. Analyze how occupational therapy practitioners can utilize culturally competent care practices to improve treatment outcomes in women's health.
6. Describe the importance of understanding the role of occupation in women's health and discuss strategies for integrating this understanding into occupational therapy practice.

Understanding Women's Health: A Global Perspective

Women's health is a universal concern that transcends geographical boundaries, cultural differences, and socioeconomic disparities. While the healthcare landscape varies significantly from one country to another, the fundamental importance of women's well-being remains constant. By examining disparities in healthcare access, outcomes, and cultural influences, we can gain a comprehensive understanding of the complex interplay between women's health and societal factors. When discussing women's health on a global scale, it is crucial to acknowledge that not all countries provide equal access to healthcare services or achieve similar health outcomes for women. Disparities in healthcare access and outcomes exist, and these discrepancies have profound implications for women's lives.

Several countries around the world face significant challenges in providing adequate healthcare for women. These challenges result from a complex interplay of factors, including limited resources, political instability, cultural norms, and gender inequality. In such countries, women's health outcomes often fall below international standards, with adverse consequences for maternal and reproductive health, as well as other aspects of well-being. Let's explore some of these regions and the specific challenges they encounter.

Sub-Saharan Africa

Sub-Saharan Africa is a region that grapples with profound healthcare challenges for women. High maternal mortality rates are a particularly concerning issue, often attributed to factors such as limited access to prenatal care, a lack of healthcare infrastructure, and sociocultural barriers. Women in this region face elevated risks during childbirth due to complications that are exacerbated by inadequate medical services. For example, obstetric fistulas, a severe childbirth-related injury, are more prevalent in Sub-Saharan Africa due to delayed or inadequate access to emergency obstetric care. Additionally, infectious diseases like HIV/AIDS disproportionately affect women in this region, further complicating their overall health and well-being.

South Asia

In countries like India and Pakistan, women encounter significant obstacles in accessing adequate healthcare services. Gender discrimination remains a pervasive issue, leading to disparities in healthcare access and outcomes. Maternal mortality rates are higher in South Asia compared to many other regions, primarily due to complications during pregnancy and childbirth. Anemia and malnutrition are prevalent among women, particularly those in lower socioeconomic strata. Limited access to education and healthcare information contributes to delayed or inadequate care-seeking behavior, impacting maternal and child health. Cultural norms surrounding early marriage and adolescent pregnancies also pose risks to young women's health.

Middle East and North Africa

Certain countries in the Middle East and North Africa (MENA) region grapple with healthcare challenges specific to their sociocultural contexts. Conservative cultural norms can restrict women's access to healthcare, particularly concerning reproductive health and family planning. In some instances, healthcare decisions may be influenced by male family members, limiting women's autonomy. This can lead to higher rates of maternal mortality, especially when women cannot make decisions about their own health or family planning. Additionally, the stigma around sexual and reproductive health discussions may discourage women from seeking necessary care.

Conflict Zones

Regions plagued by ongoing conflicts, such as Syria, Yemen, Palestine, and parts of Central Africa, present dire challenges to women's health. Conflict disrupts healthcare systems, leading to inadequate access to essential services, including maternal and reproductive healthcare. Displacement and insecurity further exacerbate these challenges, making it difficult for women to access medical facilities or receive proper care during pregnancy and childbirth. Violence against women, including sexual violence, becomes a heightened risk in such environments, causing severe physical and psychological trauma. The long-term consequences of conflict, such as malnutrition and mental health disorders, also disproportionately affect women in these areas.

Latin America and the Caribbean

In Latin America and the Caribbean, women encounter numerous healthcare challenges contributing to well-being disparities. Gender-based violence remains pervasive, posing immediate physical and mental health risks and inflicting long-term psychological trauma. Access to family planning services is inconsistent, especially in rural areas, leading to unintended pregnancies and limited reproductive choices, affecting autonomy. Healthcare quality varies widely across the region, exacerbating health outcome discrepancies, particularly in maternal and reproductive care. Maternal mortality rates fluctuate significantly, with indigenous and rural communities facing obstacles in accessing care due to geographic isolation and limited facilities. Cultural norms may influence healthcare-seeking behavior, with some relying on traditional birth attendants and home births, impacting maternal and child health. Addressing these challenges necessitates comprehensive efforts to combat gender-based violence, improve family planning access, and bolster healthcare infrastructure. Culturally sensitive practices respecting indigenous and rural traditions can mitigate healthcare disparities

Southeast Asia

Southeast Asia faces distinct healthcare challenges that impact women's well-being, particularly in countries like Myanmar and Cambodia. Limited healthcare resources and infrastructure can create significant barriers to accessing maternal and reproductive healthcare services, especially in remote areas. Women in these regions may have to travel long distances to reach healthcare facilities, and transportation options may be limited, making access to care difficult. Traditional practices, such as early marriages and home births, are prevalent in some communities. Early marriages can result in young girls becoming mothers before they are physically and emotionally prepared, leading to increased health risks for both mothers and infants. Home births, while culturally significant, can lack the necessary medical support and equipment, potentially resulting in poor maternal and child health outcomes. Inadequate access to skilled birth attendants and emergency obstetric care can further exacerbate these challenges. Complications during pregnancy and childbirth may not be promptly addressed, increasing the risk of maternal mortality and serious health issues for newborns. Efforts to improve women's healthcare in Southeast Asia must focus on expanding healthcare infrastructure, increasing access to skilled birth attendants, and promoting education on the importance of delaying early marriages and ensuring safe birthing practices. These efforts should be sensitive to the cultural contexts of the communities they serve.

Eastern Europe

Some Eastern European countries face distinct healthcare challenges that impact women's health, particularly in the context of low birth rates and limited access to infertility treatment. Low birth rates can have demographic implications, but they also reflect societal changes and women's choices regarding family planning. Limited access to infertility treatment can be a significant concern for couples struggling with fertility issues. In some

Eastern European countries, the availability and affordability of infertility treatments such as in vitro fertilization (IVF) may be restricted, limiting the options for couples seeking to start a family. Additionally, disparities in contraceptive access and education can impact family planning. Access to contraception may vary depending on location and socioeconomic status, affecting women's ability to make informed choices about their reproductive health. Comprehensive sex education can be limited in some regions, leading to gaps in knowledge about family planning options and sexual health. Efforts to address these challenges in Eastern Europe should include policies aimed at improving access to infertility treatment, promoting comprehensive sex education, and ensuring equitable access to contraception. These efforts can empower women and couples to make informed decisions about their reproductive health.

Oceania and the Pacific Islands

Women in remote Pacific Island nations often face unique barriers to accessing healthcare. Geographical isolation, limited healthcare infrastructure, and a lack of healthcare professionals can make it challenging for women to access essential services. High rates of cervical cancer in some regions of Oceania and the Pacific Islands underscore the need for improved screening and treatment. Limited access to regular Pap smears and human papillomavirus (HPV) vaccinations can contribute to higher rates of cervical cancer. Addressing this issue requires strengthening cervical cancer screening programs, increasing awareness, and ensuring access to vaccines and treatment. Efforts to improve women's healthcare in this region should focus on expanding healthcare infrastructure, training healthcare professionals, and implementing public health campaigns to raise awareness about preventable diseases like cervical cancer. Additionally, initiatives to address geographical barriers, such as telehealth services, can help improve access to care for women living in remote areas.

The Global Significance of Women's Health Disparities

Addressing women's health disparities on a global scale is not only a matter of social justice but also a matter of public health and human rights. When women's health is compromised, it has far-reaching consequences for societies and economies. Several key points illustrate the global significance of addressing these disparities:

1. **Maternal and Child Health**: High maternal mortality rates not only signify the tragic loss of women's lives but also impact children who may lose their mothers. This can lead to a cycle of poor health outcomes for generations. Furthermore, orphaned children are more likely to face adverse health and socioeconomic conditions, perpetuating a cycle of poverty and poor health. Investments in maternal health can break this cycle, improving the well-being of future generations and fostering more resilient communities.
2. **Economic Productivity**: When women's health suffers, their ability to participate in the workforce is often compromised. This can limit economic productivity and hinder a country's overall development. Healthy women are more likely to engage in income-generating activities, contributing to economic growth and stability. Additionally, improving women's health can lead to better educational outcomes for their children, creating a more skilled and productive future workforce.

3. **Public Health Emergencies**: Neglecting women's health can exacerbate public health crises, as seen during the Ebola outbreak in West Africa, where maternal mortality rates spiked due to healthcare system strain and disruptions. Strengthening women's health systems is crucial for improving overall health system resilience, enabling better responses to crises. Ensuring continuous access to reproductive health services during emergencies can mitigate long-term impacts on population health and stability.
4. **Gender Equity**: Achieving gender equity in healthcare is a crucial component of broader efforts to promote gender equality. It requires dismantling the barriers that prevent women from accessing healthcare services and participating in healthcare decision-making. Gender equity in health also promotes broader societal changes, empowering women to take on leadership roles and advocate for their rights. This shift can lead to more inclusive policies and practices, benefiting entire communities and fostering social progress.

The Relevance to Developed Nations

While the disparities in women's healthcare may appear most pronounced in developing countries, it is essential to recognize that challenges persist in developed nations as well. Even in countries with advanced healthcare systems, issues such as gender bias in medical research, disparities in access to reproductive healthcare, and the underdiagnosis of certain conditions in women persist. In the United States and the United Kingdom, for example, racial and socioeconomic disparities in maternal mortality rates highlight persistent inequalities in women's healthcare access and outcomes. Additionally, women in developed nations may still face barriers to accessing comprehensive sexual and reproductive healthcare, including contraception and family planning services. Furthermore, as developed nations become increasingly diverse due to immigration and globalization, culturally sensitive and inclusive healthcare practices become more critical to address the diverse needs of women from various backgrounds.

Occupational Therapy's Role in Addressing Disparities

Occupational therapy (OT) plays a crucial role in addressing women's health disparities globally. Occupational therapy practitioners (OTPs) are uniquely positioned to provide client-centered care, considering cultural, social, and economic factors that influence women's health. In developing countries, OTPs can collaborate with local communities to enhance healthcare access and promote health education, empowering women with the knowledge and skills to make informed health decisions. In developed nations, OTPs can advocate for gender equity in healthcare policies, contribute to gender-specific health research, and address the unique needs of diverse women.

Recognizing both progress and persistent disparities in women's health globally is essential. While some countries have improved healthcare access and outcomes, significant challenges remain in others. These disparities impact individuals, communities, and societies. The global relevance of these issues underscores the need for efforts to promote gender equity in healthcare access, research, and practice. By addressing these disparities, OTPs can ensure that all women, regardless of location or background, have the opportunity to lead healthy and fulfilling lives.

Historical Roots of Women's Health

Women's health has always been a topic of profound significance throughout human history. From ancient civilizations to modern societies, the well-being of women has been intimately tied to the broader fabric of social, cultural, and medical evolution. Throughout the annals of history, the consideration of women's health in medical research and care has evolved. It wasn't until the late 19th and early 20th centuries that women began to gain recognition within medical research, marking a pivotal turning point. Similarly, the emergence of occupational therapy as a profession, with its emphasis on addressing the unique needs of individuals, including women, took root during this transformative era.

In the United States, occupational therapy's significance in addressing women's unique needs surged during the mid-20th century. This period marked a dedicated effort toward enhancing women's health through tailored interventions, ushering in specialized care to address their distinct challenges. We delve into the historical origins of women's health and the vital role occupational therapy plays in its contemporary landscape. Exploring pivotal milestones and societal changes, we uncover the evolution of our understanding of women's health and the essential contribution of occupational therapy. Examining these historical roots offers a profound insight into the holistic approach that occupational therapy brings to women's well-being, a philosophy that continues to evolve and shape the field today.

Historical Development of Women's Health Care

When considering women's health, gynecological issues like infertility, menopause, pregnancy, childbirth, and breast health are commonly emphasized. However, women's health encompasses broader concerns, often requiring tailored approaches to diagnosis and care. For example, symptoms of a heart attack may differ in women, increasing the risk of misdiagnosis. Healthcare providers now recognize the need for customized strategies in addressing conditions such as osteoporosis, urinary disorders, sports injuries, colorectal cancer, and diabetes in women.

The World Health Organization defines health holistically, acknowledging physical, mental, and social well-being, contrasting with a narrow biomedical model. Various definitions of women's health have emerged over time, with the U.S. Public Health Service criteria being a widely accepted framework. Historically, women's healthcare primarily focused on reproductive and breast health but expanded in the mid-1980s to encompass a broader range of concerns. Women's health includes acute and chronic illnesses, lifestyle factors, access to healthcare, and participation in research. Conditions like heart disease, cancer, AIDS, HIV infection, and substance abuse may manifest differently in women than in men, necessitating adapted approaches. The Australian Ministers Advisory Council defines women's health as conditions unique to, more prevalent among, or more serious in women, considering various risk factors, interventions, or strategies. Common women's health conditions span the gynecological, obstetric, mental, cardiovascular, musculoskeletal, cancer, neurological, endocrine, sexual, and gastrointestinal domains.

Women's Health Movements: Advocating for Better Healthcare and Autonomy

The history of women's health movements stands as a testament to the enduring determination of women seeking improved healthcare, autonomy over their bodies, and recognition of their unique health needs. From the 1830s to the 2000s, these movements evolved significantly, responding to societal changes, medical advancements, and an increasing awareness of gender disparities in healthcare.

1830s–1900s: The Early Stirrings

The roots of women's health activism can be traced back to the mid-19th century when women began challenging the status quo. During this era, women were often confined to domestic roles, with limited access to education and opportunities in the medical field. Pioneering figures like Elizabeth Blackwell and Elizabeth Garrett Anderson shattered these barriers by becoming the first female physicians. Their remarkable achievements laid the foundation for women's active participation in healthcare. These early trailblazers not only became symbols of women's potential in medicine but also inspired generations of women to advocate for their health rights.

1900s–1960s: The Fight for Reproductive Rights

The early 20th century witnessed the emergence of women's health movements focused on reproductive rights. Margaret Sanger, a fearless advocate for birth control, established the first birth control clinic in the United States in 1916. Her activism paved the way for women to have greater control over their reproductive choices. By the 1960s, the modern feminist movement took center stage, demanding reproductive rights and access to safe abortion. The landmark Supreme Court decision in *Roe v. Wade* in 1973 marked a watershed moment for women's reproductive health, granting them the legal right to make choices about their own bodies.

1970s–1980s: The Women's Health Movement

The 1970s witnessed the rise of the Women's Health Movement, a powerful force advocating for a holistic approach to women's healthcare. This movement challenged the male-centric perspective prevalent in the medical establishment and championed the idea that women should have a significant say in their healthcare decisions. "Our Bodies, Ourselves," a groundbreaking publication, provided women with essential information about their bodies and health. The movement also pushed for increased research into women's health issues, shedding light on previously overlooked areas of study. It emphasized that women's health is not just a medical matter but also a social, political, and personal concern.

1990s–2000s: Advances and Challenges

The 1990s and early 2000s brought significant advancements in women's health. The Women's Health Initiative, a monumental research project, contributed crucial insights into the risks and benefits of hormone replacement therapy, guiding healthcare decisions for countless women. Breast cancer awareness campaigns, symbolized by the iconic pink ribbon, drew attention to the importance of early detection, treatment, and research funding. However, these decades also exposed persistent challenges. Disparities in healthcare access and outcomes continued to plague underserved communities and disproportionately affect women of color. The fight for equitable healthcare persisted, with organizations advocating for comprehensive sex education, improved maternal healthcare, and enhanced mental health services for women. Women's health movements confronted these issues head-on, highlighting the importance of addressing disparities in healthcare access and outcomes to achieve true gender equality in health. The journey of women's health movements from the 1830s to the 2000s is a testament to women's resilience in their pursuit of gender equality in healthcare. These movements encompassed battles for reproductive rights, raised awareness about women's unique health needs, and persistently addressed healthcare disparities.

2020–Present: Responding to Global Challenges

The onset of the COVID-19 pandemic in 2020 brought unprecedented challenges to women's health worldwide. As healthcare systems strained under the pressure of the pandemic, women faced unique vulnerabilities, including disruptions to reproductive healthcare services, increased caregiving responsibilities, and heightened risks of domestic violence and mental health issues. In response, grassroots initiatives and advocacy campaigns emerged to address these pressing concerns. Women's health advocates rallied for policies to safeguard reproductive rights, expand access to telehealth services, and provide support for maternal and mental health. Despite the challenges posed by the pandemic, women's resilience and activism continued to drive progress in advancing gender equality in healthcare.

Evolution of Occupational Therapy's Role in Women's Health

OT has undergone a remarkable transformation over the years, adapting to address the unique needs of women's health across the lifespan. From its early days in the early 20th century to the present, OT's contribution to women's health has expanded significantly, in response to changes in society, healthcare, and the roles of women.

Early 20th Century: The Emergence of Occupational Therapy

Occupational therapy emerged in the early 20th century when the healthcare landscape was still in its infancy. During this period, women were predominantly confined to domestic roles, with limited access to education and professional opportunities. Occupational therapy emerged as a profession dedicated to helping individuals, including women, regain independence and function in their daily lives. The pioneering occupational therapists of this era recognized the value of occupation in promoting health and well-being, breaking down gender norms, and empowering women to play active roles in their recovery.

World War I: A Pioneering Period for Women in OT

The outbreak of World War I created a pivotal moment for women in occupational therapy. With many men serving in the military, there was a shortage of healthcare professionals. Women stepped into these roles, providing care to wounded soldiers and helping to shape the field of occupational therapy. This period marked a significant turning point, as women demonstrated their capabilities in healthcare and made substantial contributions to the development of the profession. At this point in history, occupational therapy assistants (OTAs) were not yet part of the profession. They were introduced later in 1958 to address the growing need for occupational therapy services and to support OTPs in practice.

Post-World War I: Expanding Horizons

After World War I, occupational therapy continued to grow, and women played a central role in shaping the profession. Occupational therapists worked in various settings, including hospitals, rehabilitation centers, and mental health institutions. Their focus extended beyond physical rehabilitation to encompass the holistic well-being of their clients, which included women. This shift in perspective acknowledged that women's health was more than just the absence of illness—it was about enabling women to live fulfilling lives across various roles.

Mid-20th Century: Women's Health and Rehabilitation

As societal attitudes toward women's roles evolved in the mid-20th century, more women entered the workforce and began seeking occupational therapy services for various health-related issues. OT practitioners worked with women to address not only physical disabilities but also mental health concerns and the challenges of balancing work and family life. Occupational therapy became instrumental in helping women navigate the complexities of their changing roles in society. To support the growing demand for these services, **OTAs** were introduced in 1958. Their role was crucial in expanding the reach of occupational therapy, particularly as more women sought assistance in managing the physical and emotional challenges associated with their evolving roles.

1970s–1980s: The Women's Health Movement

The Women's Health Movement of the 1970s and 1980s ushered in a transformative shift in healthcare and the role of occupational therapy within it. This movement challenged the male-centric perspective that had long dominated the medical establishment. It advocated for a more comprehensive and woman-centered approach to healthcare, emphasizing that women should have a say in their healthcare decisions. OTPs actively participated in this movement, lending their voices to the call for women's health issues to be recognized as integral to the profession.

Reproductive Health and Maternity Care

Occupational therapy's involvement in women's health expanded to include reproductive health and maternity care. OTPs began working with women during pregnancy, labor, and postpartum recovery. They addressed the physical and psychological challenges associated with childbirth, promoting maternal well-being and supporting women in adapting to the demands of motherhood. This evolution recognized that occupational therapy had a vital role to play in empowering women to navigate the life-altering transition to motherhood.

1980s–1990s: Breast Cancer Rehabilitation

The late 20th century witnessed a growing focus on breast cancer rehabilitation within occupational therapy. As breast cancer diagnoses increased, OTPs developed specialized interventions to address the physical and emotional consequences of breast cancer treatment. They worked closely with breast cancer survivors, helping them regain function, manage lymphedema, and enhance their overall quality of life. Occupational therapy's involvement in breast cancer rehabilitation reflected the profession's commitment to addressing the specific needs of women facing this challenging journey.

21st Century: Expanding Horizons in Women's Health

OT's role in women's health in the 21st century continued to expand and diversify. OTPs began addressing a broader spectrum of women's health issues, recognizing the multifaceted nature of women's well-being. This expansion included specialized interventions for pelvic health, menopause management, osteoporosis, and gynecological conditions. OTPs also provided crucial support to women dealing with chronic pain, mental health challenges, and the consequences of gender-based violence.

Occupational Therapy in Pelvic Health

Occupational therapy's involvement in pelvic health became increasingly prominent, reflecting the recognition of the significant impact that pelvic conditions can have on women's quality of life. OTPs specialized in pelvic health helped women manage conditions such as pelvic pain, urinary incontinence, and sexual dysfunction. They embraced a holistic approach, addressing not only the physical aspects of pelvic health but also the emotional and social components. Occupational therapy became an essential part of the multidisciplinary care team for women facing these intimate and often stigmatized issues.

Mental Health and Women's Well-Being

OTPs also played a critical role in addressing women's mental health and overall well-being. They provided vital support to women confronting mental health challenges, including anxiety, depression, post-traumatic stress disorder (PTSD), and eating disorders. Occupational therapy interventions focused on equipping women with coping strategies, stress management techniques, and tools to enhance their overall mental health. Recognizing the interconnectedness of mental and physical health, OTPs worked to empower women to achieve holistic well-being.

Women's Health Across the Lifespan

Occupational therapy expanded its scope to encompass women's health across the lifespan. Practitioners recognized that women's unique health needs evolved as they progressed through different life stages. OTPs tailored their interventions to address the specific challenges faced by girls and adolescents, women in early adulthood, those in the middle years, and women in later life. This holistic approach aimed to promote healthy lifestyles, prevent chronic conditions, and enhance overall well-being at each stage of a woman's life journey.

Current Trends and Future Directions

In the present day, occupational therapy continues to adapt to the evolving landscape of women's health. OTPs integrate evidence-based practices, leverage technological innovations, and embrace interdisciplinary collaboration as they work to address the dynamic needs of women. Telehealth has emerged as a valuable tool, ensuring that women can access occupational therapy services conveniently and effectively, regardless of their location. As societal attitudes toward women's health continue to evolve, occupational therapy stands as an integral part of women's healthcare teams, offering a holistic perspective and client-centered interventions. OTPs are at the forefront of advocating for women's health, recognizing that it encompasses physical, mental, emotional, and social well-being. As they continue to adapt and innovate, OTPs empower women to lead healthier, more fulfilling lives, reflecting the profession's unwavering commitment to the changing healthcare needs of women across the lifespan. The evolution of occupational therapy in women's health serves as a testament to its dedication to improving the lives of women and promoting their well-being in a dynamic and ever-changing world.

Gender Equality and Medical Research

As we strive to understand, diagnose, and treat health conditions effectively, medical research plays a pivotal role. However, throughout history, gender disparities have persisted in the realm of medical research, often resulting in biased healthcare outcomes. Addressing these disparities and striving for gender equality in research and healthcare are essential steps toward providing equitable and effective care for all. In this chapter, we will delve into the critical issues surrounding gender equality in medical research, explore the impacts of gender bias on healthcare outcomes, and emphasize the importance of gender equality in research and healthcare.

Gender Disparities in Medical Research

The underrepresentation of women in clinical trials has long plagued medical research, stemming from concerns over hormonal fluctuations and assumptions of biological uniformity with men. This exclusion, reinforced by societal norms limiting women's roles and participation, has led to substantial gaps in understanding treatment effects and compromised healthcare quality. Medications and treatments developed primarily with male subjects may produce different outcomes or adverse effects in women, posing potentially life-threatening implications. Moreover, research traditionally fixated on reproductive health has overlooked broader health concerns disproportionately affecting women, such as autoimmune diseases and mental health disorders. Efforts to broaden the scope of women's health research in recent years aim to address these disparities and foster a more inclusive understanding of women's health needs beyond reproductive issues.

Historically, women's exclusion from clinical trials has reflected broader societal norms and expectations, restricting their roles and participation in medical research. This bias, coupled with the narrow focus on reproductive health, hindered the understanding of various health conditions impacting women differently. For example, autoimmune diseases like lupus, which predominantly affect women, received less research attention compared to conditions affecting both genders equally. Similarly, mental health disorders, despite their high prevalence among women, were often stigmatized and underexplored. Efforts to broaden women's health research aim to rectify these biases, acknowledging the need for a more comprehensive approach to address the diverse health concerns of women beyond reproductive issues.

Impacts of Gender Bias on Healthcare Outcomes

Gender bias in healthcare and research significantly impacts healthcare outcomes, spanning diagnosis, treatment, and overall health. Misdiagnosis and delayed diagnosis are critical consequences, often stemming from gendered differences in symptom presentation. For instance, women experiencing a heart attack may exhibit atypical symptoms such as shortness of breath, fatigue, or nausea, leading to underdiagnosis or delayed treatment. Similarly, conditions like rheumatoid arthritis and multiple sclerosis may manifest differently in women, resulting in overlooked symptoms and delayed interventions, thus impacting their quality of life. Mental health conditions, more prevalent in women, are also subject to underdiagnosis and undertreatment due to insufficient consideration of gender-specific factors by healthcare providers.

Furthermore, gender bias extends to treatment approaches, with medications and therapies often developed and tested primarily in male populations, leading to potential inefficacy or safety concerns for women. Clinical trial underrepresentation of women further exacerbates treatment uncertainties, hindering tailored care delivery. The lack of comprehensive research on women's health contributes to limited understanding among healthcare providers of unique physiological and psychological aspects, resulting in inadequate support for conditions such as depression, anxiety, and reproductive health issues like endometriosis and polycystic ovary syndrome. Addressing these biases is crucial for ensuring effective, equitable healthcare provision that adequately addresses the diverse health needs of women across their lifespan.

Importance of Gender Equality in Research and Healthcare

Gender equality in research and healthcare is vital for advancing medical science, improving outcomes, and promoting societal well-being. Recognizing gender differences in health experiences is crucial for tailored healthcare. Gender-sensitive practices acknowledge biological and social influences on health outcomes, ensuring personalized diagnosis and treatment plans. Precision medicine relies on inclusive research to customize healthcare decisions, optimizing medication dosages and improving early detection of conditions. Gender-specific research enhances diagnostic accuracy and intervention strategies, especially in mental health.

Inclusive medical research benefits society by providing a comprehensive understanding of health conditions and developing effective treatments applicable to diverse populations. This inclusivity reduces inequities in care, addressing health disparities among marginalized communities, including women of color and underserved populations. Gender equality in research is crucial for advancing women's health and addressing conditions that affect them differently. It enables the development of interventions across women's lifespan, including reproductive, mental, cardiovascular, and musculoskeletal health. Gender-sensitive research improves reproductive care, leading to safer childbirth practices and interventions supporting maternal well-being.

Gender Equity and Its Impact on Rehabilitation Outcomes

Gender equity in research studies related to rehabilitation and occupational therapy is a critical factor that can significantly influence rehabilitation outcomes. When women are inadequately represented in research, the resulting findings may not accurately reflect their unique needs and experiences. This section delves into the importance of gender equity in rehabilitation research and provides evidence-based examples of how the underrepresentation of women can impact rehabilitation outcomes.

The Gender Gap in Rehabilitation Research

Historically, rehabilitation research has often been characterized by a gender gap, with women being underrepresented or excluded from clinical trials and studies. This gender gap extends beyond just participant numbers; it encompasses the entire research process, including study design, data collection, and data analysis. The consequences of this underrepresentation can be profound and may lead to misinformed rehabilitation practices that do not adequately address the needs of women.

Cardiac Rehabilitation

One significant area where gender equity in research is crucial is cardiac rehabilitation. Cardiovascular disease is a leading cause of death for both men and women; however, research in this field has traditionally focused heavily on male participants. Consequently, treatment and rehabilitation protocols have often been tailored to male physiology and symptomatology. Research has shown that women can experience heart disease differently from men. For instance, women may exhibit atypical symptoms during a heart attack, such as shortness of breath, fatigue, and nausea, rather than the classic chest pain commonly associated with men. When rehabilitation interventions are primarily based on studies with male participants, they may not adequately address the unique needs and symptoms that women experience. This lack of gender equity in cardiac rehabilitation research can result in suboptimal treatment outcomes for women, including delayed diagnosis and subpar rehabilitation strategies.

Orthopedic Rehabilitation

Orthopedic rehabilitation is another field where gender equity in research is crucial for improving rehabilitation outcomes. Conditions like osteoarthritis and joint replacements are prevalent among both men and women, but the research has often skewed toward male participants. This bias can have consequences for rehabilitation strategies and interventions. For instance, the management of joint pain and post-surgical recovery may differ between men and women due to anatomical and physiological differences. Women typically have smaller joint sizes and different muscle mass distributions than men, which can impact their responses to rehabilitation exercises and post-operative care. When rehabilitation protocols are primarily based on studies with male participants, they may not effectively address these gender-specific considerations.

Pelvic Health Rehabilitation

Gender equity is particularly vital in the field of pelvic health rehabilitation, which deals with conditions like urinary incontinence, pelvic organ prolapse, and pelvic floor dysfunction. These conditions predominantly affect women, yet research and clinical studies have often overlooked their gender-specific aspects. Studies focusing on interventions for urinary incontinence, for instance, may not consider the impact of hormonal changes, pregnancy, childbirth, and menopause on women's pelvic health. The lack of gender equity in research can lead to inadequate understanding of the factors contributing to these conditions in women and result in less effective rehabilitation interventions.

The Impact of Gender Equity on Rehabilitation Outcomes

Gender equity in rehabilitation research is essential for developing effective, evidence-based interventions that cater to the diverse needs of both men and women. Below are some key ways in which gender equity positively impacts rehabilitation outcomes.

1. **Tailored Interventions**: When research includes a diverse representation of both genders, it enables the development of tailored interventions that account for physiological, anatomical, and hormonal differences. This results in rehabilitation strategies that are more effective and relevant to the specific needs of each gender.
2. **Early Detection and Diagnosis**: Gender-equitable research can help healthcare providers recognize gender-specific symptoms and risk factors earlier, leading to timely diagnosis and intervention. This is particularly critical in conditions like heart disease, where women may exhibit atypical symptoms that are not adequately addressed in male-centric research.
3. **Enhanced Recovery**: Women who receive gender-inclusive rehabilitation interventions are more likely to experience enhanced recovery and improved outcomes. Rehabilitation plans that consider gender-specific factors can lead to better physical and psychological well-being.
4. **Informed Decision-Making**: Gender-equitable research empowers healthcare providers to make informed decisions regarding rehabilitation strategies. It ensures that interventions are based on comprehensive knowledge and understanding of gender-specific health needs.

Promoting Gender Equity in Rehabilitation Research

Promoting gender equity in rehabilitation research is not only a matter of ethical responsibility but also a critical step toward improving healthcare outcomes for all. To achieve this, it's essential to implement a comprehensive approach that encompasses various strategies and initiatives. Fostering an inclusive research environment, where researchers actively collaborate with gender equity experts and engage in ongoing dialogue, can be instrumental in promoting gender equity. Furthermore, raising awareness about the importance of gender equity in research among both researchers and the public can garner support for initiatives that prioritize inclusivity. For a detailed list of strategies aimed at promoting gender equity in rehabilitation research, please refer to Table 1.1.

Gender equity in rehabilitation research is fundamental for improving rehabilitation outcomes and ensuring that interventions are relevant and effective for both men and women. Addressing the historical gender gap in research requires concerted efforts from researchers, healthcare providers, funding organizations, and policymakers. By working together to prioritize gender equity, we can enhance rehabilitation practices, leading to better outcomes and quality of life for all individuals, regardless of their gender.

Table 1.1 Strategies for promoting gender equity in rehabilitation research

Strategy	Description
Inclusive Recruitment	Actively seek diverse participants by implementing targeted outreach and recruitment efforts.
Gender-Disaggregated Data	Collect and analyze gender-specific data to identify disparities and inform gender-inclusive interventions.
Funding and Support	Allocate resources and funding to support research focusing on gender-specific rehabilitation issues.
Education and Training	Provide education and training to healthcare professionals to enhance awareness and advocacy for gender equity.
Inclusive Research Environment	Create an inclusive research environment that encourages collaboration with gender equity experts.
Public Awareness Campaigns	Raise awareness about the importance of gender equity in research among researchers and the general public.
Ongoing Dialogue and Collaboration	Foster ongoing dialogue and collaboration to continuously improve gender equity in rehabilitation research.

Employment, Gender Inequities, and Women's Health

The role of work is crucial for women, not only for their financial stability but also for their overall welfare. Beyond their jobs, women often juggle multiple responsibilities as caregivers, nurturers, and household contributors. As women progress in various professions, it's important to understand how employment, gender roles, and workplace dynamics affect their physical, mental, and social health. Exploring the impact of work on women's well-being involves recognizing persistent gender disparities in the workforce and their significant influence on women's lives.

Gender Inequities in the Workplace

Gender inequities persist in the workplace, significantly impacting women's health and well-being. These issues, such as the gender pay gap and limited access to leadership roles, affect women's professional lives. One prominent concern is the gender pay gap, where women earn less than men for equivalent work due to factors like occupational segregation and systemic biases. Organizations can address this through transparent pay policies, equity audits, and legislative advocacy. Table 1.2 highlights key disparities in the workplace.

Gender inequities in the workplace have profound effects on women's health, both physically and mentally. For instance, the gender pay gap causes financial stress and limits access to healthcare. The glass ceiling hinders women's career growth and job satisfaction by restricting leadership opportunities. Additionally, work-life imbalance, discrimination, and harassment contribute to stress and emotional distress. Inadequate maternity and family leave policies add to the strain during critical life transitions.

To address these issues and promote women's health and equity, organizations can take proactive steps. These include implementing transparent pay practices, offering leadership development and mentorship programs, promoting work-life balance, conducting anti-discrimination training, and advocating for supportive family leave policies. By addressing these issues comprehensively, workplaces can create a more inclusive and equitable environment for all employees.

Table 1.2 Gender disparities in the workplace

Inequity	Description
Gender Pay Gap	Women earn less money than men for the same work.
Glass Ceiling	Limited access for women to top leadership.
Work-Life Imbalance	Juggling work and family responsibilities.
Discrimination/Harassment	Gender-based bias and mistreatment.
Maternity/Family Leave	Insufficient support during life transitions.

OTPs can play a crucial role in addressing gender inequities in the workplace. They can raise awareness, conduct worksite assessments, support work-life balance, promote mental health, assist with return-to-work programs, advocate for inclusive environments, empower individuals with essential skills, and contribute to research and policy development. By actively participating in these roles, OTPs can advance gender equity and improve women's health and well-being in the workplace.

Work-Related Health Issues

In the realm of work-related health issues, women often face a complex web of challenges that can significantly impact their well-being. These challenges extend beyond the confines of their workplace, affecting their physical and mental health in profound ways. Understanding the severity of these issues and their underlying causes is essential. Women, as a vital part of the workforce, experience a range of health-related challenges in their professional lives. These issues encompass both physical and mental health concerns.

Musculoskeletal Disorders (MSDs)

MSDs stand out as one of the most prominent health issues affecting women in the workplace, exacerbated by their overrepresentation in jobs where such conditions are prevalent. Women tend to occupy roles requiring repetitive tasks, poor ergonomics, or prolonged periods of sitting, which significantly increases their susceptibility to MSDs. According to a study by the Bureau of Labor Statistics, women are 70% more likely than men to experience MSDs in their lifetime, reflecting the occupational disparities in job roles. Conditions like carpal tunnel syndrome, tendonitis, and back pain can significantly impact their quality of life, causing discomfort and limitations in their daily activities. Developing strategies for prevention, early intervention, and workplace ergonomics is crucial in addressing this pervasive issue.

Mental Health Challenges

Workplace stress and the pressure to balance career and family responsibilities can take a substantial toll on women's mental health. High workloads, tight deadlines, and interpersonal conflicts contribute to anxiety, depression, and burnout. Moreover, women often bear the added burden of managing household duties and caregiving responsibilities, amplifying these challenges. OTPs can play a critical role in developing mental health support programs tailored to women's needs, providing coping strategies, and advocating for work environments that prioritize employee well-being.

Occupational Hazards

Occupational hazards disproportionately affect women, particularly in industries like healthcare and manufacturing. For instance, women in healthcare professions face a higher risk of exposure to biological hazards such as infectious diseases. According to a report by the National Institute for Occupational Safety and Health (NIOSH), women healthcare workers are 1.5 times more likely than men to experience needlestick injuries, highlighting the gender-specific nature of these risks. Additionally, women are often overrepresented in roles that involve exposure to chemical hazards and ergonomic risks. Therefore, it's crucial for OTPs to collaborate with employers to assess and mitigate these hazards, implementing tailored safety measures and training programs to safeguard the health and well-being of female employees.

Workplace Violence

In sectors where women are overrepresented, such as healthcare and social services, the risk of workplace violence is notably higher. Women in these fields may experience verbal abuse, physical assault, or harassment from patients, clients, or colleagues. OTPs can contribute by developing violence prevention programs, offering strategies for conflict resolution and de-escalation, and advocating for comprehensive workplace safety policies that protect female employees from harm.

Shift Work and Sleep Disorders

According to a study published in the *American Journal of Epidemiology*, women who work rotating night shifts have a 15–18% increased risk of developing coronary heart disease compared to those who do not work night shifts. This highlights the significant impact of shift work on women's health, particularly in relation to cardiovascular outcomes. Additionally, night shifts and irregular working hours can disrupt women's circadian rhythms, leading to sleep disorders like insomnia and sleep deprivation. Sleep disturbances can result in fatigue, decreased concentration, and increased health risks. OTPs can work with employers to establish healthier shift schedules, implement strategies for managing sleep disorders, and educate employees on proper sleep hygiene practices to improve overall sleep quality and well-being.

Contributing Factors to Work-Related Health Issues for Women

Several factors contribute to the prevalence of these health issues among women in the workplace. Occupational segregation, where women are concentrated in specific industries and roles, often those with lower pay and greater health risks, plays a significant role. This segregation limits opportunities for women to access safer and more equitable workplaces. Societal expectations and traditional gender roles can impose additional stressors on women, as they are often expected to excel both in their careers and as caregivers at home. These dual roles can lead to chronic stress and mental health challenges. Awareness of work-related health issues and their prevention measures may be limited, especially among women themselves. This lack of awareness can result in delayed intervention and exacerbate health problems.

The Role of the Occupational Therapy Practitioner

OTPs are uniquely positioned to address and mitigate work-related health issues for women. Their expertise in holistic health and their focus on helping individuals engage meaningfully in their daily activities make them valuable assets in the workplace. Table 1.3 highlights key roles OTPs can play in promoting women's health and well-being at work.

Women's work-related health issues are multifaceted and can significantly impact their physical and mental well-being. OTPs are well-equipped to play a pivotal role in addressing and mitigating these challenges, making the workplace a healthier and more equitable environment for women. Through their expertise in holistic health and activity engagement, OTPs can empower women to lead healthier, more fulfilling professional lives.

Empowering Women's Professional Development

Empowering women's professional growth is vital for achieving gender equity in the workplace. Despite persistent gender inequities, promoting women's advancement in their careers is crucial. Women face unique challenges due to societal norms and biases, including the gender pay gap and limited access to leadership roles. However, they consistently demonstrate competence, resilience, and dedication. Recognizing the value of

Table 1.3 Role of the OTP in promoting women's health and well-being at work

Strategy	Description	Examples
Ergonomic Assessments	Conduct ergonomic assessments to identify and mitigate the risk of musculoskeletal disorders (MSDs). Recommend ergonomic modifications and adaptive equipment. Provide guidance on proper body mechanics.	- Analyzing workstation setups - Recommending ergonomic chairs and keyboard stands - Teaching proper lifting techniques
Stress Management Programs	Design and implement stress management programs to help women cope with workplace stress. Incorporate techniques such as mindfulness, relaxation exercises, and time management strategies to improve mental well-being.	- Offering stress reduction workshops - Teaching mindfulness meditation - Providing time management seminars
Safety Training	Provide safety training and prevention strategies in industries with high risks of violence or injury. Empower women to protect themselves and reduce workplace risks.	- Conducting self-defense classes - Developing workplace safety protocols - Training on handling potentially violent situations
Shift Work Solutions	Collaborate with employers to develop shift work schedules that minimize health impacts. Implement strategies like gradual shift changes, strategic napping, and sleep hygiene to mitigate sleep disturbances.	- Creating rotating shift schedules - Recommending strategic nap breaks - Educating on sleep hygiene best practices
Mental Health Support	Offer counseling and support for women experiencing mental health challenges related to work stress. Provide coping strategies, self-care techniques, and referrals to mental health professionals when necessary.	- Providing individual counseling sessions - Teaching stress management techniques - Referring to mental health specialists

gender diversity, organizations are increasingly investing in women's development, benefiting both individuals and workplaces. Table 1.4 presents strategies for supporting women's career growth, aiming to foster an environment where women thrive professionally while maintaining work-life balance.

The strategies in Table 1.4 aim to create an environment where women thrive in their careers while maintaining work-life balance. By offering mentorship, skill enhancement,

Table 1.4 Strategies for empowering women's professional development

Strategy	Description	Examples
Mentorship Programs	Establish mentorship programs designed to provide guidance, encouragement, and skills development to women in the workplace.	- Pairing experienced mentors with female mentees - Providing mentorship for career advancement and skill development
Networking Opportunities	Encourage women to engage in networking opportunities for knowledge sharing and career growth.	- Attending industry conferences and events - Participating in professional associations and women's networks
Skill Enhancement	Invest in skill enhancement programs tailored to women's needs, focusing on leadership, negotiation, and other vital skills.	- Leadership training workshops - Negotiation skill-building sessions - Personalized skills development plans
Work-Life Integration	Promote work-life integration by empowering women to set boundaries, allocate time efficiently, and prioritize self-care.	- Time management workshops - Stress reduction and self-care seminars - Workshops on boundary setting and assertiveness
Recognition and Advocacy	Create mechanisms for recognizing and advocating for women's contributions in the workplace.	- Celebrating achievements through awards and recognition programs - Actively promoting women's ideas and initiatives
Equal Opportunity Initiatives	Continue supporting equal opportunity initiatives that ensure accessible hiring, promotion, and leadership opportunities.	- Implementing gender-blind recruitment processes - Providing leadership development opportunities for women
Professional Development Funds	Provide access to professional development funds or scholarships to assist women in pursuing advanced education or training.	- Offering scholarships for further education - Establishing funds for women's career advancement and skill development
Leadership Training	Invest in leadership training programs specifically designed for women, focusing on building confidence and skills.	- Leadership development programs tailored to women - Building confidence through assertiveness training
Feedback and Evaluation	Establish transparent feedback and evaluation processes that provide constructive input and growth opportunities.	- Conducting regular performance evaluations with constructive feedback - Creating opportunities for career growth based on merit
Employee Resource Groups (ERGs)	Support the formation of employee resource groups dedicated to women, offering advocacy, support, and sharing experiences.	- Forming women-focused ERGs for peer support and advocacy - Organizing events and workshops for women's professional growth

and networking opportunities, organizations support women's growth. Additionally, initiatives like recognizing women's contributions, implementing equal opportunity measures, and providing professional development funds contribute to diverse and inclusive workplaces. Addressing gender inequities and prioritizing women's development moves us toward a future where women excel in their careers, free from societal biases.

Sociocultural Perspectives on Women's Health

The sphere of women's health intertwines biology, psychology, and society, with culture serving as a vital yet often overlooked component. Cultural norms influence how women perceive their health and are treated by others, enriching their health journeys. As OTPs, we delve into the intersection of cultural norms and women's well-being, striving for cultural competence in our practice and integrating cultural factors into interventions. Women's health is deeply entwined with the cultures they inhabit, impacting roles, expectations, and healthcare-seeking behaviors. Cultural beliefs shape views on motherhood, career, body image, and health conditions, influencing decisions and relationships. OTPs recognize this connection, striving for cultural competence to provide equitable services. This involves continual self-reflection, education, and sensitivity to diverse health beliefs and preferences. By fostering trust and adapting approaches to respect cultural values, therapists create a person-centered care environment for women from diverse backgrounds.

Cultural Norms and Their Impact

Cultural norms and beliefs are fundamental components within the complex landscape of women's health. These cultural constructs play a pivotal role in shaping women's choices, healthcare decisions, and overall well-being. Across diverse cultures, unique values and expectations exert a profound influence on how women perceive their roles, navigate their health journeys, and make choices regarding various aspects of their lives.

Reproductive Health and Motherhood

In some cultural contexts, motherhood assumes an elevated status, positioning it as the apex of a woman's identity and societal expectation. Consequently, women may experience substantial pressure to marry early and bear children, potentially impacting their educational and career trajectories. The cultural emphasis on motherhood can also influence women's choices regarding family planning, with expectations of fulfilling this role superseding personal aspirations. In contrast, cultures that emphasize individual autonomy and career success may lead women to postpone family planning or make different decisions about the timing of childbirth. The tension between cultural expectations and personal aspirations in matters of reproductive health can profoundly impact women's psychological well-being and life choices.

Body Image and Beauty Standards

Cultural ideals of beauty exert a significant influence on women's self-esteem and body image. Media portrayals, societal expectations, and traditional beauty standards often mold women's self-perception. These perceptions can lead to complex relationships with food, exercise, and body image, affecting both physical and mental well-being. Cultural norms surrounding beauty may promote specific body types, skin tones, or features that may not align with an individual woman's characteristics. The pressure to conform to these ideals can result in body dissatisfaction, potentially leading to unhealthy behaviors, such as extreme dieting or cosmetic procedures. Moreover, these cultural standards can impact women's mental health, contributing to issues like anxiety and depression related to body image concerns.

Gender Roles and Autonomy

Cultural norms frequently define the roles and expectations imposed on women within their families and communities. Some cultures uphold traditional gender roles, where women bear primary responsibility for caregiving and domestic duties. In such contexts, women may find themselves navigating complex dynamics, balancing their career aspirations with cultural expectations of family caregiving. Conversely, other cultures promote gender equality and women's autonomy in decision-making. These cultural norms profoundly influence women's ability to balance personal aspirations, career goals, and family responsibilities. The struggle to reconcile cultural expectations with individual aspirations can lead to stress and feelings of conflict, impacting women's overall well-being and self-fulfillment.

Stigma and Health Conditions

Cultural norms also contribute to the stigma surrounding specific health conditions, including mental health disorders and reproductive health issues. Women hailing from cultures where discussions on mental health are taboo may hesitate to seek help for conditions such as anxiety or depression, fearing judgment or ostracization. Similarly, women grappling with reproductive health challenges may contend with feelings of shame or isolation due to cultural beliefs surrounding fertility and reproduction. The stigma associated with these health conditions can prevent women from seeking timely and appropriate healthcare, exacerbating their health challenges and affecting their overall quality of life. Addressing the impact of cultural stigma on women's health requires culturally sensitive interventions that destigmatize these conditions and promote open dialogue and support.

Understanding the intricate interplay between cultural norms and women's health is a vital step for OTPs. It enables us to provide culturally sensitive care that respects individual values and preferences, recognizing the profound influence of culture on women's health and well-being.

Cultural Competence in Occupational Therapy Practice

Cultural competence is a foundational aspect of providing effective and equitable occupational therapy services in the realm of women's health. It goes beyond recognizing cultural diversity; it requires a deep understanding and appreciation of how cultural factors influence health behaviors and outcomes. As OTPs, we play a crucial role in bridging the gap between cultural norms and women's health, ensuring that our interventions are respectful, relevant, and responsive to the diverse cultural backgrounds of our clients.

Understanding the Essence of Cultural Competence

To provide meaningful care to individuals from diverse cultural backgrounds, OTPs must embrace the essence of cultural competence. It's a journey that begins with humility, as we acknowledge that we don't know everything about every culture, and every person's experience is unique. With this mindset, we delve into the essential components of cultural competence.

1. **Cultural Humility**: Cultural competence starts with self-awareness and humility—acknowledging our biases, assumptions, and stereotypes. It requires ongoing self-reflection and the recognition that we have much to learn from each client's unique perspective.
2. **Cultural Sensitivity**: Being culturally sensitive means recognizing the diversity in health beliefs, preferences, and priorities among individuals from different cultural backgrounds. It involves active listening without judgment and a genuine effort to understand each client's unique viewpoint.
3. **Effective Communication**: Cultural competence also encompasses the ability to communicate effectively across cultural boundaries. This includes recognizing the role of language, non-verbal communication, and cultural norms in shaping communication styles. OTPs must be skilled in adapting their communication to meet the needs of clients from diverse cultural backgrounds.
4. **Respect for Cultural Values**: Cultural competence involves respecting cultural values, traditions, and preferences. This may mean adapting assessment and intervention approaches to align with cultural norms and practices, always with the client's informed consent.
5. **Cultural Safety**: Creating an environment where clients from diverse backgrounds feel safe and respected is paramount. OTPs must actively work to eliminate power imbalances, discrimination, and bias in the therapeutic relationship.

Building Cultural Competence

Building cultural competence is an ongoing journey for OTPs. It requires dedication, self-awareness, and a commitment to learning. Table 1.5 lists actionable strategies that OTPs can employ to actively build cultural competence.

Developing cultural competence transcends a mere item on a checklist of professional development; it constitutes a profound commitment to delivering the highest standard of care to clients hailing from diverse backgrounds. By actively and earnestly embarking on the journey toward cultural competence, OTPs can guarantee that their interventions extend beyond mere effectiveness. Instead, these interventions become infused with the principles of respect and significance, acknowledging, and accommodating the diverse cultural contexts in which they are applied, thereby fostering a truly inclusive and equitable approach to healthcare provision.

Understanding Cultural Factors in Women's Health

In the realm of women's health, cultural factors play a pivotal role in shaping every aspect of a woman's well-being. These cultural influences extend beyond mere preferences; they can deeply impact women's health experiences, choices, and access to healthcare services. Therefore, it's essential for OTPs to explore how cultural norms and beliefs

Table 1.5 Strategies for the OTP to build cultural competence

Strategy	Description	Examples
Continuous Learning and Self-Reflection	Engage in continuous education on cultural competence, including courses, workshops, and reading. Regularly reflect on your own cultural biases and assumptions.	Attend cultural competence seminars, read books or articles on cultural sensitivity.
Cultural Resource Networks	Build networks with cultural experts and community organizations to gain insights into specific cultural practices and beliefs.	Collaborate with local cultural organizations, consult with cultural experts when needed.
Language and Communication Training	Learn basic phrases or greetings in the languages commonly spoken by your clients. Familiarize yourself with non-verbal communication norms in different cultures.	Take language courses, use translation apps, practice non-verbal communication awareness.
Client-Centered Assessment	Prioritize client-centered assessment methods that respect cultural values and preferences. Use open-ended questions to explore cultural beliefs related to health and well-being.	Incorporate cultural considerations into your assessment process, respecting client autonomy.
Cultural Competence Supervision	Seek supervision or guidance from experienced colleagues or mentors who are knowledgeable about cultural competence.	Attend supervision sessions, participate in peer consultation groups focused on cultural competence.
Cultural Immersion	Immerse yourself in diverse cultural experiences to gain firsthand insights into the perspectives, traditions, and challenges of your clients.	Attend cultural events, participate in cultural exchange programs, and engage with diverse communities.
Community Engagement	Become involved in community activities and events that celebrate different cultures. Engage with clients' communities to better understand their cultural context.	Participate in community projects, volunteer with organizations that serve diverse populations.

specifically affect women's health journeys. By doing so, therapists can create a more comprehensive and tailored approach to addressing the unique needs of their female clients. Cultural factors can come into play in various areas of occupational therapy practice, including activities of daily living (ADLs), instrumental activities of daily living (IADLs), medication management, nutrition management, habits, roles, routines, and other areas. Table 1.6 explores questions OTPs can ask clients and communication strategies to elicit information, ensuring cultural considerations are integrated into evaluations and treatment.

Understanding and addressing cultural factors in women's health interventions is crucial for equitable and effective care. Cultural norms deeply influence women's daily lives, requiring occupational therapy practitioners to navigate them sensitively. By integrating cultural insights into treatment planning, we deliver person-centered care, respecting diverse values and enhancing health outcomes. Culturally competent OT practice acknowledges the uniqueness of each woman's health journey, fostering inclusivity in women's health.

Table 1.6 Considerations for addressing cultural factors in women's health interventions

Area of Practice	Cultural Factor	Questions to Ask Clients	Communication Strategies
Activities of Daily Living (ADLs)	Cultural norms may dictate dressing, bathing, toileting, and eating practices.	- How do you prefer to dress in your cultural context? - Are there specific bathing rituals or customs you follow? - Are there dietary restrictions or preferences due to cultural beliefs?	Create a non-judgmental, open environment to discuss personal habits and preferences.
Instrumental Activities of Daily Living (IADLs)	Cultural factors can influence a person's ability to manage finances, use transportation, or shop for groceries.	- How do cultural beliefs impact your financial management? - Are there transportation barriers or preferences influenced by your culture? - Do cultural factors affect your shopping habits or food choices?	Encourage clients to share their perspectives on how culture intersects with their daily life.
Habits and Routines (Performance Patterns)	Cultural practices may dictate daily routines, exercise habits, and sleep patterns.	- What cultural habits or routines do you follow in your daily life? - How does your culture view exercise, physical activity, and rest? - Are there cultural practices related to sleep and rest that you adhere to?	Foster open dialogue about how cultural habits and routines impact daily functioning.
Roles and Expectations	Cultural norms define gender roles, family structures, and social expectations.	- How do cultural expectations shape your roles within your family or community? - Are there specific cultural roles or responsibilities you fulfill? - Do cultural norms affect your decision-making and life choices?	Encourage clients to reflect on how cultural roles and expectations influence their identity and decisions.
Spirituality and Religion	Cultural factors often intertwine with spirituality and religious beliefs.	- How does your spirituality or religion influence your health and well-being? - Are there cultural ceremonies or practices related to spirituality that are important to you? - Do you have specific beliefs regarding health and healing influenced by your culture?	Approach discussions about spirituality and religion with respect, allowing clients to share their beliefs and practices.
Medication Management	Cultural beliefs may influence whether and how individuals take medications or seek traditional remedies.	- Are there cultural beliefs regarding medication use or traditional remedies you follow? - Does your culture have specific rituals or practices related to healthcare and medication?	Approach the topic of medication management with sensitivity, allowing clients to express their beliefs and practices.
Nutrition Management	Cultural norms significantly shape dietary choices, meal preparation methods, and eating habits.	- What cultural foods or dishes are important to you? - How does your culture influence your eating habits and mealtimes? - Are there dietary restrictions based on cultural beliefs or traditions?	Create a welcoming atmosphere for discussing cultural preferences related to nutrition and food choices.

Assessments for Understanding Cultural Norms in Women's Health

In the realm of women's health, understanding cultural norms is a crucial aspect of providing holistic and effective care. To gain insights into the cultural values and beliefs that influence a client's health journey, OTPs can utilize various assessment tools and strategies. These assessments can help OTPs tailor interventions to respect and incorporate cultural factors. Here are some assessment approaches and tools that can be valuable:

1. **Cultural Genogram**: A cultural genogram is an adaptation of the traditional genogram used in family therapy. It allows therapists to visually map a client's cultural background, including their family's cultural history, traditions, and significant cultural events. This tool can help OTPs identify cultural influences on the client's health and well-being.
2. **Cultural Interviews**: Conducting cultural interviews involves asking open-ended questions about a client's cultural background, experiences, and beliefs related to health and wellness. These interviews provide a space for clients to share their unique cultural perspectives, allowing OTPs to better understand their values and preferences.
3. **Cultural Assessment Tools**: Several standardized cultural assessment tools are available for healthcare professionals. These tools often include questionnaires that explore various aspects of cultural identity, such as the Cultural Formulation Interview (CFI) and the Cultural Assessment of Risk for End-stage renal disease (CARE). These assessments can provide structured insights into a client's cultural context.
4. **Ethnographic Observations**: OTPs can engage in ethnographic observations to gain a deeper understanding of how cultural norms influence a client's daily life and health-related behaviors. Observations can provide valuable insights into routines, rituals, and cultural practices that impact women's health.
5. **Cultural Competence Self-Assessment**: OTPs can also assess their own cultural competence through self-reflection and self-assessment tools designed for healthcare professionals. This helps OTPs recognize their own biases and areas for improvement when it comes to providing culturally sensitive care.

When evaluating women's health, OTPs should integrate culturally sensitive questions and approaches. Using open-ended questions encourages clients to share cultural perspectives on health. Adjusting communication styles to match cultural norms, including non-verbal cues and respectful language, is essential. Inquire about cultural practices impacting health, including those related to women's and reproductive health. Respect cultural norms of modesty and privacy during assessments. By integrating cultural assessments and asking pertinent questions, OTPs gain a deeper understanding of clients' cultural contexts. This informs interventions aligned with cultural values, fostering trust and improving women's health outcomes. OTPs demonstrate a commitment to culturally sensitive and client-centered care, enhancing well-being in diverse cultural settings.

Women and Occupation: The Occupational Therapy Perspective

Occupational therapy (OT) provides a unique lens through which we can view and address women's health by focusing on meaningful engagement in daily activities, known as occupations. These occupations include anything people do to occupy themselves, from personal care and managing home life to professional responsibilities and leisure activities. For women, engaging in these occupations is influenced by a multifaceted array of factors, including physical capabilities, social environments, cultural expectations, and personal aspirations. Understanding how these elements intersect provides OTPs with insights into creating effective, personalized care plans that support women's health, promote their well-being, and respect their diverse life roles.

The Role of Occupations in Women's Health

Occupations are central to everyone's life, giving meaning and structure to our days. For women, these occupations can be particularly diverse, encompassing activities of daily living (ADLs), instrumental activities of daily living (IADLs), health management, rest and sleep, education, work, play, leisure, and social participation. The way women engage in these occupations is deeply influenced by their contexts, performance patterns, skills, and client factors, which collectively shape their identities and affect their overall health and well-being.

In occupational therapy, intervention plans that incorporate a focus on these occupations are crucial. They are designed not only to address participation and engagement but also to enhance the development of performance skills and patterns. This comprehensive approach ensures that women are supported in all facets of their lives, accommodating and celebrating the diversity of experiences that define women's health across different cultures and life stages.

Understanding Intersectionality in Occupational Therapy

Intersectionality is a framework that recognizes the multiple facets of identity that influence an individual's life experiences and access to resources. In the context of occupational therapy, it is particularly crucial for understanding the layered experiences of women, who often navigate compounded layers of discrimination and privilege. Factors such as race, ethnicity, socioeconomic status, age, disability, and sexual orientation intersect with gender, profoundly impacting how women experience health and engage in everyday occupations.

This multifaceted approach helps OTPs understand that the challenges faced by women are not uniform but vary greatly depending on their intersectional identities. For instance, a young African American woman with a disability faces different societal expectations and barriers than an older, affluent Caucasian woman, which in turn affects their occupational needs and health outcomes.

OTPs utilize an intersectional lens to comprehensively assess and address the unique needs of women. This involves:

- **Culturally Competent Assessments**: Ensuring that assessment tools and processes are sensitive to the cultural, linguistic, and social nuances of different women. This might involve using assessment tools developed specifically for certain cultural groups or adapting existing tools to better reflect diverse experiences.
- **Personalized Intervention Plans**: Designing interventions that acknowledge and address the specific barriers and facilitators to occupation that exist due to intersecting identities. For example, OTPs might develop specific strategies that support a Hispanic woman in managing her diabetes, considering culturally specific dietary practices and family dynamics that influence her health management.

- **Advocacy and Empowerment**: Working to advocate for changes within systems that create barriers for women. This includes advocating for workplace accommodations, accessible healthcare, and community resources that are responsive to the diverse needs of women with different intersectional identities.

Intersectionality and Women's Occupational Engagement

The application of intersectionality is particularly important in enhancing occupational engagement among women by:

- **Enhancing Work Participation**: Understanding intersectional identities helps OTPs support women in navigating the challenges they face in the workplace. This could involve advocating for policies that support pregnant women, combating workplace discrimination, or supporting women in male-dominated fields.
- **Community Life and Social Participation**: OTPs assist women in overcoming barriers to participating in community life, which may include addressing transportation issues, facilitating access to community centers that provide inclusive programs, or supporting women in roles of community leadership that reflect their cultural and social identities.
- **Health and Wellness**: Intersectionality informs how OTPs approach health promotion and wellness activities by integrating an understanding of how women's health behaviors are influenced by their cultural and social contexts. This might involve creating health education programs that respect and incorporate women's diverse health beliefs and practices.

Centering on Occupation in Women's Health Occupational Therapy

OTPs possess a unique perspective that centers on the meaningful activities—or occupations—that shape a person's life. In women's health, this focus is especially critical due to the diverse roles women assume throughout their lives and the various health challenges they may encounter. By centering on occupation, OTPs contribute significantly to enhancing women's well-being and quality of life.

Importance of Occupation-Centered Practice

Occupation-centered practice in occupational therapy is rooted in the understanding that engagement in meaningful activities is vital for health and wellness. For women, these activities can range from personal care and domestic responsibilities to professional roles and leisure pursuits. Each of these occupations contributes to a woman's sense of identity, autonomy, and well-being.

Application in Women's Health

1. **Understanding Individual Roles and Tasks**: OTPs begin by gaining a deep understanding of the daily roles and tasks that are important to each woman. This includes an assessment of how personal values, cultural influences, and life experiences impact her health and occupational engagement. By acknowledging these factors, OTPs can tailor interventions that are not only effective but also resonate deeply with the individual's life.

Example: An OTP might work with a professional woman who is also a caregiver to elderly parents. By conducting a detailed assessment that includes diary keeping and activity analysis, the OTP can identify times of day when energy levels are highest and suggest scheduling the most demanding tasks during these periods. This helps in managing energy and maintaining effectiveness in both roles.

2. **Addressing Role Overload**: Many women experience role overload due to multiple responsibilities such as caregiving, professional obligations, and household management. OTPs help women strategize to balance these roles effectively. Techniques might include time management training, prioritization strategies, and the introduction of assistive devices or technology to streamline tasks.

    Example: For a single mother juggling work and parenting, an OTP could introduce a combination of physical and digital organizational tools to help her manage household tasks, appointments, and her children's activities. Techniques such as batch cooking on weekends or setting up a shared online calendar for family activities can also be employed to reduce daily stress.

3. **Promoting Health Management and Wellness**: OTPs develop programs that integrate health management into daily routines, enhancing the accessibility and sustainability of health practices. For instance, integrating exercise into a mother's schedule while she is at the playground with her children or developing relaxation routines that can be performed during a lunch break at work.

    Example: An OTP might help a woman integrate physical activity into her routine by identifying opportunities for walking meetings at work or joining a fitness class with a friend to combine social interaction with exercise. For emotional wellness, the OTP could teach mindfulness exercises that can be practiced during short breaks in the workday.

4. **Enhancing Social Participation**: OTPs facilitate women's social participation by addressing barriers and building skills necessary for engaging in community life. This might involve social skills training, mobility training to access community resources, or modifying community environments to be more inclusive.

    Example: To assist a woman with limited mobility in participating more fully in community activities, an OTP could assess for and recommend mobility aids or adaptive transport services. Additionally, the therapist might work with local community centers to ensure that social spaces are accessible, allowing her to attend group activities or classes that interest her.

5. **Supporting Transitions**: Women experience numerous transitions such as entering or re-entering the workforce, becoming a mother, or transitioning to menopause. OTPs provide support during these transitions, helping women to adapt their occupations and manage changes in their roles and physical or emotional states.

    Example: During the transition to menopause, an OTP can help a woman manage physical symptoms that affect her daily activities, such as by suggesting ergonomic tools for work that accommodate joint discomfort or by providing education on sleep hygiene to combat insomnia. The OTP can also facilitate support groups or workshops that allow her to share experiences and strategies with other women navigating similar transitions.

Occupational therapy plays a vital role in women's health, tailoring interventions to their diverse roles and challenges. Therapists collaborate with healthcare professionals, community resources, and families to create holistic support systems. This includes advocating for adjustments in various settings and designing programs that cater to women's needs across different life stages. Additionally, OTPs address women's unique needs through culturally competent assessments and personalized interventions, advocating for system-level changes to reduce barriers and increase accessibility to healthcare and community resources.

Evaluation, Assessment, and Billing in Women's Health

Effective occupational therapy relies heavily on a structured approach to evaluation and assessment, especially within the specialized context of women's health. These foundational processes enable therapists to craft personalized, effective treatment plans that address the unique physiological, psychological, and sociocultural factors influencing women's health at various life stages. From the initial consultation through ongoing treatment, accurate and thorough assessment is vital not only for understanding a client's needs but also for measuring progress and adjusting interventions as necessary.

Moreover, understanding the intricacies of billing and coding for these services is equally crucial. It ensures that services are compensated appropriately and that clients can access the necessary care without undue financial burden. This section will explore the detailed steps involved in evaluating and assessing women in occupational therapy settings, outline effective goal-setting techniques, and discuss best practices for billing and documentation. By the end of this section, readers should have a comprehensive understanding of how these critical components are interwoven to support the delivery of high-quality occupational therapy services in women's health.

Evaluation and Assessment Process

The initial consultation serves as a foundational step in understanding the client's unique needs and formulating an effective treatment plan. This stage goes beyond mere medical history, delving into lifestyle factors, social support systems, and specific concerns pertinent to women's health. During this phase, building rapport and fostering a safe, non-judgmental atmosphere enables clients to openly share their experiences. Employing open-ended questions facilitates the gathering of comprehensive information, encompassing elements such as reproductive health history, pregnancy and childbirth experiences, menstrual patterns, and prevailing symptoms or concerns. For example, in an initial consultation with a client experiencing menopausal symptoms, thorough exploration of symptoms like hot flashes, mood changes, and sleep disturbances is essential. Additionally, understanding the efficacy of coping mechanisms and the overall impact of these symptoms on daily life aids in tailoring interventions. Similarly, when assisting a woman managing chronic pelvic pain, in-depth discussions regarding symptom onset, duration, exacerbating factors, and prior treatment experiences are crucial. Comprehending the psychosocial ramifications of pelvic pain on the client's well-being is also pivotal for devising a comprehensive treatment strategy. Throughout this process, sensitivity to cultural backgrounds, religious beliefs, and individual preferences is imperative, ensuring a client-centered approach.

Evaluation Complexity Levels in Women's Health Occupational Therapy

In women's health occupational therapy, evaluations are often categorized based on complexity levels, ranging from low to high complexity. Each complexity level corresponds to specific CPT codes, which are indicative of the depth and intensity of the evaluation performed. Understanding the nuances of each complexity level is essential for accurate billing and reimbursement, as well as for tailoring evaluation procedures to meet the unique needs of women's health clients (see Table 1.7).

By understanding the distinctions between low, moderate, and high complexity evaluations, OTPs can ensure accurate billing and reimbursement while providing high-quality

Table 1.7 Complexity levels in women's health occupational therapy evaluation, including CPT codes, descriptions, and examples

Complexity	CPT Code	Description	Examples
Low Complexity	97165	- Typically involves straightforward assessment of one to two factors, with no or minimal comorbidities, minimal interpretation & decision-making. - May not require interdisciplinary collaboration.	- Assessing a woman presenting with primary dysmenorrhea (menstrual cramps) and mild anxiety. - Conducting a basic assessment to determine the severity and duration of symptoms, the impact on daily activities, and the effectiveness of previous treatments attempted.
Moderate Complexity	97166	- Requires a comprehensive evaluation of multiple factors with moderate interpretation and decision-making. - Typically involves assessment of three to four factors, with moderate comorbidities. - May require interdisciplinary collaboration for comprehensive care.	- Assessing a woman with chronic pelvic pain, endometriosis, and depression. - Detailed assessment of onset and duration of symptoms, exacerbating and alleviating factors, impact on daily functioning, medical history, psychosocial factors, and potential coexisting conditions. - Collaboration with gynecologists and mental health professionals for integrated treatment planning.
High Complexity	97167	- Demands advanced clinical judgment, interdisciplinary collaboration, and specialized testing for intricate or multifaceted conditions. - Typically involves assessment of five or more factors, with high complexity or multiple comorbidities. - Requires interdisciplinary collaboration among various specialties for integrated care.	- Assessing a woman with complex pelvic floor dysfunction, pelvic organ prolapse, urinary incontinence, endometriosis, and anxiety disorder. - Comprehensive assessment of physical and mental health factors, alongside collaboration with urogynecologists, mental health professionals, or other specialists for integrated treatment planning.

Table 1.8 Comprehensive initial consultation checklist for women's health in occupational therapy

Area to Address	Key Points to Explore
Demographic Information	Age, ethnicity, marital status, occupation, educational background, and primary language.
Reproductive Health History	Menstrual history, pregnancies, childbirth experiences, contraceptive use, gynecological surgeries, etc.
Presenting Symptoms and Concerns	Detailed description of symptoms, onset, duration, exacerbating and alleviating factors, impact on daily life.
Psychosocial Factors	Emotional well-being, stressors, coping strategies, support networks, impact on relationships and daily functioning.
Lifestyle Habits	Diet, exercise habits, sleep patterns, substance use, smoking, alcohol consumption, and recreational activities.
Medical History	Past medical conditions, surgeries, hospitalizations, allergies, medications, and family medical history.
Occupational and Environmental Factors	Work environment, ergonomic considerations, physical demands of job, exposure to environmental toxins or hazards.
Cultural and Religious Beliefs	Cultural practices, beliefs, traditions, taboos, and their influence on health behaviors and treatment preferences.
Personal Preferences and Expectations	Client's goals, expectations from therapy, concerns, preferences for treatment modalities, and involvement in decision-making processes.

care tailored to the specific needs of women's health clients. After understanding the distinctions between low, moderate, and high complexity evaluations, OTPs can effectively navigate the assessment process to provide tailored care for women's health clients. This knowledge not only ensures accurate billing and reimbursement but also enhances the quality of care provided. A crucial aspect of this assessment process is the initial consultation and history taking checklist, which serves as the foundation for understanding the client's unique needs. By systematically exploring demographic information, reproductive health history, presenting symptoms, psychosocial factors, lifestyle habits, medical history, occupational and environmental factors, as well as cultural and religious beliefs, therapists can gain comprehensive insights into the client's health and well-being. Table 1.8 highlights key components of a comprehensive checklist, which sets the stage for effective intervention planning and personalized care.

Physical and Functional Assessments

Physical and functional assessments play a crucial role in evaluating women's health in occupational therapy. These assessments provide valuable insights into a woman's physical abilities, functional limitations, and potential areas for intervention. Key components of physical and functional assessments are listed below:

1. **Musculoskeletal Evaluation**: Assessing the musculoskeletal system involves evaluating the structure, function, and movement of muscles, bones, and joints throughout the body. This assessment encompasses a range of tests to identify impairments, such as joint range of motion, muscle strength, flexibility, and coordination. It helps pinpoint any musculoskeletal issues that may impact a woman's ability to engage in daily activities.

2. **Balance and Mobility Assessment**: Evaluating balance and mobility is essential, especially for women at risk of falls or those with neurological conditions affecting movement. Assessments may include tests like the Timed Up and Go test or the Berg Balance Scale to determine balance deficits and fall risk. Understanding a woman's balance and mobility abilities helps tailor interventions to improve safety and independence in functional tasks.
3. **Activities of Daily Living (ADLs) Assessment**: ADL assessments evaluate a woman's performance in essential self-care tasks necessary for daily living, such as dressing, bathing, grooming, toileting, and feeding. This assessment provides valuable information about her independence, functional status, and any difficulties she may encounter in performing these tasks. It guides intervention planning to enhance her autonomy and quality of life.
4. **Instrumental Activities of Daily Living (IADL) Assessment**: IADL assessments assess a woman's ability to perform more complex tasks critical for independent living, such as meal preparation, housekeeping, managing finances, and using transportation. Identifying any challenges in these areas helps tailor interventions to improve her functional independence and participation in daily life activities.
5. **Environmental Assessment**: Evaluating the woman's home and community environments helps identify any environmental barriers or facilitators that may impact her occupational engagement. This assessment includes evaluating accessibility, safety, and usability of the physical environment to ensure it supports her functional independence and participation. Identifying environmental modifications or accommodations can enhance her ability to engage in meaningful activities within her surroundings.

By conducting thorough physical and functional assessments, OTPs can gain a comprehensive understanding of a woman's health status, functional abilities, and individual needs. These assessments serve as the foundation for developing tailored intervention plans aimed at optimizing her occupational engagement and enhancing her overall well-being.

Cognitive and Emotional Assessments

Cognitive and emotional assessments are integral components of evaluating women's health in occupational therapy. These assessments provide insights into a woman's cognitive functioning, emotional well-being, and psychological factors that may impact her occupational engagement. Key components of cognitive and emotional assessments are outlined below:

1. **Cognitive Functioning Evaluation**: Assessing cognitive functioning involves evaluating various domains, including attention, memory, executive function, and problem-solving skills. Standardized assessments such as the Mini-Mental State Examination (MMSE) or the Montreal Cognitive Assessment (MoCA) may be utilized to assess cognitive abilities. Understanding a woman's cognitive strengths and weaknesses helps tailor interventions to address any cognitive impairments and enhance her ability to participate in daily activities.
2. **Emotional Well-being Assessment**: Evaluating emotional well-being involves assessing a woman's emotional state, coping mechanisms, stress levels, and mental health symptoms such as anxiety or depression. Assessment tools like the Patient Health

Questionnaire-9 (PHQ-9) or the Generalized Anxiety Disorder 7-item (GAD-7) scale may be used to screen for mental health conditions. Identifying emotional concerns enables OTPs to incorporate strategies for emotional regulation and stress management into intervention plans.

3. **Psychosocial Assessment**: A psychosocial assessment examines various psychosocial factors that may impact a woman's health and well-being, including social support networks, family dynamics, cultural influences, and life stressors. This assessment helps identify sources of support as well as potential barriers to occupational engagement. Understanding a woman's psychosocial context informs intervention planning and facilitates the development of strategies to address psychosocial needs. For example, during an assessment, the occupational therapy practitioner may inquire about:

    - **Family Structure**: Understanding the composition of the woman's family, including relationships with partners, children, and extended family members.
    - **Social Support**: Assessing the presence of social support networks, such as friends, neighbors, or community organizations, and how they provide assistance or emotional support.
    - **Cultural Influences**: Exploring the woman's cultural background, traditions, beliefs, and values, and how they influence her health behaviors and attitudes toward occupations.
    - **Life Stressors**: Identifying any significant life events, such as job loss, relocation, financial difficulties, or interpersonal conflicts, that may impact her emotional well-being and occupational engagement.

    Based on the findings of the psychosocial assessment, the occupational therapist can collaboratively develop interventions that address social support needs, cultural considerations, and stress management strategies to support the woman's overall well-being.

4. **Self-Perception and Identity Assessment**: Assessing self-perception and identity involves exploring a woman's sense of self, body image, self-esteem, and personal values. This assessment provides insights into how she perceives herself and her roles within various contexts, including family, work, and community. Understanding a woman's self-perception and identity helps tailor interventions to promote a positive self-image and empower her to engage in meaningful occupations. For example, the occupational therapy practitioner may:

    - **Explore Body Image**: Discuss the woman's feelings and attitudes toward her body, including any concerns or dissatisfaction with physical appearance.
    - **Assess Self-Esteem**: Inquire about the woman's sense of self-worth, confidence, and beliefs about her abilities and achievements.
    - **Explore Personal Values**: Discuss the values and beliefs that are important to the woman, such as independence, autonomy, spirituality, or cultural identity.
    - **Evaluate Roles and Responsibilities**: Identify the various roles and responsibilities the woman holds within her family, work, and community, and how they contribute to her sense of identity and fulfillment.

5. **Functional Emotional Assessment Scale (FEAS)**: The FEAS is a tool specifically designed to assess emotional functioning in relation to daily life activities. It evaluates emotional expression, regulation, and communication within the context of occupational performance. This assessment aids in identifying emotional barriers to engagement in occupations and guides intervention planning to address emotional concerns effectively.

34 Occupational Therapy and Women's Health

By conducting comprehensive cognitive and emotional assessments, OTPs gain a holistic understanding of a woman's psychological well-being and emotional functioning. These assessments inform goal setting and treatment planning, allowing therapists to develop personalized interventions that address cognitive and emotional needs, enhance coping strategies, and promote overall well-being.

Goal Setting and Treatment Planning

Goal setting and treatment planning are fundamental aspects of occupational therapy practice in women's health. These processes involve collaboratively establishing specific, measurable, achievable, relevant, and time-bound (SMART) goals and designing interventions to address the unique needs and priorities of each woman. Effective goal setting and treatment planning promote overall well-being by empowering women to achieve meaningful outcomes and enhance their quality of life.

Goal Setting

Goal setting begins with a comprehensive assessment of the woman's needs, strengths, and challenges. This assessment includes evaluating her physical, cognitive, emotional, and social functioning, as well as considering environmental factors that may impact her occupational engagement. Based on this assessment, SMART goals are identified in collaboration with the woman.

Examples of SMART goals in women's health occupational therapy may include:

- **Empowering Pregnancy**: Develop and implement three strategies to manage prenatal discomfort, such as breathing techniques, relaxation exercises, and birthing positions, aiming to reduce discomfort from 6/10 to 3/10 by the end of the second trimester, enabling the client to actively participate in household chores and childcare activities without discomfort.
- **Reclaiming Postpartum Health**: Restore pelvic floor strength and stability by completing pelvic floor home exercises daily, aiming to improve strength by one half-grade on the Modified Oxford Scale within six weeks postpartum, facilitating the client's ability to engage in activities such as lifting and carrying her newborn without pelvic discomfort.
- **Navigating Menopause**: Explore and practice two coping skills, such as mindfulness meditation and progressive muscle relaxation, to manage symptoms of menopause, aiming to reduce the frequency and intensity of hot flashes by 50% within eight weeks, allowing the client to maintain focus and concentration at work or during leisure activities.
- **Balancing Work and Caregiving**: Develop and implement a time management plan to balance professional responsibilities with caregiving duties, utilizing calendar scheduling and task prioritization techniques, aiming to reduce stress levels and improve work-life balance by increasing leisure time by two hours per week within four weeks, enabling the client to engage in enjoyable hobbies or social activities with friends.
- **Thriving with Chronic Conditions**: Identify and engage in two leisure activities or hobbies that provide enjoyment and relaxation, such as painting or gardening, aiming to increase overall satisfaction and sense of well-being by 25% within four weeks, fostering a sense of purpose and fulfillment in the client's daily life.

Treatment Planning

Once goals are established, treatment plans are developed to outline the interventions and strategies that will be implemented to achieve those goals. Treatment plans are tailored to the woman's unique needs, preferences, and circumstances, and may incorporate a variety of therapeutic approaches and modalities.

Interventions in women's health occupational therapy are designed to address specific goals and may include the following:

1. **Therapeutic Exercises and Activities (CPT code range 97110–97530)**
   - Strengthening exercises to improve muscle tone and function.
   - Range of motion exercises to enhance flexibility and joint mobility.
   - Balance and coordination exercises to reduce fall risk and improve stability.

2. **Manual Therapy (CPT code 97140)**
   - Soft tissue mobilization techniques to address muscle tightness and trigger points.
   - Joint mobilization techniques to improve joint mobility and reduce pain.

3. **Patient Education and Self-Care Training (CPT code range 98960–98962, 97535)**
   - Education on proper body mechanics and ergonomic principles to prevent injury and promote safety during daily activities.
   - Instruction on self-care techniques and home exercises to reinforce treatment goals and facilitate independence.

4. **Modalities (CPT code range 97010–97028)**
   - Heat and cold therapy to manage pain and inflammation.
   - Electrical stimulation to reduce muscle spasms and promote muscle re-education.
   - Ultrasound therapy to enhance tissue healing and reduce scar tissue formation.

5. **Functional Training (CPT code 97530)**
   - Task-specific training to improve performance in activities of daily living, such as dressing, bathing, and cooking.
   - Community reintegration activities to facilitate participation in social and leisure activities outside the home environment.

6. **Cognitive-Behavioural Interventions (CPT code 97129)**
   - Cognitive restructuring to challenge negative thought patterns and promote positive coping strategies.
   - Stress management techniques such as relaxation training and mindfulness meditation to reduce anxiety and improve emotional well-being.

7. **Environmental Modifications (CPT code 97535)**
   - Home assessments and modifications to improve accessibility and safety, such as installing grab bars in the bathroom or removing tripping hazards.
   - Workplace ergonomic assessments and recommendations to optimize workstation setup and prevent musculoskeletal injuries.

8. Community/Work Integration Activities (CPT code 97537)

- Participation in community-based programs and activities to promote social engagement and enhance quality of life.
- Leisure and recreational therapy interventions to facilitate participation in hobbies and interests that promote emotional well-being and satisfaction.

By implementing a comprehensive treatment plan that combines these interventions, OTPs empower women to achieve their goals, enhance their functional independence, and improve their overall well-being. Ongoing assessment and modification of the treatment plan ensure that interventions remain effective and responsive to the woman's changing needs and priorities.

Billing Practices in Occupational Therapy

Billing for occupational therapy services involves several key considerations to ensure accurate reimbursement and compliance with insurance regulations. OTPs must navigate insurance policies, document services appropriately, and advocate for their clients to receive the coverage they need.

Navigating Insurance and Coverage Issues

Understanding insurance policies and coverage criteria is essential for OTPs to provide optimal care while maximizing reimbursement for their services. This includes being knowledgeable about different insurance plans, coverage limitations, and authorization requirements. Therapists may need to advocate for their clients to receive the necessary services by communicating with insurance providers and providing supporting documentation when required.

Documentation for Billing

Accurate and detailed documentation is crucial for billing purposes and ensuring reimbursement for occupational therapy services. Documentation should include thorough assessments, treatment plans, progress notes, and any other relevant information that supports the medical necessity of the services provided. OTPs must adhere to specific documentation guidelines outlined by insurance companies and regulatory bodies to ensure compliance and facilitate successful billing. To ensure successful reimbursement for occupational therapy services, avoiding common billing mistakes is essential. Table 1.9 outlines typical errors and provides strategies for OTPs to navigate the billing process effectively.

Accurate and detailed documentation is crucial for billing purposes and ensuring reimbursement for occupational therapy services. OTPs must adhere to specific documentation guidelines outlined by insurance companies and regulatory bodies to ensure compliance and facilitate successful billing. By implementing these strategies and maintaining meticulous documentation practices, OTPs can streamline the billing process, maximize reimbursement, and continue providing essential services to their clients.

Table 1.9 Common billing mistakes and mitigation strategies

Common Billing Mistake	Mitigation Strategies
Incomplete or Inaccurate	Ensure all required fields in the billing documentation are completed accurately. Double-check codes, dates, and patient information before submitting claims.
Lack of Medical Necessity	Clearly document the medical necessity of occupational therapy services in the patient's records. Include thorough assessments, treatment plans, and progress notes to justify the need for ongoing therapy.
Incorrect Coding	Stay up-to-date with current coding guidelines and use the most appropriate CPT codes for the services provided. Avoid unbundling services or using codes that do not accurately reflect the interventions performed.
Missing Prior Authorization	Verify whether prior authorization is required for occupational therapy services and obtain approval from the insurance company before initiating treatment. Keep detailed records of authorization requests and approvals.
Failure to Follow-Up	Regularly monitor the status of submitted claims and follow up promptly on any denials or delays in reimbursement. Address any issues or discrepancies with the insurance company in a timely manner to expedite payment.
Insufficient Documentation	Ensure documentation is comprehensive and includes all necessary information to support the billed services. Include detailed assessments, treatment plans, progress notes, and any additional documentation requested by the insurance provider.

Further Reading

Agner, J. (2020). Moving from cultural competence to cultural humility in occupational therapy: Aparadigm shift. *American Journal of Occupational Therapy* July/August 2020, *74*(4), 7404347010p1–7404347010p7. https://doi.org/10.5014/ajot.2020.038067

Halle, A. D., Mroz, T. M., Fogelberg, D. J., & Leland, N. E. (2018). Occupational therapy and primary care: Updates and trends. *The American Journal of Occupational Therapy: Official Publication of the American Occupational Therapy Association, 72*(3), 7203090010p1–7203090010p6. https://doi.org/10.5014/ajot.2018.723001

Institute of Medicine (US) Committee on Women's Health Research. (2010). *Women's health research: Progress, pitfalls, and promise*. National Academies Press (US).

Jones, J., Domanico, J., Peek, H., Lee, T. E., & Kern, L. A. (2020). Promoting women's health and wellness. *AOTA OT Practice Magazine, 23*(7), 56–61.

Leland, N. E., Crum, K., Phipps, S., Roberts, P., & Gage, B. (2015). Advancing the value and quality of occupational therapy in health service delivery. *The American Journal of Occupational Therapy: Official Publication of the American Occupational Therapy Association, 69*(1), 6901090010p1–6901090010p7. https://doi.org/10.5014/ajot.2015.691001

Muñoz, J. P. (2007). Culturally responsive caring in occupational therapy. *Occupational Therapy International, 14*(4), 256–280. https://doi.org/10.1002/oti.238

Nichols, F. H. (2000). History of the women's health movement in the 20th century. *Journal of Obstetric, Gynecologic, and Neonatal nursing: JOGNN, 29*(1), 56–64. https://doi.org/10.1111/j.1552-6909.2000.tb02756.x

Office of Research on Women's Health, National Institutes of Health, U.S. Department of Health & Human Services. (2010). Strategic plan moving into the future with new dimensions and strategies: A vision for 2020 for women's health research. Retrieved from https://orwh.od.nih.gov/about/trans-nih-strategic-plan-womens-health-research/vision-2020-womens-health-research

Pergolotti, M., Lavery, J., Reeve, B. B., & Dusetzina, S. B. (2018). Therapy caps and variation in cost of outpatient occupational therapy by provider, insurance status, and geographic region. *The American Journal of Occupational Therapy: Official Publication of the American Occupational Therapy Association, 72*(2), 7202205050p1–7202205050p9. https://doi.org/10.5014/ajot.2018.023796

Spiers, M. V., Geller, P. A., & Kloss, J. D. (Eds.). (2013). *Women's health psychology, Illustrated Edition*. CRC Press.

United Nations. (2020). The world's women 2020: Trends and statistics. Retrieved from https://unstats.un.org/unsd/gender/worldswomen.html

Witt, A., Womersley, K., Strachan, S., Hirst, J., & Norton, R. (2024). Women's health needs beyond sexual, reproductive, and maternal health are missing from the government's 2024 priorities. *BMJ (Clinical Research ed.), 384*, q679. https://doi.org/10.1136/bmj.q679

World Health Organization. (2019). Women's health: Data and statistics. Retrieved from https://www.who.int/health-topics/women-s-health#tab=tab_1

2 Occupational Therapy in Gynecological Health Management

> **Chapter Objectives**
>
> Upon completion of this chapter, the reader will be able to:
>
> 1. Describe the anatomy of the female pelvis, including the bony pelvis, ligaments, joints, vascular supply, and innervation, and their relevance to occupational therapy practice.
> 2. Explain the role of female reproductive hormones and their impact on occupational therapy considerations during different stages of fetal development.
> 3. Identify occupational therapy assessments and interventions specific to gynecological conditions such as urinary incontinence, fecal incontinence, and chronic pelvic pain.
> 4. Illustrate practical applications of occupational therapy in managing gynecological conditions through case studies, including endometriosis.
> 5. Discuss occupational therapy strategies for managing gynecological surgical care, emphasizing holistic and client-centered approaches.

Clinical Anatomy of the Female Pelvis and Perineum

Understanding the anatomy of the female reproductive system provides a solid foundation to managing gynecological conditions. In this comprehensive overview, we will explore the female pelvis, its supporting structures, and the external and internal reproductive organs, shedding light on their significance in occupational therapy practice.

The Bony Pelvis

The pelvis is a strong bony framework reinforced with ligaments and lined with muscles. These muscles form a supportive diaphragm, essential for maintaining the health and function of pelvic organs, including those of the digestive, urinary, and reproductive systems, along with their nerves and blood vessels.

Figure 2.1 shows the components of the female bony pelvis. As shown, it is an irregular but complete bony ring formed by the right and left hip bones anterolaterally, and the sacrum and coccyx posteriorly. Each hip bone is formed by the fusion of three bones: The ilium, ischium, and pubis. The hip bones connect anteriorly via the pubic symphysis and

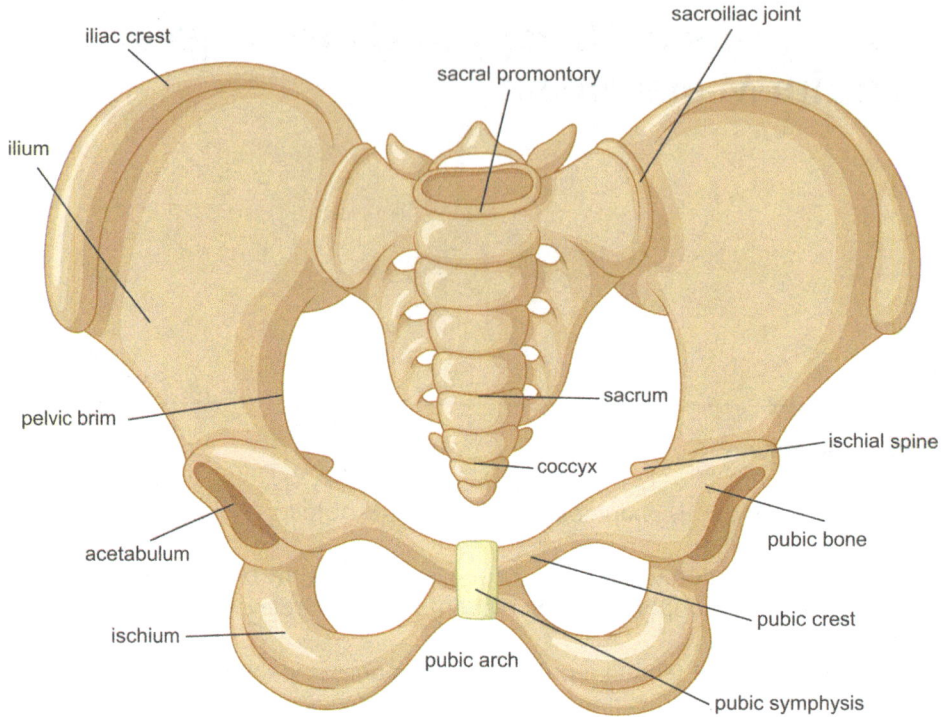

Figure 2.1 The bony pelvis.

posteriorly through the two sacroiliac joints, forming the pelvic girdle. The pelvic girdle articulates with the femoral heads to form the hip joint. The coccyx, attached to the sacrum, consists of fused vertebrae and connects to the caudal end of the sacrum by sacrococcygeal ligaments. The pelvis is separated by an oblique plane into the greater (false) pelvis and the lesser (true) pelvis. The boundary between the true and false pelvis is called the pelvic inlet or brim.

The ilium is the largest and most superior part of the hip bone, forming the upper third of the acetabulum. It consists of the body and wing (ala), with the iliac crest making its superior border. The iliac fossa is the concave inner surface of the wing, separated from the true pelvis by the arcuate line. The ilium's posterior surface, where the gluteal muscles originate, plays a crucial role in stability and mobility, aiding in hip extension and abduction, which are essential for functional mobility and maintaining balance.

The ischium forms the posteroinferior part of the acetabulum and the posterior border of the obturator foramen. The ischial tuberosities support body weight when seated, contributing to postural stability. The ischial spine serves as a landmark for the greater sciatic notch, which is important for the passage of the sciatic nerve, affecting lower limb coordination and movement.

The pubis contributes to the anterior acetabulum and completes the obturator foramen. The pubic symphysis provides anterior stability to the pelvis. The pectineal line runs from the pubic tubercle to the arcuate line of the ilium, playing a role in the attachment of muscles that assist in thigh movement and stabilization during activities like walking and climbing.

OT in Gynecological Health Management 41

The sacrum, made of five fused vertebrae, forms the posterior pelvic wall and articulates with the lumbar vertebrae and coccyx. It provides a strong foundation for the pelvis, supporting the weight of the upper body and contributing to overall postural stability. The female pelvis is typically wider due to a shorter and broader sacrum, accommodating pregnancy and childbirth.

The coccyx, consisting of four fused vertebrae, provides attachment points for several ligaments and muscles, including the sacrotuberous and sacrospinous ligaments, as well as the gluteus maximus, levator ani, and coccygeus muscles. These structures are important for pelvic floor stability and function, supporting activities like sitting, bowel and bladder control, and core stability.

The pelvic inlet is bounded by the iliopectineal lines, pubic symphysis, and sacral promontory, while the pelvic outlet is defined by the pubic symphysis, pubic rami, ischial tuberosities, sacrotuberous ligaments, and coccyx apex. The space between the pelvic inlet and outlet, known as the pelvic cavity, is crucial for supporting and protecting internal organs, and its configuration impacts activities requiring lower body coordination and mobility.

The differences between the male and female pelvis play crucial roles in various functional activities and physical capacities. The male pelvis is typically characterized by a narrower pelvic cavity and a sub-pubic angle of approximately 90 degrees, designed for supporting a heavier build and larger muscle attachments. Conversely, the female pelvis is adapted for childbirth, featuring a wider pelvic cavity and a sub-pubic angle of about 120 degrees. This structure not only supports the reproductive process but also affects everyday activities by providing stability and mobility, critical for maintaining balance and facilitating movement. The shallower pelvic cavity in females enhances lower body coordination and mobility, which is essential during pregnancy as the body undergoes significant physiological changes to accommodate and support fetal development. These anatomical distinctions are pivotal for OTPs in addressing health management activities related to pregnancy and childbirth (see Figure 2.2).

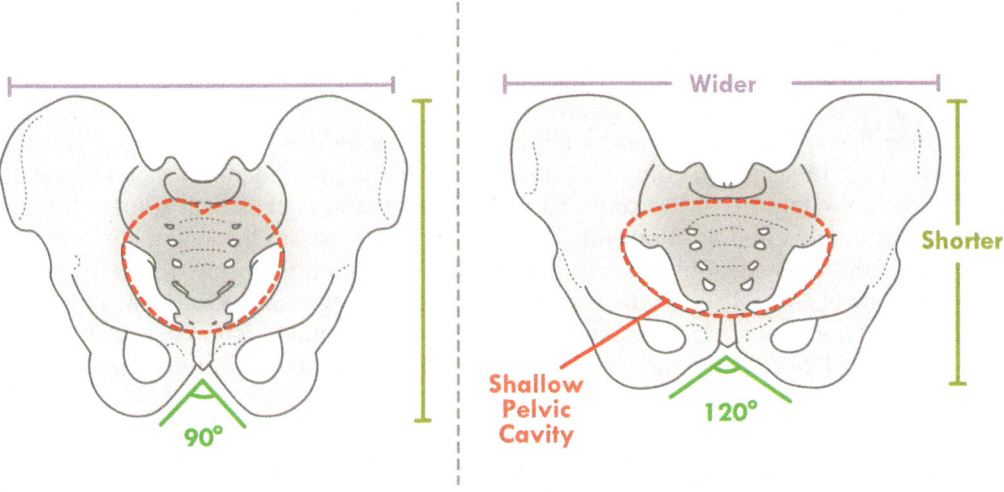

Figure 2.2 The male pelvis (left) compared to female (right) pelvis.

Joints and Ligaments of the Pelvis

The joints in the pelvis include the symphysis pubis and the lumbosacral, sacroiliac, and sacrococcygeal joints. The bony pelvis as an entity articulates with the femur laterally to form the hip joint. The symphysis pubis is a cartilaginous joint formed by the anterior articulation of the two pubic bones. It is capable of minimal movement and is secured by the superior and arcuate pubic ligaments. The sacroiliac joint is a compound joint formed by the articulation of the ilium and sacrum. It permits minimal movement and transmits some weight from the upper limbs and trunk to the lower limbs. The joints in the pelvis are reinforced by ligaments such as the sacrospinous, sacrotuberous, and iliolumbar ligaments. These ligaments help to stabilize the pelvic joints. The ligaments attached to the symphysis pubis are flexible and further loosen during pregnancy via the action of hormones to facilitate separation of the pelvic bones at childbirth.

Pelvic fascia and ligaments provide structural support to the pelvic organs and contribute to their stability. The parietal pelvic fascia covers the deep surfaces of the pelvic wall and floor muscles, while the visceral pelvic fascia forms an investing layer around the pelvic viscera. Continuous bands of connective tissue, such as the tendinous arch of the pelvic fascia, anchor the bladder anteriorly and the vagina and rectum posteriorly.

Pelvic Organs

The pelvic cavity houses key components of the urinary, reproductive, and digestive systems, all of which play significant roles in daily activities and occupational performance. The pelvic viscera include the bladder and proximal urethra, rectum, the distal third of the sigmoid colon, uterus, fallopian tubes, ovaries, and the pelvic portion of the vagina.

The urinary bladder is situated anteriorly in the pelvis, just behind the symphysis pubis. The bladder is supported by pubovesical ligaments in females. This structure is critical for continence and influences activities like toileting. The urethra extends from the bladder, passing through the pelvic floor to the vaginal vestibule in females, affecting urinary function and control. The vagina, located just behind the bladder, is supported by the uterus above it. The uterus, with its forward tilt, rests on the bladder, impacting its stability and function. The uterine tubes extend from the uterus towards the ovaries, which are anchored by suspensory and broad ligaments. These reproductive organs are essential for functions related to fertility, pregnancy, and childbirth, which OTPs address when working with clients on reproductive health and maternal care. In a subsequent section, we shall consider in detail the female reproductive system.

The digestive system components within the pelvis include the sigmoid colon, rectum, and anal canal. The sigmoid colon transitions into the rectum at the third sacral segment, and the rectum conforms to the contours of the sacrum and coccyx as it approaches the pelvic floor. The rectum transitions into the anal canal as it passes through the pelvic diaphragm, controlled by the puborectalis portion of the levator ani muscle. This transition is crucial for bowel control and impacts activities of daily living, such as toileting and maintaining bowel continence. Understanding these anatomical and functional aspects is vital for occupational therapy practitioners to address issues related to gastrointestinal health and its impact on daily occupations.

Blood Vessels and Nerves of the Pelvis

The blood supply and innervation of the pelvic organs are integral to their function and have significant implications for occupational therapy. The bladder receives blood from branches of the internal iliac arteries, specifically the superior, middle, and inferior vesical arteries, and is innervated by the vesical nerve plexus. This innervation includes parasympathetic fibers that stimulate muscle contraction for urine release and sympathetic fibers that help maintain continence by inhibiting the internal sphincter. Efficient bladder function is crucial for continence management, which is a key focus in occupational therapy interventions related to toileting and personal care.

The ovaries and uterus also have a rich blood supply and nerve network. The ovaries are supplied by the ovarian arteries from the abdominal aorta, with venous drainage into the left renal vein and inferior vena cava. The uterine arteries, branching from the internal iliac arteries, provide blood to the uterus, while venous drainage occurs through plexuses that join the internal iliac veins. Innervation to the uterus is from sympathetic and afferent fibers, which are important for reproductive health and managing pain during menstrual cycles. Other female genitalia receive innervation from a complex network of nerves, including branches of the pelvic plexus, pudendal nerve, and hypogastric nerve. The rectum and anal canal receive blood from the superior, middle, and inferior rectal arteries, with venous drainage following similar pathways. The pelvic splanchnic nerves innervate the rectum, providing motor control for bowel movements.

Lymphatic vessels transport lymphatic fluid away from pelvic organs to lymph nodes in the pelvis and inguinal region. Lymphatic drainage is integral to maintaining fluid balance and immune function within the female reproductive system.

OTPs need to understand these systems to effectively address issues related to reproductive health, bowel management, and overall pelvic health in their clients. Understanding the vascular anatomy within the pelvis is crucial, especially in the context of gynecological surgeries, where minimizing the risk of hemorrhage is paramount. Additionally, patients with vascular conditions like deep vein thrombosis (DVT) may require special considerations for activity recommendations to optimize healing and pain management. Also, OTPs may need to address lymphatic system dysfunction such as lymphedema following cancer treatment.

OTPs should also consider neural innervation when assessing patients with neuropathic pain or neurological conditions affecting the pelvic region, such as pelvic floor dysfunction or urinary incontinence.

The Female Reproductive System

The female reproductive system is made up of the internal and external reproductive organs.

The external female genitalia, collectively known as the vulva, consist of the mons pubis, labia majora, labia minora, clitoris, urethra, vulva vestibule, Bartholin's glands, Skene's glands, vestibular bulbs, and vaginal opening. It serves a dual purpose—reproduction and urination. The external female reproductive anatomy plays a significant role in various aspects of daily functioning and quality of life.

The **mons pubis** is a rounded fatty area over the pubic bone containing sweat and scent glands and contributes to sexual arousal and lubrication. Occupational therapy practitioners may encounter clients experiencing pain or discomfort in this area, impacting their ability to engage in activities such as sitting, exercising, or sexual intercourse. The **labia majora** and **labia minora** protect inner vulvar structures and are involved in sensory and protective functions. Discomfort or irritation in these areas can hinder participation in daily activities, including personal hygiene, clothing choices, and sexual activities. The **clitoris** is a highly sensitive organ. It is central to sexual pleasure, and clients may report issues related to clitoral pain or hypersensitivity, which can affect sexual functioning and overall well-being.

The **vestibule** houses the urethral opening and vaginal orifice, playing a critical role in urinary and reproductive functions (see Figure 2.3). Pain or discomfort in the vestibular area can disrupt activities such as urination, sexual intercourse, and tampon use. The **vaginal orifice** is essential for sexual intercourse, childbirth, and menstruation. Concerns related to pain or discomfort during these activities can significantly impact a woman's quality of life. OTPs are equipped to address these issues through targeted interventions, education, and therapeutic exercises, thereby enhancing clients' participation in meaningful activities and improving their overall well-being.

The internal female reproductive organs include the vagina, cervix, uterus, fallopian tubes, and ovaries.

The **vagina**, a muscular canal connecting the external genitalia to the cervix, is essential for sexual intercourse, childbirth, and menstrual flow. Conditions such as vaginismus or vulvodynia can cause significant pain and discomfort, affecting a woman's ability to engage in intimate activities or use tampons, thereby impacting her daily functioning and quality of life.

The **cervix**, the lower part of the uterus, connects the vagina to the uterine cavity and plays a vital role in reproductive health by allowing sperm transport, enabling menstruation, and acting as a barrier during pregnancy. Women experiencing cervical pain or discomfort may find it challenging to engage in physical activities or maintain a healthy sexual life.

The **uterus** is a muscular organ where a fertilized egg implants and develops into a fetus during pregnancy. Although it is primarily a pelvic organ, during pregnancy, it

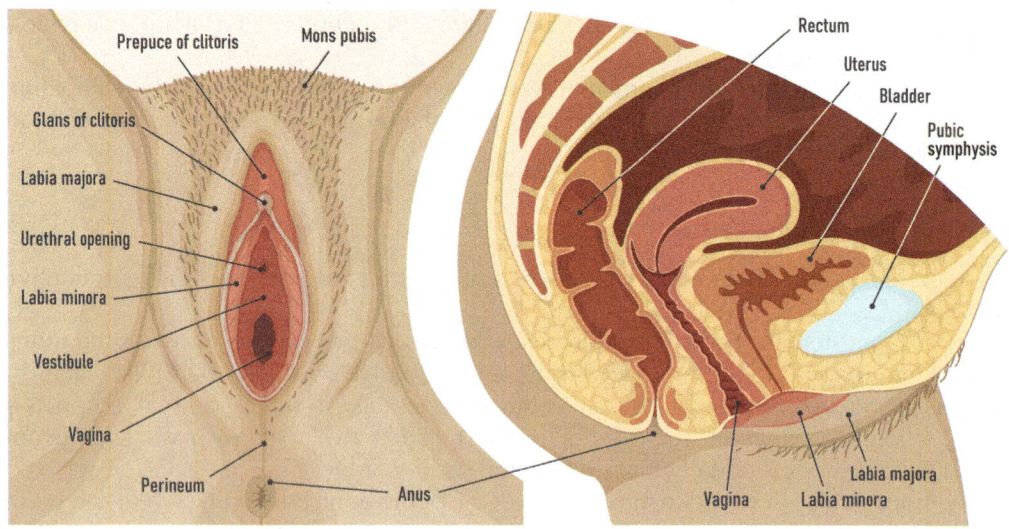

Figure 2.3 The female external genitalia.

OT in Gynecological Health Management 45

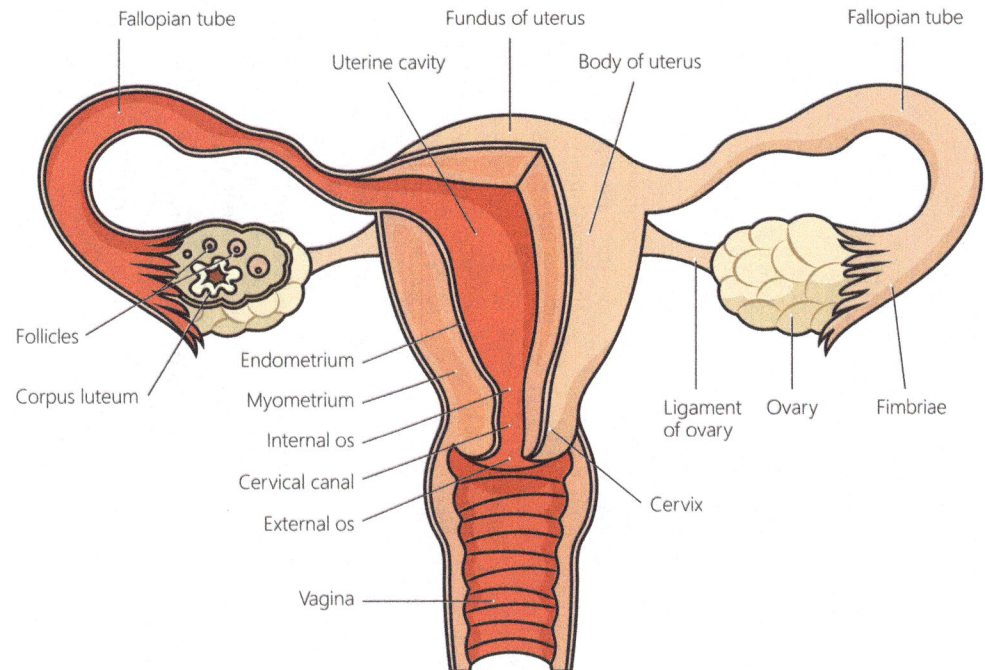

Figure 2.4 The female internal reproductive organs.

hypertrophies and can extend up to the epigastric region in the third trimester. The uterus may be affected by conditions like uterine fibroids or endometriosis, causing significant pain and discomfort. This pain can interfere with a woman's ability to perform daily tasks, work, and engage in social activities.

The **ovaries**, responsible for producing ova and hormones like estrogen and progesterone, play a critical role in a woman's reproductive and hormonal health. Hormonal imbalances can lead to emotional disturbances and affect daily routines.

Pelvic Floor Muscles

The muscles of the pelvis form the pelvic diaphragm which is integral to daily functioning and well-being. The pelvic diaphragm consists of the pubococcygeus, iliococcygeus, coccygeus, and puborectalis muscles. The pelvic floor plays a crucial role in supporting organs within the pelvis, particularly when the intrabdominal pressure rises, e.g., when coughing or straining. They also facilitate essential bodily functions such as urination, defecation, and sexual activity. Importantly, other muscles which attach to the bony pelvis also contribute to pelvic function and stabilization. As OTPs, understanding the anatomy of the pelvic floor is vital, as these muscles contribute significantly to our clients' ability to engage in meaningful activities and occupations. See Table 2.1 below for a detailed overview of the pelvic floor muscles and other muscles of the pelvis.

Table 2.1 The muscles of the pelvis

Muscle	Origin (Proximal Attachment)	Insertion (Distal Attachment)	Innervation	Main Action	Blood Supply	Muscle Group
Iliacus	Superior two-thirds of iliac fossa, ala of sacrum, anterior sacro-iliac ligaments	Lesser trochanter of femur and shaft inferior to psoas major tendon	Femoral nerve	Flexes thigh at hips and stabilizes hip joint, acts with psoas major	Iliac branches of iliolumbar artery	Anterior thigh
Obturator Internus	Pelvic surface of obturator membrane and surrounding bone	Medial surface of greater trochanter of femur	Nerve to obturator internus	Laterally rotates extended thigh, abducts flexed thigh at hip	Internal pudendal and obturator arteries	Gluteal region
Piriformis	Anterior surface of sacral segments 2–4, sacrotuberous ligament	Superior border of greater trochanter of femur	Ventral rami of S1, S2	Laterally rotates extended thigh, abducts flexed thigh at hip	Superior and inferior gluteal arteries, internal pudendal artery	Gluteal region
Coccygeus (Ischiococcygeus)	Ischial spine, sacrospinous ligament	Inferior sacrum, coccyx	Ventral rami of lower sacral nerves	Supports pelvic viscera, draws coccyx forward	Inferior gluteal artery	Pelvic floor
Levator ani	Body of pubis, tendinous arch of obturator fascia, ischial spine	Perineal body, coccyx, anococcygeal raphe, walls of prostate or vagina, rectum, anal canal	Ventral rami of lower sacral nerves, perineal nerve	Supports pelvic viscera, raises pelvic floor	Inferior gluteal artery, internal pudendal artery and its branches (inferior rectal and perineal arteries)	Pelvic floor
Puborectalis	Lower part of pubic symphysis, superior fascia of urogenital diaphragm	Loops around rectum; no distal attachment	Nerve to levator ani muscle	Maintains fecal continence	Inferior gluteal, inferior vesical and pudendal arteries	Pelvic floor
Bulbospongiosus	Perineal body in females	In females, dorsum of clitoris, inferior fascia of urogenital diaphragm, bulb of vestibule, pubic arch	Deep branch of perineal nerve from pudendal nerve	In females, constricts vaginal orifice, assists in expressing secretions of greater vestibular gland, forces blood into body of clitoris	Internal pudendal artery and its branch (perineal artery)	Perineal

Muscle	Origin	Insertion	Nerve	Action	Artery	Region
Compressor urethrae (female only)	Ischiopubic ramus	Anterior aspect of urethra	Perineal branches of pudendal nerve	Sphincter of urethra	Perineal branch of internal pudendal artery	Perineal
Deep transverse perineal	Inner surface of inferior ischial rami	The sides of vagina in females	Perineal branches of pudendal nerve	Stabilizes perineal body, supports vagina	Perineal branch of internal pudendal artery	Perineal
External anal sphincter	Tip of coccyx, anococcygeal ligament	Deeper fibers surround anal canal, attach posteriorly to coccyx and anteriorly to central point of perineum	Perineal and inferior rectal branches of pudendal nerve	Closes anal orifice	Inferior rectal and transverse perineal artery	Perineal
Ischiocavernosus	Inferior internal surface of ischiopubic ramus, ischial tuberosity	Crus of the clitoris	Deep branch of perineal nerve from pudendal nerve	Forces blood into body of penis and clitoris during erection	Internal pudendal artery and its branch (perineal artery)	Perineal
Sphincter urethrae	External fibers from junction of inferior pubic and ischial rami and adjacent fascia; internal fibers pass medially to surround membranous urethra	Encloses urethra, attaches to sides of vagina in females	Perineal branches of pudendal nerve	Compresses urethra at end of micturition. Also compresses the distal vagina	Perineal branch of internal pudendal artery	Perineal
Sphincter urethrovaginalis (female only)	Perineal body	Passes forward and anterior around urethra	Perineal branches of pudendal nerve	Sphincter of urethra and vagina	Perineal branch of pudendal artery	Perineal
Superficial transverse perineal	Ischial rami and tuberosities	Central tendon (perineal body)	Perineal branches of pudendal nerve	Stabilizes central tendon	Perineal branch of internal pudendal artery	Perineal

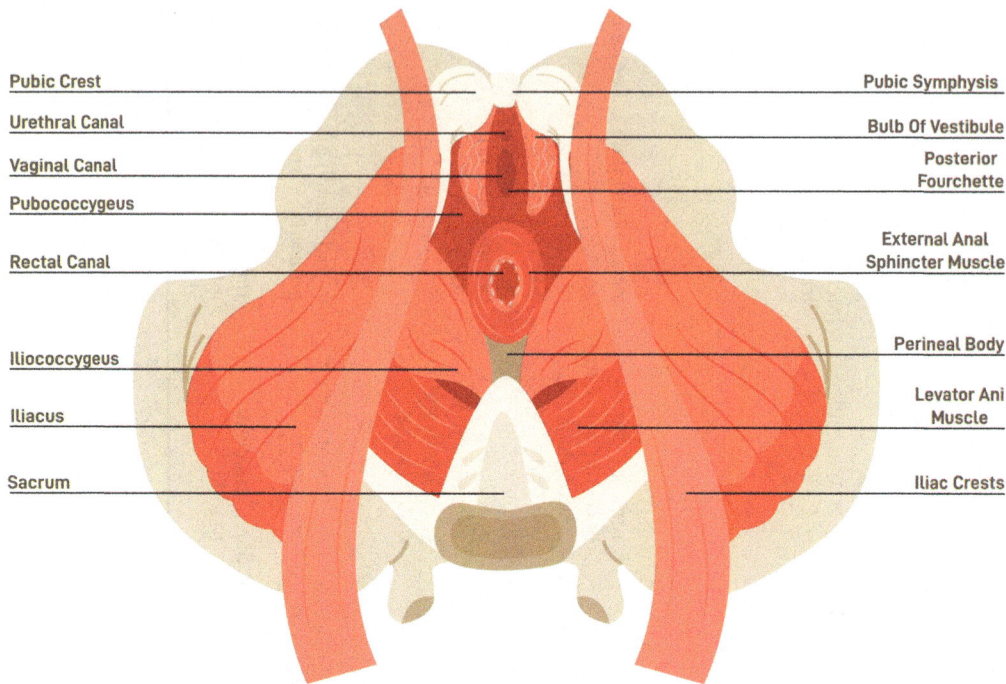

Figure 2.5 Female pelvic floor muscles.

Persons Assigned Male at Birth: Pelvic Floor Considerations

Pelvic floor muscles play a crucial role in supporting bodily functions such as urination, defecation, and sexual activity. The functionality and health concerns related to these muscles can vary significantly depending on one's reproductive anatomy, which is influenced by whether they were assigned female at birth (AFAB) or assigned male at birth (AMAB). See Table 2.2 for pelvic floor muscle functions by gender assigned at birth. For AMAB individuals, including cisgender men, some transgender women, and nonbinary individuals with penises, pelvic floor muscle considerations often differ from those of AFAB individuals. Understanding these differences is essential for OTPs specializing in pelvic rehabilitation.

Table 2.2 Pelvic floor muscle functions by gender assigned at birth

Pelvic floor muscles in people who are AFAB	Pelvic floor muscles in people who are AMAB
Support bladder, urethra, vagina, uterus, bowel (large intestine), rectum, anus	Support bladder, urethra, bowel (large intestine), rectum, anus
Control urination and defecation	Control urination and defecation
Help with blood flow and vaginal contractions during sex and orgasm	Help with erection and ejaculation during sex
Support vaginal delivery during childbirth	

AMAB pelvic floor muscles primarily support the bladder, urethra, bowel (large intestine), rectum, and anus, and are involved in controlling urination and defecation, as well as aiding in erection and ejaculation during sexual activity. It is important for OTPs to consider the unique aspects of pelvic health in AMAB individuals, especially for those who may undergo hormone replacement therapy (HRT) or gender-affirming surgeries. These treatments can alter muscle tone, tissue elasticity, and overall pelvic floor function. For instance, testosterone therapy can lead to changes in muscle mass and strength, while surgical procedures like phalloplasty or orchiectomy can impact pelvic floor integrity and necessitate specialized rehabilitative strategies.

This nuanced understanding aids in developing targeted interventions that address specific pelvic health issues, from incontinence to sexual dysfunction, while also ensuring respectful and culturally competent care. OTPs must be adept at adjusting therapeutic approaches based on individual anatomical and hormonal backgrounds to effectively support the pelvic health and well-being of AMAB individuals.

The Perineum

The perineum, situated between the thighs, is defined by lines connecting the pubic symphysis, ischial tuberosities, and coccyx. It consists of an anterior urogenital triangle and a posterior anal triangle. The urogenital triangle contains the external genitalia and urethral orifice, while the anal triangle houses the anal canal and ischioanal fossa, a fat-filled space. The urogenital (UG) diaphragm, composed of skeletal muscle and covered by fascia, spans between the ischiopubic rami, closing the anterior half of the pelvic outlet while allowing passage of the urethra and vagina. The perineal body, located centrally between the anal and urogenital triangles, serves as an anchor for the vagina and anal canal, contributing to urinary and fecal continence. The pudendal nerve supplies the perineum, originating from spinal nerves S2-S4 and providing sensory and motor innervation.

The perineal body, described as a complex fibromuscular mass, plays a crucial role in maintaining urinary and fecal continence by serving as an anchor for both the vagina and anal canal. Its integrity prevents the expansion of the urogenital hiatus and acts as a physical barrier between the rectum and vagina. Damage to the perineal body, often occurring during childbirth, can lead to weakness of perineal muscles and subsequent incontinence issues. Furthermore, injury to the pudendal nerves during labor may result in compromised muscle function, highlighting the importance of perineal health in functional activities related to bowel and bladder control.

Additionally, the pudendal nerve, which supplies the perineum, contributes to the innervation of pelvic floor muscles involved in maintaining urinary continence. Understanding the physiology of micturition and the role of pelvic floor muscles in maintaining urinary continence is essential for OTPs when addressing functional impairments related to bladder control in their clients. By targeting interventions aimed at strengthening pelvic floor muscles and optimizing nerve function, OTPs can support individuals in maintaining independence and participation in essential daily activities.

Female Reproductive Hormones

Hormonal regulation in the female reproductive system involves key hormones such as estrogen, progesterone, and gonadotropins (including luteinizing hormone (LH) and follicle-stimulating hormone (FSH). These hormones are crucial for maintaining gynecological health and have significant impacts on a woman's overall well-being, daily routines, and activities of daily living (ADLs). Understanding these hormonal influences is essential for OTPs when addressing the unique needs of female patients.

Estrogen is a primary hormone responsible for the development of secondary sexual characteristics, regulation of the menstrual cycle, and maintenance of reproductive tissues. It is released by the ovaries. Estrogen also impacts mood, bone density, and cardiovascular health. Fluctuations in estrogen levels, e.g., during menopause, can lead to gynecological symptoms like vaginal dryness, hot flashes, and irregular menstrual cycles. These changes can affect a woman's ability to engage in daily activities and maintain a consistent routine.

Progesterone, also secreted by the ovaries, functions in conjunction with estrogen to regulate the menstrual cycle and support pregnancy. It prepares the endometrium for a fertilized egg and maintains pregnancy. Low levels of progesterone can lead to gynecological issues such as irregular menstrual cycles, which may cause mood changes and sleep disturbances, impacting overall well-being and daily functioning.

The gonadotropins are the luteinizing hormone (LH) and follicle stimulating hormone (FSH). They are produced by the pituitary gland in the brain. LH triggers ovulation, while FSH promotes the growth of ovarian follicles. Imbalances in these hormones can result in conditions such as polycystic ovary syndrome (PCOS), characterized by irregular menstrual cycles, infertility, and metabolic issues. Symptoms of PCOS, such as weight gain, acne, and excessive hair growth, can affect self-esteem and participation in daily activities.

Pelvic Health and Pelvic Floor Dysfunction in Occupational Therapy

Pelvic floor dysfunction encompasses a spectrum of conditions affecting the pelvic floor muscles and connective tissues, which play a crucial role in supporting pelvic organs and maintaining continence. Despite the prevalence of these conditions, particularly among older adult women and those who have undergone pelvic surgeries such as caesarean sections or vaginal births, it is critical to recognize that these dysfunctions are not normal aspects of aging or post-surgical recovery. Evidence indicates that pelvic floor dysfunction can manifest in various ways, with urinary and fecal incontinence being prominent examples. These conditions can significantly impact daily activities, psychological well-being, and quality of life, but they can be managed effectively with appropriate interventions.

Urinary and fecal incontinence are among the most common forms of pelvic floor dysfunction, and while often associated with aging or as standard postpartum experiences, they should not be considered normal or inevitable. Research highlights that these are treatable conditions, not merely unavoidable consequences of life changes. They significantly impede occupational functioning by restricting individuals' ability to engage in daily activities, work, social interactions, and even leisure due to fear of incontinence episodes. Occupational therapy plays an indispensable role in managing these conditions through evidence-based interventions like pelvic floor muscle training, therapeutic activities, lifestyle education, adaptive strategies, and biofeedback. These therapeutic strategies aim not only to promote health of the pelvic floor but also to restore confidence and enable individuals to participate more fully in their desired occupations and activities, thus improving their overall quality of life.

Urinary Incontinence

Urinary incontinence (UI) has a significant impact on occupation, activities of daily living, and overall mental health. It is associated with depression, loss of self-esteem, hopelessness, and anxiety. Women with UI further experience restrictions in social interactions, relationships, and sexual activity. The psychosocial impact of urinary incontinence spreads across the individual, family members, caregivers, and the community as a whole. OTPs are key players in assisting individuals with UI to regain control of their lives and resume their daily occupations, ensuring an improvement in their quality of life.

There are three main types of urinary incontinence:

1. **Stress Urinary Incontinence (SUI)**: This type of incontinence predominantly affects women due to both physiological and anatomical factors. While childbirth is a common cause, with potential complications such as the use of forceps, damage to the pudendal nerve, episiotomies, and prolonged labor weakening the pelvic floor muscles and internal urethral sphincter, women who have not given birth can also be susceptible. Factors like hormonal fluctuations, particularly the decrease in estrogen during menopause, can weaken pelvic tissues and exacerbate SUI. Additionally, women's broader pelvic structure inherently places more stress on the pelvic floor, increasing the risk of SUI during activities that raise intra-abdominal pressure, such as coughing, sneezing, or exercising.
2. **Urge Incontinence**: Although both men and women can suffer from urge incontinence, women may experience it more acutely due to structural and hormonal differences. The prevalence of overactive bladder syndrome is notably higher in women, particularly after menopause, which can lead to involuntary contractions of the bladder muscle and sudden, difficult-to-control urges to urinate. These symptoms are often exacerbated by hormonal changes that affect the stability and responsiveness of the urinary tract, making management and treatment a crucial aspect of women's healthcare.
3. **Mixed Incontinence**: Mixed incontinence, which combines symptoms of both stress and urge incontinence, poses a significant challenge for women. This condition can greatly impact a woman's ability to engage in daily activities and maintain social or occupational roles due to the unpredictability of leakage and the need for frequent bathroom visits. Women with mixed incontinence face both the involuntary muscle contractions characteristic of urge incontinence and the weakened pelvic support associated with SUI. Effective management of mixed incontinence in women often requires a comprehensive approach that addresses hormonal balance, strengthens pelvic floor muscles, and modifies lifestyle factors to mitigate symptoms.

Fecal Incontinence

Fecal continence is maintained by several factors such as adequate transit time and consistency of feces, normal storage capacity in the rectum, functioning anal sphincters, adequate contraction of the puborectalis muscle, and sensory awareness of feces in the rectum. Impairment of any of these factors may result in fecal incontinence. Common causes of fecal incontinence include trauma from childbirth, surgical repairs, neurological impairments, and rectal prolapse. Managing fecal incontinence requires a comprehensive evaluation to ascertain the cause and provide effective and individualized therapy for clients. Important assessments to be conducted when evaluating fecal incontinence include:

- **Digital Rectal Examination:** This involves placing the index finger in the rectum to manually test the resting tone and strength of the external anal sphincters. It may also be done to test for tenderness in the anal canal.
- **Anorectal Manometry:** This examines the integrity of the anal sphincters, rectal sensations, and patterns of expulsion within the anal canal. A flexible pressure-sensitive catheter is inserted into the rectum to evaluate reflexes, contractions, and measure rectal pressures.
- **Balloon Expulsion Test:** This tests the client's perception of feces within the rectum using a balloon. The balloon is gradually inflated with air, and the first sensation, first urge to defecate, and maximum tolerable volume are recorded.

Management of urinary and fecal incontinence may involve surgical, pharmacological, or behavioural interventions. Behavioural therapy is recommended as the first-line approach for managing UI and FI, and OTPs help provide this treatment to clients.

Client Education and Lifestyle Modification

Client education and lifestyle adjustments are crucial for a successful pelvic rehabilitation program. Clients may be educated on the anatomy of the pelvic floor, triggers to avoid, and beneficial habits. Key lifestyle changes include:

- Adequate hydration to prevent the formation of concentrated urine.
- Modification of fluid intake patterns, especially at night.
- Intentional weight loss for individuals with a body mass index above 25 kg/m^2.
- Smoking cessation.
- Elimination or reduction in intake of bladder irritants, such as alcohol, caffeine, spicy meals, carbonated drinks, chocolate, coffee, and tea.
- Dietary modification with increased consumption of high-fiber meals to encourage adequate bowel movements. Constipation worsens bladder symptoms as a distended rectum exerts pressure on the bladder, and straining further stresses the pelvic floor muscles.
- Timed voiding and double voiding. Scheduling toileting helps with bladder training. Clients should avoid straining while urinating to prevent stressing the pelvic floor muscles. If there is a feeling of incomplete voiding, clients may sit back again (double voiding).
- The use of incontinence pads may be associated with excoriations and irritations around the pelvic region; hence, clients using these pads may be advised to apply barrier skincare products.
- Consuming fiber-rich diets can help increase stool bulk and bowel movement beneficial for FI. Avoidance of bowel irritants may also be advised.

Pelvic Floor Muscle Exercises

Weak pelvic floor muscles can be strengthened through pelvic floor contractions, also known as Kegel exercises. It is important for these contractions to be done consistently and frequently to yield results—around 60 to 80 squeezes per day are generally recommended. However, the specific set of repetitions should be individually prescribed after a pelvic floor examination. The contractions can be spaced out, for example, to 20 contractions thrice daily to improve adherence and can be performed during daily activities such as showering or brushing teeth. Clients need to be taught to maintain a normal breathing rhythm while doing the exercises.

When performing Kegel exercises, individuals should be cued to "imagine stopping the flow of urine and holding in gas," which helps understand the motion of pulling the pelvic floor muscles up and in. There are two main types of Kegel exercises:

- **Short Holds**: These involve contracting the pelvic floor muscles for about 2 seconds, then relaxing. This targets the Type II muscle fibers, which are fast-twitch fibers responsible for quick, powerful contractions.
- **Endurance Contractions**: These involve holding the contraction for about 10 seconds before relaxing, aiming to build endurance in the Type I muscle fibers, which are slow-twitch fibers designed for stamina and sustained activities.

These exercises are crucial because they strengthen all aspects of the pelvic floor muscles, accommodating their mixed muscle fiber composition, which is essential for both rapid responses and sustained support.

Additionally, the squeezes should not be performed while urinating as this can lead to voiding dysfunctions. **On the contrary, if hypertonicity (overactive or excessively tense pelvic floor muscles) is the contributing factor to pelvic floor dysfunction, Kegel exercises might exacerbate symptoms**. In cases of hypertonicity, relaxation exercises are recommended instead. These focus on relaxing the pelvic floor muscles rather than strengthening them, aiming to reduce muscle tension and improve functional outcomes. Detailed instructions for pelvic muscle strengthening and relaxation exercises are described in Table 2.3. Sample relaxation and strengthening exercises are shown in Figures 2.6 and 2.7. In cases of FI, a deficient external anal sphincter can be strengthened via squeezes assisted by EMG biofeedback. Kegel exercises are also recommended to strengthen the pelvic floor muscles in cases of FI.

Table 2.3 Do's and don'ts of an effective pelvic floor muscle exercise program

Do's	*Don'ts*
Lie in a supine or lateral recumbent position.	Avoid using your stomach, buttocks or thigh muscles when performing the exercise.
Contract and relax the pelvic floor, as if preventing the flow of urine	Avoid holding your breath while performing the squeezes
Begin by doing brief 1 second squeezes and gradually increases the duration of the squeezes as tolerated.	Avoid performing pelvic floor contractions during urination. Instead, perform them while washing your hands and after drying your hangs.
Contract and hold your pelvic floor muscles before sneezing, coughing or lifting.	
Squeeze and hold your pelvic floor when getting out of bed or standing from a sitting position.	

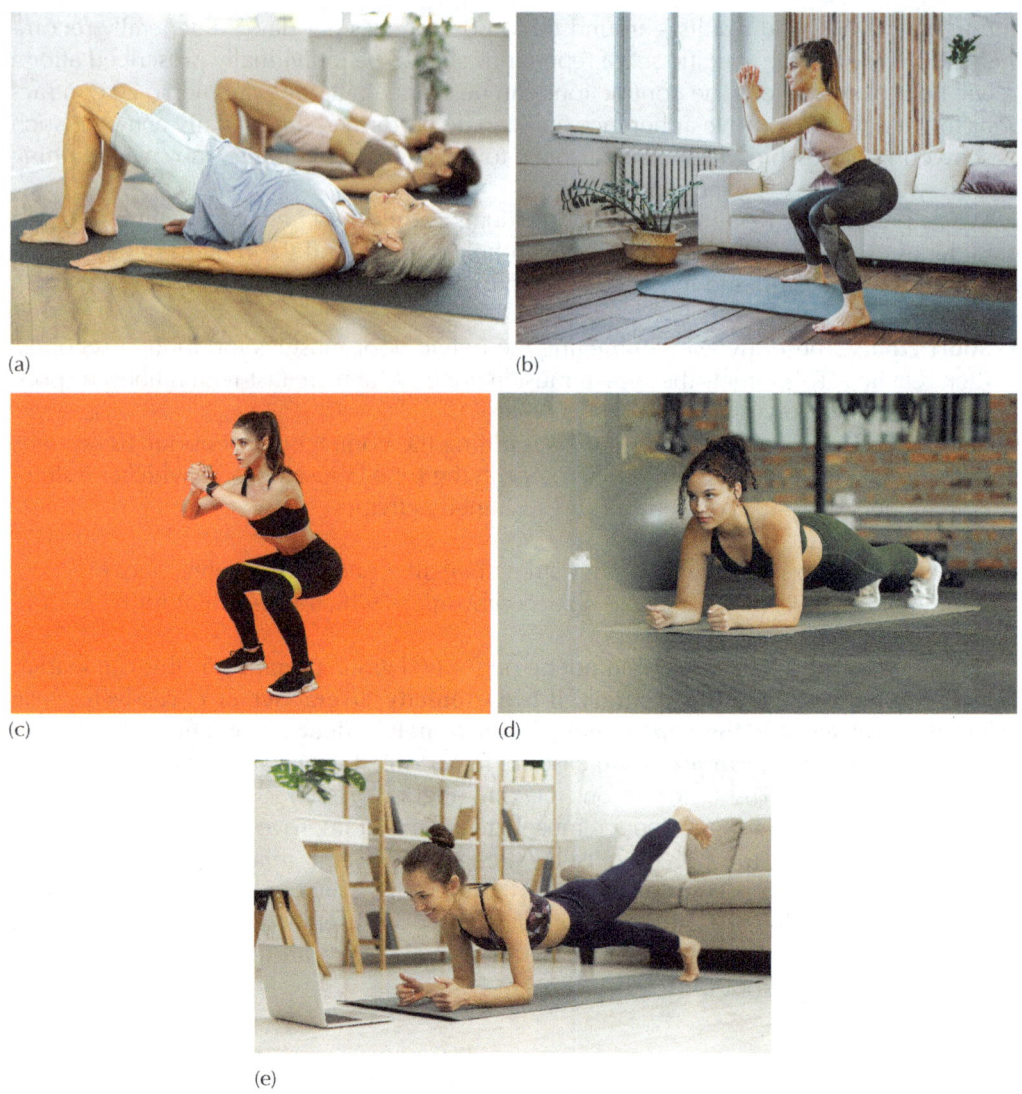

Figure 2.6 Pelvic floor strengthening exercises: (a) Glute bridge; (b) Squat; (c) Squat graded up with resistance band for adductor activation; (d) Plank; (e) Plank graded up with single leg raise.

Biofeedback

Biofeedback is a technique that utilizes electronic monitoring with electromyography to provide real-time feedback about pelvic floor muscle activity. In a biofeedback session, sensors are placed vaginally or rectally, and clients can observe the contractions and relaxations of the pelvic floor muscles on a screen. It is a useful tool that can help clients learn how to effectively perform the exercises. Sensory training with manometry biofeedback can be used to address sensory deficits.

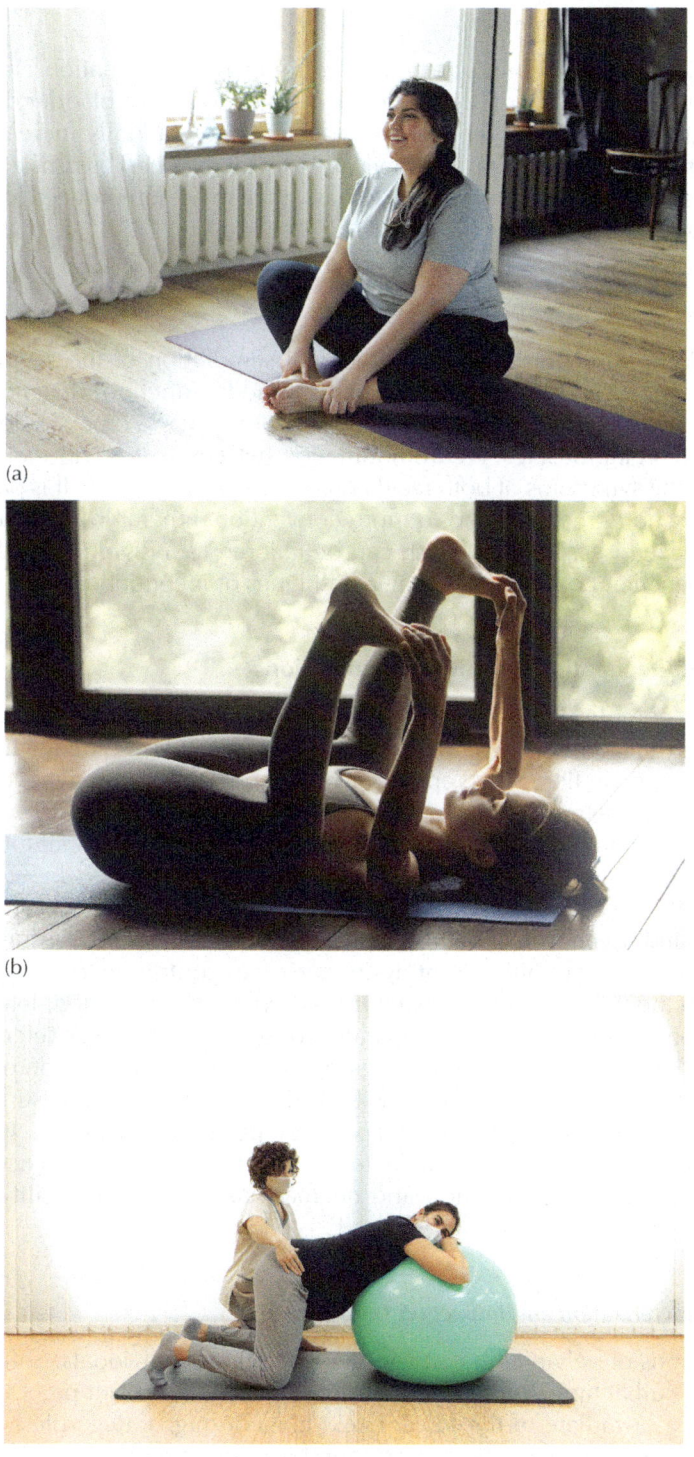

Figure 2.7 Pelvic floor relaxation exercises: (a) Seated adductor stretch; (b) Hip opening and pelvic alignment stretch; (c) Pregnant pelvic stretch and breathing exercise.

Bladder Training and Urge Suppression

The goal of bladder training is to decrease the frequency of urination and increase the storage capacity of the bladder. Clients are encouraged to keep a bladder diary, recording the time of urination. The interval between voids can be gradually increased over time. Clients may also be taught to suppress their urges by taking deep breaths and doing some Kegel squeezes. After waiting for the urge to pass, they may then proceed to the bathroom at a regular pace.

Neuromodulation

Neuromodulation, particularly through electrical stimulation of the sacral nerve, is an effective treatment for regulating both bowel and bladder function. This method works by sending mild electrical pulses to the sacral nerves, which play a crucial role in controlling the bladder and rectal muscles. Neuromodulation helps to restore normal nerve activity, thereby improving symptoms of both fecal and urinary incontinence. It is particularly useful for patients who do not respond to more conventional therapies such as medications or pelvic floor exercises. This approach can be tailored to individual needs, making it a versatile and beneficial option for managing all types of incontinence.

Pelvic Pain and Occupational Therapy Interventions

Pelvic pain is a complex and often debilitating condition that can significantly affect an individual's daily life. It refers to pain experienced in the pelvic region, which includes the lower abdomen, pelvic floor, and reproductive organs. It occurs in gynecological conditions such as endometriosis, uterine fibroids, and pelvic inflammatory disease (PID). Understanding the causes and manifestations of pelvic pain is essential for OTPs seeking to provide effective care.

Pelvic pain may also arise from musculoskeletal issues, neurological factors, inflammatory disorders, and psychosocial factors. Conditions like pelvic floor dysfunction, myofascial pain syndrome, or sacroiliac joint dysfunction can contribute to ongoing pain in the area. Nerves in the pelvic region can become compressed or irritated, leading to neuropathic pain. Conditions like pudendal neuralgia or sciatica may cause referred pain in the pelvic area. Inflammation in the pelvic region, whether due to infection or autoimmune conditions, can result in significant pain. Disorders like interstitial cystitis and irritable bowel syndrome (IBS) often feature pelvic pain as a prominent symptom. It's essential not to overlook the impact of psychosocial factors on pelvic pain. Stress, anxiety, and depression can exacerbate pain perception and decrease an individual's ability to cope with discomfort.

Pelvic Pain Characterization and Impact on Daily Life

The manifestations of pelvic pain can vary widely among individuals. Some may experience constant, dull aching, while others endure sharp, intermittent pain. It can be localized to one area or radiate to the lower back, hips, or thighs. Regardless of the specific characteristics, pelvic pain can have a profound impact on daily life. OTPs often witness how pelvic pain can affect a person's ability to engage in essential activities and areas of occupation, as outlined in the Occupational Therapy Practice Framework.

- **Activities of Daily Living (ADLs)**: Simple tasks like getting dressed, bathing, and using the restroom can become challenging and painful for individuals with pelvic pain. This can lead to a loss of independence and a need for assistance.
- **Instrumental Activities of Daily Living (IADLs)**: More complex activities such as meal preparation, housekeeping, and managing finances may be compromised due to pelvic pain. Individuals may struggle to maintain their homes or perform tasks related to their jobs.
- **Rest and Sleep**: Pelvic pain can disrupt comfortable sleeping positions, leading to poor sleep quality and fatigue, which affects overall health and ability to function during the day.
- **Education**: Pelvic pain may affect concentration and physical ability, impacting a person's participation in educational environments.
- **Work**: This pain can hinder a person's ability to perform job-related tasks, especially those requiring physical activity or prolonged sitting, potentially leading to decreased productivity or absence from work.
- **Play, Leisure, and Social Participation**: Pelvic pain can lead to isolation and reduced participation in social, leisure, and recreational activities. Individuals may avoid gatherings or events due to discomfort, impacting their social well-being.

Understanding the causes and manifestations of pelvic pain is crucial for OTPs. Additionally, the chronic nature of pelvic pain can lead to emotional distress, including anxiety and depression, which can further exacerbate pain perception and disrupt daily routines. OTPs should be aware of the various types of pelvic pain commonly encountered in clinical practice. These distinct types of pelvic pain can arise from different sources and may require tailored approaches for effective management. Table 2.4 highlights common types of pelvic pain and occupational therapy strategies to address them.

Pelvic Pain Assessment and Evaluation

When working with clients experiencing pelvic pain, effective assessment and evaluation are crucial components of providing patient-centered care. OTPs must gather comprehensive information to understand the unique factors contributing to a client's pain experience and tailor interventions accordingly.

Interviewing and Assessing the Client with Pelvic Pain

- **Pain Characteristics**: Begin by asking the client to describe their pain. Inquire about the location, intensity, and nature of the pain (e.g., sharp, dull, burning). Ask if the pain is constant or intermittent, and whether it radiates to other areas like the lower back or thighs.
- **Onset and Duration**: Explore when the pain first began and if there were any triggering events or patterns associated with it. Determine how long the client has been experiencing pelvic pain and if there have been any changes in its intensity or frequency.
- **Aggravating and Alleviating Factors**: Investigate factors that exacerbate or relieve the pain. Encourage clients to share activities, positions, or movements that worsen their symptoms and those that provide relief.
- **Impact on Daily Life**: Assess how pelvic pain affects the client's ability to perform activities of daily living (ADLs) and instrumental activities of daily living (IADLs). Inquire about any modifications or assistive devices they have used to manage daily tasks.

Table 2.4 Types of pelvic pain and corresponding occupational therapy strategies

Type of Pelvic Pain	Description	OT Strategies
Adenomyosis	Adenomyosis occurs when the tissue that normally lines the uterus grows within its muscular walls. This can cause severe menstrual cramps and heavy, prolonged bleeding, affecting ADLs and IADLs due to pain and fatigue.	Pain management, ADL/IADL retraining techniques, ergonomic advice, adaptive equipment for daily tasks.
Dysmenorrhea	Dysmenorrhea refers to painful menstrual cramps experienced by some women during their menstrual periods.	Teaching relaxation techniques, heat therapy application, ergonomic positioning for pain relief during menstruation, adaptive strategies for comfort.
Dyspareunia	Dyspareunia is characterized by persistent or recurrent genital pain experienced by women before, during, or after sexual intercourse.	Emotional support, sexual health education, pain management techniques, adaptive equipment for comfort during sexual activity.
Endometriosis	Endometrial tissue grows outside of the uterus, leading to pain during menstruation or at other times, which may impact all areas of occupation including work, education, and social participation.	Lifestyle modifications, stress management, self-management techniques, ADL/IADL retraining for pain minimization during daily activities.
Fibroids	Benign masses on the uterine walls that can cause discomfort or pain, impacting ADLs and IADLs during menstruation or between periods.	Symptom management strategies, pelvic floor strengthening, adaptive strategies for managing heavy menstrual flow and pain, ADL/IADL task simplification.
Interstitial Cystitis	A chronic bladder condition causing pain and frequent urination which can disrupt sleep and daily activities.	Bladder training techniques, dietary modifications, adaptive equipment for bladder control, education on managing pain during ADLs/IADLs.
Neuropathic Pelvic Pain	Neuropathic pelvic pain is caused by irritation or compression of nerves in the pelvic region, leading to sensations of burning, tingling, or sharp pain.	Pain management strategies, sensory desensitization, sensory integration therapy.
Ovarian Cysts	Fluid-filled sacs on the ovaries that can cause pain, impacting daily and recreational activities, and may require surgery.	Pain relief strategies, ADL/IADL adaptation techniques, education on surgical options, adaptive equipment for managing pain during activities.
Pelvic Congestion Syndrome	Enlarged veins in the pelvis causing chronic pain, often worsening in certain positions, impacting rest, sleep, and physical activities.	Positional strategies, venous flow improvement exercises, adaptive equipment for positional comfort, relaxation techniques.
Pelvic Inflammatory Disease (PID)	An infection of the reproductive organs that can cause severe pain and affect all areas of occupation, often stemming from untreated STIs.	Education on infection management, stress reduction techniques, support for emotional well-being, adaptive strategies for managing pain during ADLs/IADLs.

(Continued)

Table 2.4 (Continued)

Type of Pelvic Pain	Description	OT Strategies
Pelvic Organ Prolapse	Weakening of the pelvic muscles causing organs to slip out of place, affecting physical activity and potentially causing pain during social and intimate activities.	Pelvic floor rehabilitation, education on proper lifting techniques, ADL/IADL adaptation, adaptive equipment for support during functional activities.
Psychosocial Pelvic Pain	Psychological factors, including stress, anxiety, and depression, can exacerbate pelvic pain perception.	Psychosocial counseling, stress management, supportive group therapy participation.

- **Medical History**: Gather information about the client's medical history, including any gynecological conditions, surgeries, or chronic illnesses that may be relevant to their pelvic pain. Inquire about medications, treatments, or therapies they have tried in the past.
- **Psychosocial Factors**: Recognize the emotional toll of pelvic pain. Ask about the client's emotional well-being, stressors, and any symptoms of anxiety or depression. Explore their social support system and coping mechanisms.
- **Bladder and Bowel Function**: Pelvic pain can sometimes be associated with bladder and bowel dysfunction. Inquire about urinary and fecal symptoms, such as urgency, frequency, incontinence, or constipation.
- **Sexual Function**: Discuss any changes in sexual function and discomfort during sexual activity, as well as any associated emotional concerns. Use open and non-judgmental language to facilitate dialogue.

Pelvic pain assessments serve as invaluable tools in the realm of occupational therapy for several compelling reasons. First and foremost, these assessments enable OTPs to pinpoint the underlying causes and contributing factors of pelvic pain. By delving into the specifics of muscle function, coordination, and structural anomalies, OTPs gain a comprehensive understanding of the client's condition. This, in turn, facilitates the development of highly targeted and individualized treatment plans.

Furthermore, assessments provide objective data to complement the client's subjective reports of pain and discomfort. This objective information is critical for tracking progress and adjusting interventions as needed. It also helps in identifying any potential red flags or contraindications that may impact the course of treatment. Incorporating various pelvic pain assessments into the evaluation process empowers OTPs to offer evidence-based interventions. By systematically assessing muscle tone, strength, and coordination, as well as identifying areas of tenderness or dysfunction, OTPs can tailor interventions to address specific deficits. This holistic approach not only enhances the effectiveness of treatment but also helps clients regain control over their pelvic health and overall well-being. Table 2.5 highlights common assessments for the pelvic pain client.

Additionally, the utilization of pelvic pain assessments fosters collaboration and shared decision-making between OTPs and clients. Engaging clients in the assessment process not only empowers them with knowledge about their pelvic health but also encourages active participation in their treatment journey. Clients become partners in their care,

Table 2.5 Pelvic floor pain assessments and contraindications

Pelvic Floor Pain Assessment	Description	Contraindications
Digital Pelvic Floor Examination	Conducted by a trained healthcare provider, this examination assesses pelvic floor muscle tone, strength, coordination, and the presence of trigger points or areas of tenderness.	Severe pelvic pain, acute infections, recent pelvic surgery, known malignancy in the pelvic area, pregnancy (requires caution).
Surface Electromyography (sEMG)	Non-invasive and informative. sEMG measures the electrical activity of pelvic floor muscles, revealing data on muscle function, coordination, and potential dysfunctions.	Open wounds, skin infections in the area where electrodes are applied, severe pelvic pain.
Pelvic Floor Ultrasound	Utilized for visualizing pelvic floor muscles, this assessment can assess muscle thickness, identify injuries, and evaluate muscle contractions during exercises.	Early pregnancy, cases of acute infection, open wounds, recent pelvic surgery, known malignancy.
Biofeedback	Using sensors and cues, biofeedback helps individuals gain control over their pelvic floor muscles, assesses muscle tone and coordination, and provides real-time feedback.	Severe pelvic pain, acute infections, skin irritation where sensors are applied.
Perineometry	Measures pressure in the vaginal or rectal canal, offering insights into the resting and maximal squeeze pressure of pelvic floor muscles.	Severe pelvic pain, acute infections, recent surgery in the vaginal or rectal area, known malignancy.
Pelvic Organ Prolapse Quantification (POP-Q)	Though primarily for pelvic organ prolapse assessment, POP-Q can provide insights into pelvic floor function by measuring pelvic organ descent, aiding in identifying contributing factors to pelvic pain.	Severe pelvic pain, acute infections, recent pelvic surgery.
Pain Mapping	This assessment involves using a pain diagram to pinpoint specific areas of discomfort within the pelvic region, helping to identify pain triggers.	None specific, but caution is needed if mapping exacerbates pain.
Pelvic Floor Trigger Point Assessment	Identifies trigger points or myofascial trigger points within pelvic floor muscles through palpation and evaluation of tender areas.	Severe pelvic pain, acute infections, recent pelvic surgery, known malignancy.

making informed decisions alongside their therapists and setting goals that align with their priorities and preferences.

Occupational Therapy for Managing Pelvic Pain

Client-centered care lies at the heart of occupational therapy, and it is especially relevant in the context of pelvic pain. OTPs recognize that each individual's experience of pelvic pain is unique, shaped by factors such as the underlying cause, pain intensity, duration, and its impact on daily life. Therefore, treatment approaches are tailored to meet the specific needs and goals of the client. Pain management is a primary focus of occupational

OT in Gynecological Health Management   61

therapy in the treatment of pelvic pain. OTPs employ a variety of strategies to help individuals alleviate pain and discomfort, regain function, and improve their overall quality of life.

Education

Education is a foundational component of occupational therapy for managing pelvic pain. OTPs provide clients with detailed information about the underlying causes of their pelvic pain, potential triggers, and the importance of self-care. This knowledge empowers clients to take an active role in their treatment. For example, an OTP might explain how certain postures or activities exacerbate pain and provide strategies to avoid these triggers. Clients are also educated on the anatomy and function of the pelvic floor muscles, which can help demystify their condition and reduce anxiety. Incorporating education into daily routines, OTPs might suggest keeping a pain diary to identify patterns and triggers, and teach clients how to use this information to make informed decisions about their activities.

Relaxation Techniques

Relaxation techniques are critical in managing pelvic pain, as stress and muscle tension can exacerbate symptoms. The science behind relaxation techniques lies in their ability to activate the parasympathetic nervous system, which counteracts the body's stress response. When the body is stressed, the sympathetic nervous system is activated, leading to muscle tension and increased pain perception. By engaging the parasympathetic nervous system, relaxation techniques help reduce muscle tension and lower stress hormones like cortisol, thereby alleviating pain.

OTPs teach various relaxation methods, such as deep breathing, progressive muscle relaxation, and mindfulness. For instance, an OTP might guide a client through diaphragmatic breathing exercises, encouraging them to breathe deeply into their abdomen and exhale slowly. This technique helps to relax the pelvic floor muscles by promoting a more relaxed state throughout the body. Progressive muscle relaxation involves tensing and then slowly relaxing different muscle groups, including the pelvic floor, which helps reduce overall muscle tension. Mindfulness practices can include guided imagery or meditation, focusing on relaxation and body awareness. These techniques are incorporated into the client's daily routine by practicing them during moments of high stress or before bed to improve sleep quality and reduce pain.

Biofeedback

Biofeedback is a valuable tool that helps clients gain awareness and control over their pelvic floor muscles. OTPs use sensors to monitor muscle activity and provide real-time feedback, helping clients learn how to properly contract and relax their pelvic floor muscles. For example, during a biofeedback session, an OTP might place sensors on the pelvic floor and show the client a visual representation of their muscle activity on a screen. This visual feedback allows clients to see the immediate effects of their efforts to relax or contract their muscles, promoting better control. Biofeedback sessions are often combined with pelvic floor exercises and can be practiced at home using portable biofeedback devices, making it an integral part of daily routines for managing pelvic pain.

Pain Medication Management

While OTPs do not prescribe medications, they play a crucial role in pain medication management by collaborating with healthcare providers and educating clients. OTPs help clients understand their medication regimens, potential side effects, and the importance of adherence. For instance, an OTP might work with a client to develop a medication schedule that fits their daily routine and ensures they take their medications consistently. Additionally, OTPs educate clients on non-pharmacological pain management strategies that can complement their medication regimen, such as using heat therapy or engaging in gentle exercise. By integrating medication management into their overall treatment plan, OTPs help clients achieve more effective pain relief and improved function.

Cognitive-Behavioural Strategies

Cognitive-behavioural strategies are essential for addressing the emotional aspects of pelvic pain. OTPs help clients identify and challenge negative thought patterns related to pain, which can significantly impact their perception of pain and overall well-being. For example, an OTP might work with a client to recognize catastrophizing thoughts, such as "I will never be pain-free," and replace them with more positive and realistic thoughts, like "I can manage my pain with the right strategies." OTPs also teach coping strategies, such as stress management techniques and positive self-talk, to help clients manage their emotional responses to pain. Incorporating these strategies into daily life, OTPs might suggest practicing cognitive-behavioural techniques during moments of pain flare-ups or when feeling overwhelmed.

Energy Conservation Techniques

Fatigue often accompanies chronic pelvic pain, making energy conservation techniques vital. OTPs help clients develop strategies to conserve energy and prioritize essential activities, allowing them to accomplish more with less discomfort. For example, an OTP might teach a client to break tasks into smaller, manageable steps and take frequent breaks to avoid overexertion. They may also suggest using adaptive equipment, such as a rolling cart for carrying heavy items, to reduce physical strain. By incorporating energy conservation techniques into daily routines, clients can manage their activities more efficiently and reduce the impact of fatigue on their pelvic pain.

Pacing and Activity Modification

Pacing and activity modification are crucial for the effective management of pelvic pain. OTPs collaborate with clients to establish activity levels that are manageable and sustainable, ensuring they do not overexert themselves, which can worsen pain. For instance, an OTP might work with a client to create a daily schedule that balances activity and rest, preventing overexertion. They might also suggest modifying activities to reduce strain on the pelvic area, such as using a raised toilet seat to minimize bending or using a stool while cooking. By teaching clients to pace themselves and modify their activities, OTPs help them maintain function and reduce pain flare-ups.

Functional Rehabilitation and Adaptations

OTPs are skilled in addressing functional limitations caused by pelvic pain. These limitations can affect an individual's ability to perform ADLs and IADLs. OTPs work closely with clients to find solutions that optimize their independence and quality of life. For example:

- **Assistive Devices**: OTPs evaluate and recommend devices like reachers, dressing aids, or adaptive kitchen utensils to aid daily tasks. These devices can help clients perform activities more comfortably and independently.
- **Ergonomic Recommendations**: OTPs assess the ergonomics of the client's home and work environments to identify potential pain triggers. They provide recommendations for modifications, such as adjusting chair heights or using supportive cushions, to reduce discomfort and strain.
- **Adaptive Techniques**: OTPs teach clients adaptive techniques and strategies for completing ADLs and IADLs, such as dressing, grooming, cooking, and cleaning. This might include teaching alternative methods for tasks that minimize pain and strain on the pelvic area.
- **Home Safety**: OTPs conduct home safety assessments and make recommendations to reduce fall risks and enhance overall safety, considering that pain episodes can affect balance and mobility.

Pelvic Floor Muscle Training

For many individuals with pelvic pain, pelvic floor muscle dysfunction is a contributing factor. OTPs play a vital role in addressing these muscle-related issues through pelvic floor muscle training and relaxation exercises. Common pelvic floor relaxation exercises include:

- **Diaphragmatic Breathing**: Clients practice deep, diaphragmatic breathing to release tension in the pelvic floor muscles. They inhale deeply through the nose, allowing the diaphragm to expand, and exhale slowly through pursed lips.
- **Pelvic Floor Drops**: Clients learn to consciously relax the pelvic floor muscles by visualizing them dropping like an elevator descending. This exercise promotes muscle relaxation and relief from tension.
- **Pelvic Floor Stretching**: Gentle stretches help release tight pelvic floor muscles. Clients perform controlled stretches, focusing on relaxing and lengthening the muscles.
- **Reverse Kegels**: Reverse Kegel exercises focus on relaxation rather than contraction. Clients learn to release tension in the pelvic floor by actively relaxing the muscles during exhalation.
- **Yoga and Mindfulness**: Incorporating yoga and mindfulness practices into daily routines can promote pelvic floor relaxation. These practices emphasize body awareness and relaxation techniques that are beneficial for pelvic pain management.
- **Hot Baths and Warm Compresses**: The application of heat to the pelvic area can soothe tense muscles and provide relief from pain. Clients are encouraged to use hot baths or warm compresses as needed.

By employing these targeted strategies, occupational therapy practitioners can help clients manage pelvic pain effectively, improve their functional abilities, and enhance their overall quality of life.

Occupational Therapy Management of Gynecological Conditions

Gynecological conditions are common and often debilitating aspects of women's health, encompassing a wide spectrum of diagnoses, each with unique challenges and impacts on daily life. From adolescence to menopause, women may experience chronic pain, discomfort, fertility issues, emotional distress, and limitations in performing daily activities.

The impact of gynecological conditions extends beyond the physical symptoms. They can affect a woman's emotional well-being, self-esteem, social participation, and overall quality of life. Gynecologists and other medical specialists play a crucial role in diagnosing and managing these conditions, often utilizing medical, surgical, or pharmaceutical interventions. However, the journey to healing and improved function is not solely about addressing the medical aspects of these conditions. It is also about empowering women to regain control over their lives, engage in meaningful occupations, and live fully.

OTPs are uniquely positioned to address the multifaceted challenges women face with gynecological conditions. They bring a holistic and client-centered approach that focuses on enhancing an individual's functional independence, quality of life, and overall well-being. OTPs work collaboratively with individuals to develop tailored interventions that consider physical, emotional, environmental, and societal factors.

Comprehensive Assessment of Gynecological Conditions

In the realm of women's health occupational therapy, a profound understanding of the female reproductive system's anatomy goes hand in hand with effective clinical practice. Comprehensive assessment is crucial and a holistic approach is essential as pelvic pain and other gynecological conditions can significantly impact various aspects of a woman's life. Addressing these factors ensures a more thorough and effective intervention plan, fostering overall well-being and improving quality of life.

Assessing Range of Movement and Manual Muscle Testing in the Pelvis

A comprehensive assessment of the range of movement (ROM) can help to identify limitations in mobility and flexibility, which can impact activities of daily living such as walking, bending, or sitting. Also, manual muscle testing (MMT) is important for diagnosing muscle weakness or spasticity that may contribute to pelvic pain or instability. These objective assessments can assist OTPs in developing personalized and effective intervention strategies for their clients, as well as monitor treatment progress. See Tables 2.6 and 2.7 for ROM and MMT norms.

Anatomical Correlates of Common Signs and Symptoms

As OTPs, our mission extends beyond the mere recognition of anatomical structures; it encompasses a profound awareness of how these structures relate to daily functioning, well-being, and quality of life for our clients. By bridging the gap between anatomical knowledge and functional relevance, we empower ourselves to provide holistic, client-centered care, addressing the unique needs and challenges that women may encounter

Table 2.6 Functional assessment of the muscles of the pelvis

Muscle Group	Normal ROM	Functional Assessment
Pelvic Floor Muscles	N/A	Assess for ability to initiate and maintain a pelvic floor contraction; observe for coordinated movement during tasks such as coughing, sneezing, or lifting. Specific muscles include: Pubococcygeus, iliococcygeus, puborectalis, coccygeus. Functional tasks include bladder and bowel control, and sexual activity.
Hip Flexors	0–120 degrees	Evaluate for strength and coordination during activities such as standing, walking, and stair climbing. Specific muscles include: Iliopsoas, rectus femoris, sartorius. Functional tasks include transferring from sitting to standing, functional mobility, stepping into a bathtub, and lifting leg to don pants.
Hip Extensors	0–30 degrees	Assess strength during activities like sit-to-stand and stair climbing. Specific muscles include: Gluteus maximus, hamstrings (biceps femoris, semitendinosus, semimembranosus). Functional tasks include getting up from a chair, climbing stairs, walking uphill, standing from a low surface, lifting objects from the ground, pushing objects while walking, and moving from sitting to standing.
Hip Abductors	0–45 degrees	Assess for balance and stability during single-leg stance and lateral movements. Specific muscles include: Gluteus medius, gluteus minimus, tensor fasciae latae. Functional tasks include side-stepping, getting into and out of a car, maintaining balance while walking and moving sideways to reach for objects in the home environment, workplace, or store.
Hip Adductors	0–30 degrees	Assess for balance and coordination during activities such as crossing legs or side-stepping. Specific muscles include: Adductor longus, adductor brevis, adductor magnus, gracilis, pectineus. Functional tasks include crossing legs while sitting, moving sideways to reach for objects, and stabilizing during walking.
Hip Internal Rotators	0–45 degrees	Evaluate for coordination and strength during activities such as pivoting and turning. Specific muscles include: Gluteus medius, gluteus minimus, tensor fasciae latae. Functional tasks include turning while walking, pivoting to change directions, adjusting foot position while standing, and donning socks or shoes.
Hip External Rotators	0–45 degrees	Evaluate for coordination and strength during activities such as crossing legs or turning out the feet. Specific muscles include: Piriformis, obturator internus, obturator externus, gemellus superior, gemellus inferior, quadratus femoris. Functional tasks include putting on shoes and socks, crossing legs while sitting, turning the feet while walking, and adjusting foot position when seated.

Table 2.7 Manual muscle testing grading scale

MMT Grade	Description	Muscle Strength
0	No contraction	The muscle shows no visible or palpable contraction.
1	Trace contraction	A slight contraction is felt, but there is no visible movement of the joint.
2	Poor	The muscle can move the joint when gravity is eliminated (horizontal plane).
3	Fair	The muscle can move the joint against gravity, but cannot hold against any resistance.
4	Good	The muscle can move the joint against gravity and hold against moderate resistance, but not full resistance.
5	Normal	The muscle can move the joint against gravity and hold against full resistance without any signs of fatigue or weakness.

throughout their health journey. Table 2.8 offers a concise yet comprehensive overview of anatomical insights, abnormal observable signs, functional implications, and treatment considerations to bear in mind.

Occupational Therapy Interventions for Gynecological Conditions

While there are disease-specific interventions in women's health, certain treatment modalities are applicable across numerous conditions and encompass a holistic approach to care. Pain management is a critical component, where OTPs teach relaxation techniques such as deep breathing and guided imagery, use modalities like heat therapy or transcutaneous electrical nerve stimulation (TENS), and recommend ergonomic adjustments to reduce discomfort during daily activities. Education and lifestyle modifications are also essential; OTPs provide comprehensive education on disease management, nutrition, and exercise, advising clients on lifestyle changes to manage symptoms effectively, such as dietary adjustments for PCOS.

Emotional and psychological support is another vital aspect of care, with OTPs offering counseling and support groups, teaching coping mechanisms to deal with stress and anxiety, and using cognitive-behavioural techniques to address negative thoughts and emotions. Activity modification and energy conservation are integral to managing daily activities, where clients learn to modify activities to reduce symptom exacerbation, implement energy conservation techniques, and understand the importance of pacing activities to prevent fatigue. For instance, using adaptive equipment to simplify tasks or scheduling rest breaks during the day can make a significant difference in managing energy levels.

Pelvic floor rehabilitation involves conducting pelvic floor strengthening and relaxation exercises to manage symptoms of pelvic organ prolapse and other related conditions. OTPs may collaborate with pelvic floor physical therapists to ensure comprehensive care, addressing both the physical and functional aspects of pelvic floor dysfunction. Additionally, health promotion and preventive care are emphasized through the development of programs aimed at preventing complications, such as fall prevention strategies for women with osteoporosis or educational programs on cervical cancer screening.

ADL and IADL adaptation strategies are woven throughout these interventions. For example, OTPs might suggest using reachers or dressing aids to make dressing easier, recommend shower chairs to conserve energy during bathing, or provide ergonomic kitchen tools to reduce strain during meal preparation. These adaptations help clients maintain independence and improve their quality of life by enabling them to perform

Table 2.8 Overview of occupational therapy considerations for key signs and symptoms in women's health

Anatomical/ Pathological Context	Signs and Symptoms	Functional Implications	Treatment Considerations
Pelvic Floor Muscles & Pelvic Organ Support	Visible bulge or protrusion in the vaginal area; complaints of incontinence or pelvic pain; difficulty initiating urination or defecation.	Weakened pelvic floor muscles and compromised pelvic organ support; difficulty with bladder and bowel control; pain during intercourse.	- Discuss urinary or fecal incontinence management. - Implement pelvic floor strengthening exercises. - Use biofeedback for muscle retraining. - Educate on proper lifting techniques and postures during functional activities. - Educate on pelvic organ prolapse management and lifestyle modifications.
Structural Variations	Observation of prolapsed structures during a visual examination; palpable masses or irregularities in pelvic exams; asymmetry or abnormal positioning of pelvic organs.	Altered reproductive function; discomfort during daily activities; potential impact on sexual function.	- Consider consulting physician for surgical consult for structural abnormalities. - Evaluate and address functional impact on daily activities and sexual function. - Educate on lifestyle modifications.
Inflammation	Redness and inflammation in the vulvar or vaginal area; sensation of burning or irritation; increased urinary frequency.	Pain and discomfort; potential impact on sexual function and daily activities due to discomfort.	- Implement pain management strategies (topical creams, medications). - Educate on reducing potential irritants and lifestyle modifications. - Recommend sitz baths and anti-inflammatory medications.
Dryness	Dry, flaky skin or mucous membranes in the genital area; complaints of itching or discomfort during intercourse; reduced vaginal lubrication.	Pain and discomfort; decreased sexual function; potential for skin irritation or damage.	- Recommend moisturizers or lubricants. - Address potential hormonal causes with lifestyle recommendations. - Educate on hydration and use of vaginal moisturizers. - Consider impact on menstrual hygiene and sexual functioning.
Neural Innervation of Reproductive Structures	Sensations of numbness, tingling, or pain experiences; altered sensation during pelvic exams; decreased sensation in the genital area.	Altered sensory and motor function, and pain experiences; impact on daily activities and sexual function.	- Assess sensory and motor function. - Implement sensory re-education and pain management strategies. - Adapt activities accordingly. - Use desensitization techniques and graded exposure to activities.

(Continued)

Table 2.8 (Continued)

Anatomical/ Pathological Context	Signs and Symptoms	Functional Implications	Treatment Considerations
Vascular Anatomy and Postoperative Care	Localized swelling, discoloration, surgical incisions; signs of infection or poor wound healing; edema in the lower extremities.	Potential postoperative vascular complications; impact on mobility and daily activities; risk of lymphedema.	- Monitor postoperative clients and refer as needed. - Focus on pain management, edema control, and gradual mobility progression. - Educate on postoperative care and signs of complications.
Lymphatic Drainage	Visible edema, swelling, discomfort, restricted mobility; heaviness or tightness in the pelvic region.	Impact on daily activities and functional limitations; potential risk of chronic lymphedema.	- Assess extent of edema. - Teach manual lymphatic drainage. - Provide compression garment education. - Promote self-management for edema control. - Implement gentle exercise programs to promote lymphatic flow.

daily tasks with less discomfort and greater efficiency. By integrating these comprehensive strategies, OTPs can provide holistic, client-centered care that addresses the unique needs and challenges faced by women with gynecological conditions.

Utilizing Occupational Therapy Frameworks for Gynecological Conditions

Additionally, OTPs use a variety of frameworks and models to address the multifaceted challenges posed by gynecological conditions. These models provide a structured approach to understanding the complex interplay between a client's physical, emotional, and environmental factors, enabling OTPs to design comprehensive and client-centered interventions that focus on enhancing functional independence, quality of life, and overall well-being. Below are practical ways to apply relevant models to treating gynecological conditions:

Person-Environment-Occupation (PEO) Model: Emphasize the dynamic relationship between the person, their environment, and their occupations. Tailor interventions to improve occupational performance by modifying the environment, adapting activities, and enhancing personal skills.

Example: For a woman experiencing menopausal symptoms, interventions might include modifying her home environment to reduce heat (e.g., using fans and light bedding) and adapting her work schedule to accommodate periods of fatigue. She can be taught personal skills such as stress management techniques to help her cope with mood swings.

Model of Human Occupation (MOHO): Focus on understanding the motivations, routines, performance capacity, and environment of the individual. Design interventions that are meaningful and motivating for the client, develop new habits and routines, and enhance volition through engagement in valued activities.

Example: For a woman with PCOS, interventions might include developing a structured exercise routine that aligns with her interests and motivations. This could involve creating a daily schedule that incorporates physical activities she enjoys, which can help improve her performance capacity and overall well-being.

Biopsychosocial Model: Consider the biological, psychological, and social aspects of health. Integrate physical rehabilitation with psychological support, stress management, and social participation enhancement.

Example: When addressing the multifaceted impacts of uterine fibroids, an OTP might combine physical rehabilitation exercises to manage pain, psychological support to address anxiety and depression, and strategies to enhance social participation, such as joining a support group.

Canadian Model of Occupational Performance and Engagement (CMOP-E): Address the client's occupational performance through the lens of their engagement in meaningful activities. Focus on the interaction between person, environment, and occupation, and tailor interventions to enhance overall well-being and participation.

Example: For a woman recovering from gynecological cancer, the focus might be on re-engaging in meaningful leisure activities and adapting her home environment to support her recovery and participation in daily life activities.

Occupational Adaptation (OA) Model: Help clients adapt to their changing circumstances by focusing on their ability to meet occupational challenges. Develop adaptive strategies to enhance performance and satisfaction in daily activities.

Example: When assisting a woman with endometriosis, the OTP might develop adaptive strategies for managing work tasks during flare-ups, ensuring she can maintain productivity while managing pain. This could include flexible scheduling and ergonomic adjustments at her workstation.

Kawa Model: Use the metaphor of a river to understand the client's life flow and the barriers they face. Develop interventions that enhance the flow of their life by addressing physical, social, and environmental obstacles.

Example: For a client dealing with infertility, the OTP might help reduce stressors (represented as rocks in the river) and improve social support (represented as riverbanks) to enhance her overall life flow and well-being. This could involve connecting her with a support group and developing stress-reduction strategies.

Ecological Model of Human Performance (EMHP): Focus on the interaction between the individual and their environment to enhance performance. Modify the environment or task to better fit the individual's needs and capabilities.

Example: For a woman experiencing pelvic organ prolapse, the OTP might recommend environmental modifications such as ergonomic adjustments at home and work to reduce strain during daily activities. This could include using supportive seating and modifying workstations to prevent exacerbation of symptoms.

By employing these diverse frameworks and models, OTPs can create tailored, holistic interventions that address the complex needs of women with gynecological conditions, ultimately enhancing their quality of life and overall well-being.

Common Gynecological Conditions

Within the realm of women's health, OTPs may frequently encounter and provide care for a diverse range of gynecological conditions. Table 2.9 details common gynecological conditions that significantly affect women's quality of life and daily functioning, their clinical presentation, and OT treatment considerations.

Table 2.9 Common gynecological conditions and occupational therapy interventions

Condition	Etiology	Clinical Presentation	Occupational Therapy Interventions
Endometriosis	Growth of endometrial tissue outside the uterus	Pelvic pain, dysmenorrhea, potential infertility	Pain management strategies (heat therapy, TENS), myofascial release, trigger point release, lifestyle modifications, support for emotional well-being, ergonomic adjustments, energy conservation techniques, postural training, pelvic floor rehabilitation.
Polycystic Ovary Syndrome	Hormonal disorder with small cysts on the ovaries	Irregular menstrual cycles, excess hair growth, metabolic issues	Support in managing symptoms (heat therapy, TENS), myofascial release, trigger point release, therapeutic exercises (gentle stretching, strengthening), lifestyle habit development, stress management techniques, addressing emotional challenges, ergonomic adjustments, energy conservation techniques, skincare routine education for hirsutism.
Uterine Fibroids	Noncancerous growths in the uterus	Pelvic pain, pressure, changes in menstrual patterns	Assistance in managing pain (heat therapy, TENS), optimizing sleep, addressing the impact of fibroids on daily life, ergonomic adjustments, energy conservation techniques, postural training.
Menstrual Disorders	Range of conditions from heavy menstrual bleeding (menorrhagia) to the absence of menstruation (amenorrhea)	Prolonged or heavy bleeding, irregular periods, or complete absence of menstruation	Assistance in managing the impact of menstrual disorders on daily routines, pain management strategies (heat therapy, TENS), ergonomic adjustments, energy conservation techniques.
Ovarian Cysts	Fluid-filled sacs developing on the ovaries	Lower abdominal pain, bloating, changes in menstrual patterns	Support in managing pain (heat therapy, TENS), optimizing movement, addressing the impact of cysts on daily life, ergonomic adjustments, energy conservation techniques.
Cervical Dysplasia	Abnormal changes in cervical cells linked to human papillomavirus infection (HPV)	Typically asymptomatic, may lead to emotional distress and concerns about cancer risk	Emotional support, education about HPV and cervical health, strategies to reduce anxiety related to cervical dysplasia.
Gynecological Cancers	Includes cancers of the ovaries, cervix, uterus, vagina, and vulva	Abnormal bleeding, pelvic pain, weight loss, fatigue	Support in managing treatment side effects (heat therapy, TENS), energy conservation techniques, emotional support, postural training, ergonomic adjustments.

(Continued)

Table 2.9 (Continued)

Condition	Etiology	Clinical Presentation	Occupational Therapy Interventions
Pelvic Organ Prolapse	Weakening of the pelvic floor muscles leading to descent of pelvic organs	Sensation of pressure, urinary incontinence, discomfort	Pelvic floor strengthening exercises, myofascial release, trigger point release, education on bladder management, lifestyle modifications, ergonomic adjustments, energy conservation techniques.
Premenstrual Syndrome	Hormonal changes before menstruation	Mood swings, bloating, headaches, fatigue	Stress management techniques, education on lifestyle modifications, support for emotional well-being, pain management strategies (heat therapy, TENS), ergonomic adjustments, energy conservation techniques.
Menopause-Related Symptoms	Hormonal changes associated with the end of menstrual cycles	Hot flashes, night sweats, vaginal dryness, mood swings	Education on lifestyle modifications, strategies to manage hot flashes and night sweats, support for emotional well-being, recommendations for managing vaginal dryness, ergonomic adjustments, energy conservation techniques.
Infertility	Various causes including hormonal imbalances, structural issues, and lifestyle factors	Difficulty conceiving, emotional distress	Emotional support, stress management strategies, education on fertility treatments, lifestyle modifications, ergonomic adjustments, energy conservation techniques.

Rehabilitative Strategies in Gynecological Surgery: An Occupational Therapy Perspective

Gynecological surgeries are medical procedures performed on the female reproductive system to diagnose, treat, or manage various conditions and diseases. These surgeries can range from minimally invasive procedures to complex and major surgeries. While gynecological surgeries aim to improve a woman's health and quality of life, they can also pose physical, emotional, and functional challenges. OTPs play a vital role in enhancing the overall surgical experience and facilitating a smoother recovery process.

Gynecological surgeries encompass a wide range of procedures, each with its own set of indications, surgical techniques, and potential risks. Some of the common gynecological surgeries include hysterectomy, myomectomy, oophorectomy, salpingectomy, and pelvic organ prolapse repairs. These surgeries may be performed via laparoscopy, hysteroscopy, robotic-assisted techniques, or traditional open surgery, depending on the patient's condition and surgical goals.

While gynecological surgeries have advanced significantly in terms of safety and minimally invasive approaches, they are not without challenges. Patients undergoing these surgeries often experience physical discomfort, pain, limitations in daily activities, emotional distress, and uncertainty about their postoperative recovery. It is in these areas that OTPs play a crucial role in optimizing the surgical experience and promoting a successful recovery.

Preoperative Preparation and Education by OTPs

Preoperative preparation and education are integral components of a woman's journey towards gynecological surgery. These processes serve multiple essential purposes, ensuring that patients are well-informed, physically prepared, and emotionally supported as they approach their surgical procedures. One of the primary goals of preoperative preparation and education is to empower women with comprehensive information about their impending surgery. This knowledge equips them to make informed decisions regarding their treatment options. By understanding the surgical procedure, potential risks, benefits, and alternatives, women can actively participate in the decision-making process alongside their healthcare providers. This shared decision-making approach promotes a sense of autonomy and allows patients to align their treatment choices with their personal preferences and values.

The period leading up to surgery can be emotionally challenging for patients. Anxiety and stress are common emotional responses. Preoperative preparation and education play a crucial role in addressing these emotional aspects. By providing patients with clear explanations of what to expect before, during, and after surgery, healthcare professionals can help alleviate uncertainty and fear. Furthermore, relaxation techniques and coping strategies are often taught during preoperative education sessions, enabling patients to manage pre-surgery anxiety more effectively.

Depending on the type of gynecological surgery, there may be physical preparations required to enhance surgical outcomes and minimize complications. Preoperative education includes guidance on specific pre-surgery preparations, such as fasting or bowel preparation, to ensure that patients adhere to these essential steps. Additionally, patients may be advised to discontinue certain medications or supplements in the days leading up to surgery to reduce the risk of adverse interactions.

Gynecological surgeries can bring about significant changes in a woman's life, including temporary or permanent alterations to daily activities and routines. Preoperative education serves to set realistic expectations for patients regarding the immediate postoperative period and the recovery process. This includes discussions about potential limitations, such as lifting restrictions, modifications to exercise regimens, and changes in daily routines. By providing this information beforehand, patients can better prepare themselves both physically and mentally for the challenges they may encounter.

Adequate preoperative preparation enables patients to actively participate in their own care and recovery. Patients who are well-informed and prepared are more likely to adhere to pre-surgery instructions and postoperative recommendations. They become active partners in their healthcare journey, working collaboratively with their healthcare providers to optimize surgical outcomes and overall well-being.

Hysterectomy

A hysterectomy involves the removal of the uterus and may be performed for various reasons, such as treating fibroids, endometriosis, or cancer. OTPs can provide preoperative preparation by assessing the woman's functional status and addressing any existing physical limitations. After a hysterectomy, women are typically advised to avoid heavy lifting for a specific period, usually several weeks to a few months, depending on the type of surgery and individual factors. Heavy lifting can strain the surgical site, potentially leading to complications or delayed healing. Therefore, it is crucial for women to understand and adhere to these restrictions. OTPs can provide guidance on alternative strategies for managing daily activities that involve lifting, such as using assistive devices, asking for assistance from family members or friends, or modifying their environment to minimize the need for heavy lifting.

Additionally, OTPs can help women plan and organize their living spaces to optimize safety and independence during the recovery period. For instance, if the woman experiences pain and discomfort due to her condition, OTPs can teach pain management techniques and introduce adaptive strategies to maintain independence in daily activities. They can also educate her on what to expect post-surgery, including limitations in bending.

Ovarian Cystectomy

Ovarian cystectomy is the surgical removal of ovarian cysts. OTPs can prepare women for this surgery by discussing the potential impact on their daily activities and providing strategies to manage pain and discomfort. They can educate the woman on the importance of following postoperative restrictions and gradually resuming activities. For ovarian cystectomy, OTPs can emphasize the importance of following medical advice and adhering to postoperative restrictions, such as limitations on lifting heavy objects or engaging in strenuous physical activities. They can provide practical strategies to help manage pain and discomfort during the recovery phase, such as recommending specific positions or techniques for pain relief. Furthermore, OTPs can offer relaxation techniques to alleviate pre-surgery anxiety and stress, promoting emotional well-being before the procedure.

Pelvic Organ Prolapse Repair

Surgery for pelvic organ prolapse aims to restore the positioning of pelvic organs, which may have shifted or descended. OTPs play a vital role in helping women prepare for this surgery by providing comprehensive education and support. OTPs assist women in understanding how the surgery may affect their daily activities and routines. They discuss potential limitations that may arise post-surgery, such as restrictions on lifting heavy objects or participating in strenuous exercises. Additionally, OTPs educate patients on proper body mechanics to prevent strain and promote optimal healing. By teaching techniques for safe movement and activity modification, OTPs empower women to navigate their postoperative period with confidence. Furthermore, OTPs address emotional concerns that may accompany this surgical experience. They provide coping strategies to manage anxiety or stress related to the procedure, ensuring that women are emotionally prepared for their pelvic organ prolapse repair.

Endometriosis Excision

Surgical excision of endometrial tissue outside the uterus is a common procedure for women with endometriosis. OTPs offer valuable support during the preoperative phase by addressing both physical and emotional aspects of the surgery. OTPs engage in discussions with patients about potential functional limitations they may encounter post-surgery.

74 *Occupational Therapy and Women's Health*

These limitations can include pelvic pain, bloating, fatigue, and discomfort. OTPs provide practical strategies for managing these symptoms, helping patients maintain a balanced routine during their recovery period. This may involve teaching pain management techniques, introducing adaptive strategies, and promoting self-care practices. OTPs also address emotional concerns related to fertility and overall well-being. They offer emotional support and provide guidance on navigating the emotional aspects of the surgical journey. By addressing the holistic needs of women with endometriosis, OTPs play a crucial role in ensuring their successful preparation for surgical excision.

Fibroid Embolization

Uterine fibroid embolization (UFE) is a minimally invasive procedure aimed at treating fibroids. OTPs contribute to women's preparedness for UFE by providing them with essential knowledge and guidance. OTPs educate women on what to expect during and after the UFE procedure, emphasizing the importance of rest and proper self-care. They offer insight into managing potential postoperative symptoms, such as cramping and discomfort, by teaching pain management techniques and relaxation strategies. OTPs also help women plan for a gradual return to their usual activities following UFE. By providing guidance on activity resumption and suggesting modifications, OTPs ensure a safe and effective recovery. Overall, OTPs empower women undergoing UFE to take an active role in their recovery and well-being, setting the stage for a successful and comfortable postoperative experience.

Postoperative Rehabilitation and Recovery Support

Recovery from gynecological surgeries involves tailored postoperative care to address individual needs. OTPs play a crucial role in facilitating recovery and minimizing complications. While general precautions include refraining from sexual intercourse for 6–12 weeks and adhering to lifting restrictions (typically 5–10 lbs for 6–12 weeks), specific considerations vary based on the type of surgery. Table 2.10 provides an overview of these postoperative restrictions and ADL considerations for each surgery type.

Physical Rehabilitation

The type and extent of physical rehabilitation required may vary depending on the specific surgical procedure, the woman's overall health, and any pre-existing conditions. OTPs collaborate closely with patients to create customized exercise programs that focus on regaining strength, flexibility, and overall physical well-being. For example, following a hysterectomy, women may experience abdominal weakness and discomfort. OTPs guide them through gentle abdominal exercises that gradually rebuild core strength without causing strain on the surgical site. After ovarian cystectomy or pelvic organ prolapse repair, exercises may emphasize pelvic floor muscle rehabilitation and techniques to maintain proper body mechanics during daily activities.

Pain Management

Effective pain management is essential to ensure that women can comfortably engage in their postoperative rehabilitation and recovery process. OTPs work collaboratively with healthcare teams to develop individualized pain management strategies that may include

OT in Gynecological Health Management 75

Table 2.10 Postoperative rehabilitation and recovery considerations for gynecological surgeries

Surgery Type	Postoperative Restrictions and OT Considerations
Abdominal Hysterectomy	**Lifting Restrictions**: Avoid lifting items heavier than 5–10 lbs to prevent strain on the incision site. **Functional Tasks**: Minimize bending and twisting during activities to reduce strain on the abdomen. Use adaptive equipment like reachers for lower-reaching tasks. **Bed Mobility Technique**: Use LOG rolling technique when changing positions to minimize strain on the abdominal muscles. **Driving**: Delay driving until discomfort or pain subsides and mobility improves, typically 4–6 weeks post-surgery. **Sexual Intercourse**: Refrain from sexual intercourse for 6–12 weeks post-surgery. Avoid positions that put pressure on the abdominal incision. **Bathing**: Use a shower chair and avoid bending at the waist. Consider a handheld showerhead for easier bathing. Use a long-handled sponge or reacher if needed. **Dressing**: Use adaptive equipment like a dressing stick or sock aid to avoid bending. **Toileting**: Consider raised toilet seats and grab bars for support.
Cesarean Section (C-section)	**Lifting Restrictions**: Avoid lifting items heavier than 5–10 lbs to prevent strain on the C-section incision. **Functional Tasks**: Avoid bending at the waist to reduce strain on the incision. Use a reacher for lower-reaching tasks. **Driving**: Delay driving until discomfort or pain subsides and mobility improves, typically 4–6 weeks post-surgery. **Bathing**: Use a shower chair and avoid strenuous movements. Consider a handheld showerhead for easier bathing. Use a long-handled sponge or reacher if needed. **Dressing**: Use adaptive equipment like a dressing stick or sock aid to avoid bending. **Toileting**: Consider raised toilet seats and avoid straining.
Pelvic Organ Prolapse Repair	**Lifting Restrictions**: Avoid lifting items heavier than 5–10 lbs to prevent strain on the pelvic floor. **Functional Tasks**: Minimize activities that stress the pelvic floor. Use side-lying techniques for bed mobility. **Sexual Intercourse**: Refrain from sexual intercourse for 6–12 weeks post-surgery. **Bathing**: Use a shower chair and avoid strenuous movements. Consider a long-handled sponge or reacher for easier bathing. **Dressing**: Use adaptive equipment like a dressing stick or sock aid to avoid bending. **Toileting**: Consider raised toilet seats and avoid straining.
Endometriosis Excision	**Lifting Restrictions**: Avoid lifting items heavier than 5–10 lbs to prevent strain on the surgical site. **Functional Tasks**: Minimize bending and twisting movements to reduce strain on the surgical site. Use adaptive equipment like reachers for lower-reaching tasks. **Driving**: Delay driving until discomfort or pain subsides and mobility improves, typically 4–6 weeks post-surgery. **Bathing**: Use a shower chair and avoid strenuous movements. Consider a handheld showerhead for easier bathing. Use a long-handled sponge or reacher if needed. **Dressing**: Use adaptive equipment like a dressing stick or sock aid to avoid bending. **Toileting**: Consider raised toilet seats and avoid straining.

medication management, relaxation techniques, and recommendations for positioning and movement. For instance, women recovering from surgery for endometriosis excision may experience pelvic pain and discomfort. OTPs teach them specific pain management techniques, such as guided relaxation and deep breathing exercises, to alleviate discomfort and improve overall well-being. OTPs may also recommend ergonomic adjustments in sitting or lying positions to minimize pressure on the surgical site and reduce pain.

ADL and IADL Retraining

Gynecological surgeries can significantly impact a woman's ability to perform everyday tasks, including basic self-care activities (ADLs) and more complex tasks (IADLs). OTPs address these challenges by providing training and adaptive strategies to promote independence and functional recovery. For example, women recovering from pelvic organ prolapse repair may initially find ADLs like dressing and bathing challenging due to discomfort or postoperative restrictions. OTPs teach them modified techniques and suggest adaptive equipment, such as long handled reachers or dressing aids, to make these activities more manageable. Similarly, IADLs such as meal preparation, housekeeping, and managing finances may become daunting during the recovery period. OTPs collaborate with women to develop energy conservation strategies, simplify tasks, and adapt their home environments to promote independence.

Emotional Support and Coping Strategies

The emotional impact of gynecological surgery should not be underestimated. Women may experience a wide range of emotions, including anxiety, depression, frustration, and fear, during their recovery journey. OTPs offer emotional support and provide coping strategies to help women navigate these challenges. Through active listening and therapeutic communication, OTPs create a safe and non-judgmental space for women to express their emotions and concerns. This practice helps women process their feelings and develop effective coping mechanisms. Coping strategies may involve relaxation techniques, stress management strategies, and referrals to mental health professionals when needed.

Reintegration into Daily Life

As women progress in their recovery, OTPs assist them in reintegration into their daily lives. This phase involves gradually resuming activities, work, and social participation. OTPs work closely with women to develop step-by-step plans for re-engaging in activities they enjoy while ensuring their safety and comfort. For example, women who have undergone fibroid embolization may initially need support in planning their return to work or resuming physical activities like exercise. OTPs help set realistic goals, provide guidance on activity modification, and monitor progress to ensure a smooth transition back to their routine.

Collaborative Care with Surgical Teams

Effective collaboration between OTPs and surgical teams is paramount for providing comprehensive care to women undergoing gynecological surgeries. OTPs work in tandem with surgeons, nurses, and other healthcare professionals to ensure that every aspect of a woman's care is considered and optimized. Clear and open communication between

OTPs and surgical teams is essential to coordinate care effectively. OTPs stay informed about the surgical procedure, postoperative restrictions, and potential complications. This information allows OTPs to tailor their rehabilitation plans to each woman's unique needs and circumstances.

Postoperative care is dynamic, and women's needs may change as they progress in their recovery. OTPs continually assess the woman's progress and adjust rehabilitation plans accordingly. They communicate any changes or concerns to the surgical team, ensuring that the woman receives timely and appropriate care. In recent years, there has been a growing emphasis on enhanced recovery programs (ERPs) for surgical patients. ERPs are evidence-based protocols designed to optimize the perioperative care of patients and enhance their recovery outcomes. OTPs play a crucial role in ERPs by contributing their expertise in functional rehabilitation, pain management, and emotional support. Collaborative care between OTPs and surgical teams is fundamental to promoting the holistic well-being of women undergoing gynecological surgeries. By working together to address physical, emotional, and functional aspects of recovery, healthcare professionals can enhance the overall experience and outcomes for women on their journey to restored health and vitality.

Case Studies in Gynecological Health

CASE A

Background and Past Medical History: The client is a 27-year-old woman presenting with severe dysmenorrhea, pain with intercourse (dyspareunia), and bowel-related pain during menstruation. She works as an office administrator, is physically active and enjoys social activities with friends. A laparoscopy revealed significant endometriosis behind the uterus (Pouch of Douglas) extending to the vagina. Despite these findings, the client opted not to proceed with surgery at this time. Her diagnosis has significantly impacted her daily life, affecting her ability to perform various ADLs and IADLs.

Prior Level of Function:

- Worked as an office administrator.
- Drove to work independently.
- Independent in all ADLs and IADLs.
- Regularly participated in physical and social activities.
- Managed household tasks independently.

Household Living Arrangements and Social History:

- Lives alone in a single-level apartment.
- Has a supportive network of friends and family.
- No use of assistive equipment prior to her current condition.

Change in Functional Status and Challenges:

The client reports significant pelvic pain and fatigue, impacting her ability to perform daily activities. Specific areas that have become difficult include:

- **Sexual functioning**: Dyspareunia has led to avoidance of sexual activity, causing strain in her intimate relationships.

- **Basic self-care (menstrual care)**: Experiences difficulty with menstrual care, such as inserting tampons, due to severe dysmenorrhea and pelvic pain.
- **Bathing and dressing**: Pain and discomfort, particularly during menstruation, make tasks requiring bending and reaching challenging.
- **Maintaining the home**: Difficulty with household chores like vacuuming, mopping, and other tasks requiring bending and lifting due to pelvic pain and fatigue.
- **Driving**: Experiences pain while sitting for extended periods, making it difficult to drive to work or other places.
- **Social activities**: Avoids social gatherings due to discomfort and emotional distress related to chronic pain.

OT Assessments:

- **Pain Mapping**: Pinpointed specific areas of discomfort in the pelvic region, with the most severe pain located in the lower abdomen and pelvic floor.
- **Endometriosis Health Profile-30 (EHP-30)**: Scores indicated a significant impact on the client's quality of life, with high levels of pain, feelings of control and powerlessness, and reduced emotional well-being and social support.
- **Pelvic Pain Impact Questionnaire (PPIQ)**: Results showed a significant impact on daily activities, work, and social interactions, with the client reporting difficulties in all areas assessed.

Physical Assessments:

- **Observation**: Forward shoulders, anterior pelvic tilt, and reduced hip mobility observed.
- **Palpation**: Tenderness noted in lower abdominal and pelvic areas.
- **Range of Motion (ROM)**: Limited hip internal and external rotation.
- **Manual Muscle Testing (MMT)**: Reduced strength in hip flexors and extensors.

Occupational Therapy Plan of Care and Goals:

The client will receive skilled occupational therapy once a week for 8 weeks to increase independence with ADLs, IADLs, and other functional activities.

Goals:

1. Client will manage household tasks independently without experiencing significant pelvic pain or fatigue, as measured by self-report and 75% improvement in PPIQ scores within 8 weeks.
2. Client will safely and comfortably engage in social activities without pain or anxiety, as measured by increased participation and satisfaction within 8 weeks.
3. Client will drive for at least 30 minutes without experiencing pelvic pain, as observed and self-reported within 8 weeks.
4. Client will demonstrate a reduction in depressive symptoms, with EHP-30 scores increasing by 50% within 8 weeks.
5. Client will identify and incorporate two stress management techniques into her daily routine within 4 weeks.
6. Client will encounter a 30–50% reduction in pain during sex, as measured by self-report and pain scale, within 8 weeks.
7. Client will independently manage menstrual hygiene, including tampon insertion, without significant pain, as observed and self-reported within 8 weeks.

Interventions:

The following interventions will be implemented to address the client's specific needs and goals:

Pain Management Strategies:

- Teaching relaxation techniques such as deep breathing, progressive muscle relaxation, and guided imagery to help reduce pelvic pain and tension.
- Using modalities like heat therapy and TENS for pain relief, focusing on the lower abdomen and pelvic region.
- Ergonomic adjustments to reduce discomfort during daily activities, including proper seating and posture recommendations for work and driving.

Activity Modification and Energy Conservation:

- Educating the client on how to modify activities to reduce symptom exacerbation, such as using a rolling cart for heavy items and avoiding prolonged standing or sitting.
- Implementing energy conservation techniques, such as pacing activities, scheduling rest breaks, and planning high-energy tasks during peak energy times.
- Advising on the use of assistive devices like reachers and dressing aids to minimize strain during self-care tasks.

Menstrual Hygiene Management:

- Educating the client on alternative menstrual products that may be easier to manage with dysmenorrhea, such as menstrual cups or pads.
- Providing strategies for comfortable tampon insertion, including relaxation techniques and positioning advice.
- Teaching the use of a perineal mirror to aid in visualization and reduce anxiety during tampon insertion.

Pelvic Floor Rehabilitation:

- Conducting pelvic floor muscle relaxation exercises to alleviate pain associated with endometriosis and dyspareunia.
- Incorporating biofeedback and manual therapy as indicated.
- Teaching techniques to manage bowel-related pain during menstruation, such as gentle stretching and pelvic floor relaxation exercises.
- Incorporating postural training and exercises to strengthen back muscles, addressing the forward shoulders and anterior pelvic tilt observed in the physical assessment.

Emotional and Psychological Support:

- Offering psychosocial counseling and support groups to help the client manage emotional distress related to chronic pain and social isolation.
- Teaching coping mechanisms to deal with stress and anxiety, including mindfulness practices and cognitive-behavioural techniques to address negative thought patterns.
- Providing resources for mental health professionals if additional psychological support is needed.

ADL and IADL Adaptation Strategies:

- Suggesting home modifications to facilitate safer lifting and task performance, such as organizing frequently used items within easy reach and using ergonomic kitchen tools.
- Providing adaptive techniques for dressing, grooming, and meal preparation to reduce pain and improve efficiency.
- Educating the client on effective menstrual care techniques, such as the use of alternative menstrual products that may be easier to manage with dysmenorrhea.

Sexual Functioning Interventions:

- Addressing pain during sex by teaching relaxation and breathing techniques to reduce muscle tension.
- Providing education on different sexual positions that may reduce pain and discomfort, considering the location of endometriosis pain:
  - **For deep pelvic pain**: Suggest positions that limit deep penetration, such as side-lying or woman-on-top positions, allowing the client to control depth and angle of penetration.
  - **For lower abdominal pain**: Recommend positions that reduce pressure on the abdomen, such as rear-entry positions where the woman can control the angle and depth.
  - **For pain in the back or hips**: Encourage positions that provide support and stability, such as spooning or using pillows to support the hips and back.
- Recommending the use of lubricants to minimize friction and discomfort during intercourse.
- Offering counseling on communication strategies with partners to address intimacy concerns and improve sexual health.

Outcomes:

Post Treatment:

- Reduced pelvic pain and improved pain management skills, with the client reporting a significant decrease in daily pain levels.
- Increased participation in social activities and improved emotional well-being, evidenced by the client's return to regular social gatherings and reported reduction in anxiety and depression.
- Ability to drive for at least 30 minutes without experiencing pelvic pain, as observed and self-reported.
- Decreased depressive symptoms, with EHP-30 scores increasing by 50%, indicating a notable improvement in emotional health and quality of life.
- Enhanced independence in managing household tasks and daily activities, with the client successfully completing chores such as vacuuming, mopping, and meal preparation without significant pain or fatigue.
- Reduction in pain during sex by 30–50%, improving sexual functioning and overall quality of life, with the client reporting increased comfort and satisfaction during intimate activities.
- Improved posture and alignment:

- Noticeable improvement in forward shoulder posture and correction of anterior pelvic tilt, as observed in follow-up physical assessments.
- Reduced tenderness in the lower abdominal and pelvic areas during palpation, with the client reporting decreased sensitivity.
- Improved hip internal and external rotation ROM, as measured during physical assessments.
- Increased strength in hip flexors and extensors, with manual muscle testing showing strength improvements from 3/5 to 4/5.

Follow-Up Visits:

Two additional visits will focus on reinforcing the client's progress in addressing pain management and functional issues related to her endometriosis. During these visits, the following will be emphasized:

- **Pain Management Techniques**: Reinforcement and practice of relaxation and breathing techniques to manage pain, particularly during activities of daily living and sexual intercourse.
- **Functional Mobility and Endurance**: Progression of exercises to improve her endurance for daily activities, including driving and social engagements.
- **ADL and IADL Adaptations**: Continued adaptation and modification strategies for self-care, household tasks, and work-related activities to minimize pain and maximize function.
- **Sexual Functioning**: Reinforcement of relaxation techniques and adaptive strategies for pain reduction during intercourse, including education on positioning and the use of lubricants.

The client exhibited significant improvement in managing her pelvic pain and overall function, including a reduction in dysmenorrhea and dyspareunia. She is now able to independently perform various ADLs and IADLs, such as cooking, cleaning, driving, dressing, and participating in social activities, without experiencing significant discomfort or pain. Notably, the reduction in pain during sexual activity enhanced her sexual functioning and intimate relationships. Her ability to drive for extended periods without pain further improved her independence and quality of life. The comprehensive, occupation-based approach in managing gynecological conditions like endometriosis, demonstrates the profound impact of holistic occupational therapy care on clients' daily lives and well-being.

CASE B

Background and Past Medical History: The client is a 30-year-old woman presenting with irregular menstrual cycles, weight gain, and hirsutism (excessive hair growth). She works as a nurse in a hospital and enjoys participating in community theater. Her diagnosis of PCOS has significantly impacted her daily life, affecting her ability to perform various ADLs and IADLs. The client has a past medical history of insulin resistance and a family history of type 2 diabetes. She has been on metformin to manage her insulin levels for the past two years and has attempted several lifestyle changes, including diet and exercise modifications, with limited success in managing her symptoms. She also has a history of anxiety, which has been exacerbated by her PCOS symptoms.

Prior Level of Function:

- Worked as a nurse in a hospital.
- Drove to work independently.
- Independent in all ADLs and IADLs.
- Regularly participated in physical and social activities.
- Managed household tasks independently.

Household Living Arrangements and Social History:

- Lives with her partner in a two-story house.
- Has a supportive network of friends and family.
- No use of assistive equipment prior to her current condition.

Change in Functional Status and Challenges: The client reports significant fatigue and emotional distress, impacting her ability to perform daily activities. Specific areas that have become difficult include:

- **Physical Activity**: Struggles to maintain a regular exercise routine due to fatigue and joint pain.
- **Diet and Nutrition**: Difficulty with meal planning and preparation, leading to unhealthy eating habits despite her professional knowledge.
- **Self-Esteem**: Emotional distress related to weight gain and hirsutism, affecting her self-esteem and social interactions.
- **Professional Responsibilities**: Experiences difficulty standing for long periods and managing patient interactions due to fatigue.
- **Household Tasks**: Difficulty with household chores like cleaning and organizing due to lack of energy.
- **Driving**: Experiences fatigue and discomfort, making it challenging to drive long distances.

OT Assessments:

Pain Mapping: Identified areas of discomfort, including:

- Dull, aching pain in the lower pelvis, particularly around the ovaries and uterus.
- Intermittent sharp pain in the lower back and hip areas.
- Generalized joint pain in the knees and ankles.

PCOS Health Questionnaire: Scores indicated a significant impact on the client's quality of life, with high levels of fatigue, emotional distress, and physical discomfort.

Physical Assessments:

- **Observation**: Forward shoulders and rounded back posture observed.
- Asymmetrical lateral pelvic tilt when seated, with the right hip higher than the left.
- **Palpation**: Tenderness noted in the lower back and pelvic areas, particularly around the iliac crest and sacroiliac joints.
- **Range of Motion (ROM)**: Limited hip and knee flexion, with the client experiencing discomfort during full range movements.
- **Manual Muscle Testing (MMT)**: Reduced strength in hip flexors and extensors, graded at 3/5.
- Weakness in the abdominal muscles, affecting overall core stability.

Occupational Therapy Plan of Care and Goals: The client will receive skilled occupational therapy once a week for 8 weeks to increase independence with ADLs, IADLs, and other functional activities.

Goals:

1. Client will manage household tasks independently without experiencing significant fatigue, as measured by self-report and 75% improvement in PCOS Health Questionnaire scores within 8 weeks.
2. Client will safely and comfortably engage in social activities without anxiety related to her condition, as measured by increased participation and satisfaction within 8 weeks.
3. Client will drive for at least 30 minutes without experiencing fatigue, as observed and self-reported within 8 weeks.
4. Client will demonstrate a reduction in depressive symptoms, with PCOS Health Questionnaire scores increasing by 50% within 8 weeks.
5. Client will identify and incorporate two stress management techniques into her daily routine within 4 weeks.
6. Client will report a 30–50% reduction in joint pain, as measured by self-report and pain scale, within 8 weeks.
7. Client will develop and follow a personalized skincare routine to manage hirsutism, resulting in improved self-esteem and reduced emotional distress within 8 weeks.

Interventions: The following interventions will be implemented to address the client's specific needs and goals:

Pain Management Strategies:

- Teaching relaxation techniques such as deep breathing, progressive muscle relaxation, and guided imagery to help reduce joint pain and tension.
- Using modalities like heat therapy and TENS for pain relief, focusing on the lower back and knee areas.
- Ergonomic adjustments to reduce discomfort during daily activities, including proper seating and posture recommendations for work and driving.

Activity Modification and Energy Conservation:

- Educating the client on how to modify activities to reduce symptom exacerbation, such as using a rolling cart for heavy items and avoiding prolonged standing or sitting.
- Implementing energy conservation techniques, such as pacing activities, scheduling rest breaks, and planning high-energy tasks during peak energy times.
- Advising on the use of assistive devices like reachers and dressing aids to minimize strain during self-care tasks.

Pelvic Floor Rehabilitation:

- Conducting pelvic floor muscle relaxation exercises to alleviate pain associated with PCOS.
- Incorporating biofeedback and manual therapy as indicated.
- Utilizing myofascial release techniques to reduce tension and pain in the pelvic and lower back regions.

- Teaching techniques to manage joint-related pain during physical activity, such as gentle stretching and pelvic floor relaxation exercises.
- Incorporating postural training and exercises to strengthen back muscles, addressing the forward shoulders and rounded back posture observed in the physical assessment.

Emotional and Psychological Support:

- Offering psychosocial counseling and support groups to help the client manage emotional distress related to her condition and social isolation.
- Teaching coping mechanisms to deal with stress and anxiety, including mindfulness practices and cognitive-behavioural techniques to address negative thought patterns.
- Providing resources for mental health professionals if additional psychological support is needed.

ADL and IADL Adaptation Strategies:

- Suggesting home modifications to facilitate safer lifting and task performance, such as organizing frequently used items within easy reach and using ergonomic kitchen tools.
- Providing adaptive techniques for dressing, grooming, and meal preparation to reduce pain and improve efficiency.
- Educating the client on effective dietary and nutritional strategies to manage PCOS symptoms, such as balanced meal planning and healthy eating habits.

Hirsutism Management:

- Developing a personalized skincare routine to manage excessive hair growth, including recommendations for gentle hair removal techniques such as waxing, threading, or the use of depilatory creams.
- Teaching skin care practices to prevent irritation and maintain skin health.
- Providing education on potential medical treatments for hirsutism, such as topical creams or laser hair removal, and facilitating discussions with healthcare providers.

Outcomes:

Post Treatment:

- Reduced joint pain and improved pain management skills, with the client reporting a significant decrease in daily pain levels.
- Increased participation in social activities and improved emotional well-being, evidenced by the client's return to regular community theater activities and reported reduction in anxiety and depression.
- Ability to drive for at least 30 minutes without experiencing fatigue, as observed and self-reported.
- Decreased depressive symptoms, with PCOS Health Questionnaire scores increasing by 50%, indicating a notable improvement in emotional health and quality of life.
- Enhanced independence in managing household tasks and daily activities, with the client successfully completing chores such as cleaning and organizing without significant fatigue.
- Reduction in joint pain by 30–50%, improving physical functioning and overall quality of life, with the client reporting increased comfort and satisfaction during physical activities.

Improved posture and alignment:

- Noticeable improvement in forward shoulder posture and correction of rounded back, as observed in follow-up physical assessments.
- Reduced tenderness in the lower back and knee areas during palpation, with the client reporting decreased sensitivity.
- Improved hip and knee flexion ROM, as measured during physical assessments.
- Increased strength in hip flexors and extensors, with manual muscle testing showing strength improvements from 3/5 to 4/5.

Improved self-esteem and reduced emotional distress related to hirsutism, with the client following a consistent skincare routine and reporting increased confidence in her appearance.

Follow-Up Visits:

Two additional visits will focus on reinforcing the client's progress in addressing pain management and functional issues related to her PCOS. During these visits, the following will be emphasized:

- **Pain Management Techniques**: Reinforcement and practice of relaxation and breathing techniques to manage pain, particularly during activities of daily living and physical activity.
- **Functional Mobility and Endurance**: Progression of exercises to improve her endurance for daily activities, including driving and social engagements.
- **ADL and IADL Adaptations**: Continued adaptation and modification strategies for self-care, household tasks, and work-related activities to minimize pain and maximize function.

The client exhibited significant improvement in managing her joint pain and overall function, including a reduction in symptoms of PCOS. She is now able to independently perform various ADLs and IADLs, such as cooking, cleaning, driving, dressing, and participating in social activities, without experiencing significant discomfort or pain. Notably, the reduction in pain during physical activity enhanced her quality of life. Her ability to drive for extended periods without fatigue further improved her independence and quality of life. The comprehensive, occupation-based approach in managing gynecological conditions like PCOS demonstrates the profound impact of holistic occupational therapy care on clients' daily lives and well-being.

Further Reading

American Occupational Therapy Association. (2020). Occupational therapy practice framework: Domain and process (4th ed.). *American Journal of Occupational Therapy, 74*(Supplement 2), 7412410010. https://doi.org/10.5014/ajot.2020.74S2001

Bordeianou, L. G., Thorsen, A. J., Keller, D. S., Hawkins, A. T., Messick, C., Oliveira, L., Feingold, D. L., Lightner, A. L., & Paquette, I. M. (2023). The American Society of Colon and Rectal Surgeons clinical practice guidelines for the management of fecal incontinence. In *Diseases of the colon & rectum* (Vol. 66, Issue 5, pp. 647–661). Ovid Technologies (Wolters Kluwer Health). https://doi.org/10.1097/dcr.0000000000002776

Cho, S. T., & Kim, K. H. (2021). Pelvic floor muscle exercise and training for coping with urinary incontinence. *Journal of Exercise Rehabilitation, 17*(6), 379–387. https://doi.org/10.12965/jer.2142666.333

Cunningham, R., & Valasek, S. (2019). Occupational therapy interventions for urinary dysfunction in primary care: A case series. *The American Journal of Occupational Therapy: Official Publication of the American Occupational Therapy Association, 73*(5), 7305185040p1–7305185040p8. https://doi.org/10.5014/ajot.2019.038356

Elliott-Sale, K. J., Bostock, E. L., Jackson, T., Wardle, S. L., O'Leary, T. J., Greeves, J. P., & Sale, C. (2022). Investigating the efficacy of an 18-week postpartum rehabilitation and physical development intervention on occupational physical performance and musculoskeletal health in UK servicewomen: Protocol for an independent group study design. *JMIR Research Protocols, 11*(6), e32315. https://doi.org/10.2196/32315

Fraga, M. V., Oliveira Brito, L. G., Yela, D. A., de Mira, T. A., & Benetti-Pinto, C. L. (2021). Pelvic floor muscle dysfunctions in women with deep infiltrative endometriosis: An underestimated association. *International Journal of Clinical Practice, 75*(8), e14350. https://doi.org/10.1111/ijcp.14350

Gordon, D. A., & Katlic, M. R. (Eds.). (2021). *Pelvic floor disorders: A multidisciplinary textbook* (2nd ed.). StatPearls Publishing.

Huang, Y. C., & Chang, K. V. (2023). Kegel exercises. In *StatPearls*. StatPearls Publishing.

Occupational Therapy Association of California. (n.d.). Vision & Mission: Pelvic Health. Retrieved from https://www.otaconline.org

Quaghebeur, J., Petros, P., Wyndaele, J. J., & De Wachter, S. (2021). Pelvic-floor function, dysfunction, and treatment. *European Journal of Obstetrics, Gynecology, and Reproductive Biology, 265*, 143–149. https://doi.org/10.1016/j.ejogrb.2021.08.026

Raizada, V., & Mittal, R. K. (2008). Pelvic floor anatomy and applied physiology. *Gastroenterology Clinics of North America, 37*(3), 493–509. https://doi.org/10.1016/j.gtc.2008.06.003

Role of Occupational Therapy in Primary Care. (2020). The American journal of occupational therapy: Official publication of the American Occupational Therapy Association, *74*(Supplement_3), 7413410040p1–7413410040p16. https://doi.org/10.5014/ajot.2020.74S3001

Scott, K. (2014). Pelvic floor rehabilitation in the treatment of fecal incontinence. *Clinics in Colon and Rectal Surgery, 27*(3), 99–105. https://doi.org/10.1055/s-0034-1384662

Song, S. Y., Jung, Y. W., Shin, W., Park, M., Lee, G. W., Jeong, S., An, S., Kim, K., Ko, Y. B., Lee, K. H., Kang, B. H., Lee, M., & Yoo, H. J. (2023). Endometriosis-related chronic pelvic pain. *Biomedicines, 11*(10), 2868. https://doi.org/10.3390/biomedicines11102868

Speer, L. M., Mushkbar, S., & Erbele, T. (2016). Chronic pelvic pain in women. *American Family Physician, 93*(5), 380–387.

Twiddy, H., Lane, N., Chawla, R., Johnson, S., Bradshaw, A., Aleem, S., & Mawdsley, L. (2015). The development and delivery of a female chronic pelvic pain management programme: A specialised interdisciplinary approach. *British Journal of Pain, 9*(4), 233–240. https://doi.org/10.1177/2049463715584408

Vasilyev, V., Borisov, V., & Syskov, A. (2019). Biofeedback methodology: A narrative review. In *2019 International Multi-Conference on Engineering, Computer and Information Sciences (SIBIRCON)*. IEEE. https://doi.org/10.1109/sibircon48586.2019.8958019

Wood, L. N., & Anger, J. T. (2014). Urinary incontinence in women. *BMJ, 349*, (Sep 15 4), g4531–g4531). BMJ. https://doi.org/10.1136/bmj.g4531

Xu, P., Wang, X., Guo, P., Zhang, W., Mao, M., & Feng, S. (2022). The effectiveness of eHealth interventions on female pelvic floor dysfunction: A systematic review and meta-analysis. *International Urogynecology Journal, 33*(12), 3325–3354. https://doi.org/10.1007/s00192-022-05222-5

3 Occupational Therapy in Obstetric Health Management

> **Chapter Objectives**
>
> Upon completion of this chapter, the reader will be able to:
>
> 1. Describe the physiological and anatomical changes during pregnancy and their implications for occupational therapy practice.
> 2. Identify occupational therapy assessments and interventions specific to different stages of pregnancy, including prenatal and postnatal care.
> 3. Discuss the management strategies for high-risk pregnancies within the scope of occupational therapy.
> 4. Illustrate the role of occupational therapy in providing psychosocial support to pregnant women.
> 5. Evaluate environmental adaptations in the home and workplace to support pregnant women's health and occupational engagement.

Physiological and Anatomical Changes During Pregnancy

Pregnancy triggers complex physiological and anatomical changes that are essential for supporting fetal development and significantly impact occupational engagement and participation, as it relates to the Occupational Therapy Practice Framework (OTPF). Hormonal fluctuations, including increased levels of hCG, progesterone, and estrogen, drive these changes, affecting various body systems. The cardiovascular system adapts with increased blood volume and cardiac output, while the respiratory system experiences higher tidal volume and oxygen consumption. Musculoskeletal changes, such as ligamentous laxity and altered posture, can lead to discomfort and affect mobility. These changes may disrupt daily occupations, including ADLs, IADLs, rest and sleep, and social participation. Understanding these changes is crucial for OTPs to provide effective support and interventions, helping expectant mothers maintain comfort, functionality, and overall well-being throughout pregnancy.

Changes in the Body During Pregnancy

Physiological changes during pregnancy impact multiple systems, most notably the endocrine system, which supports and sustains the pregnancy. Key hormonal changes include the secretion of human chorionic gonadotropin (hCG), which begins within 10 days of conception and peaks between the eighth and tenth weeks. This hormone stimulates the production of progesterone and estrogen, essential for maintaining the uterine lining and preventing menstruation. As the placenta develops, it becomes the primary source of these hormones.

Estrogen, produced at levels up to 30 times higher than before pregnancy, enlarges the uterus and breasts and contributes to ligament relaxation. Relaxin, another hormone, peaks in the first trimester and remains elevated until after delivery, inhibiting uterine contractions and softening the cervix. Progesterone causes smooth muscle relaxation throughout the body, impacting the gastrointestinal tract and respiratory system. This relaxation can lead to constipation, varicose veins, and hyperventilation of pregnancy.

Cortisol, an adrenal hormone, rises throughout pregnancy and influences stress response and immune function. Prolactin, essential for lactation, increases during pregnancy and stimulates milk production and various hypothalamic functions. Aldosterone helps regulate blood pressure and fluid balance, which can cause swelling and increased blood pressure.

Understanding these hormonal changes and their impacts can help OTPs support pregnant women in managing their daily activities and maintaining their health and well-being (see Table 3.1). Figure 3.1 illustrates the fluctuating levels of estrogen, progesterone, and hCG throughout pregnancy, highlighting their pivotal roles during this period. This visualization highlights the dynamic nature of hormonal changes and sets the stage for discussing other physiological changes, such as musculoskeletal and tissue adaptations, that occur during pregnancy.

Embryological and Fetal Development Stages

Understanding the embryological development of the female reproductive system is crucial for OTPs working with pregnant women. This knowledge can guide the

Table 3.1 Key pregnancy hormones, their functions, and impact on daily activities

Hormone	Function	Impact on Daily Activities
Human Chorionic Gonadotropin (hCG)	Stimulates production of progesterone and estrogen	May cause nausea and vomiting (morning sickness)
Estrogen	Enlarges uterus and breasts, relaxes ligaments	Can cause fatigue, breast tenderness, and changes in physical activity due to ligament laxity
Progesterone	Relaxes smooth muscle, maintains uterine lining	Leads to constipation, varicose veins, and changes in breathing patterns (hyperventilation)
Relaxin	Inhibits uterine contractions, softens cervix	Increases joint laxity, potentially impacting physical stability and comfort
Cortisol	Influences stress response and immune function	May affect sleep patterns, stress levels, and overall energy
Prolactin	Stimulates milk production and hypothalamic functions	Can cause breast tenderness and changes in sleep due to its impact on hypothalamic-pituitary axis
Aldosterone	Regulates blood pressure and fluid balance	Can cause swelling and increased blood pressure

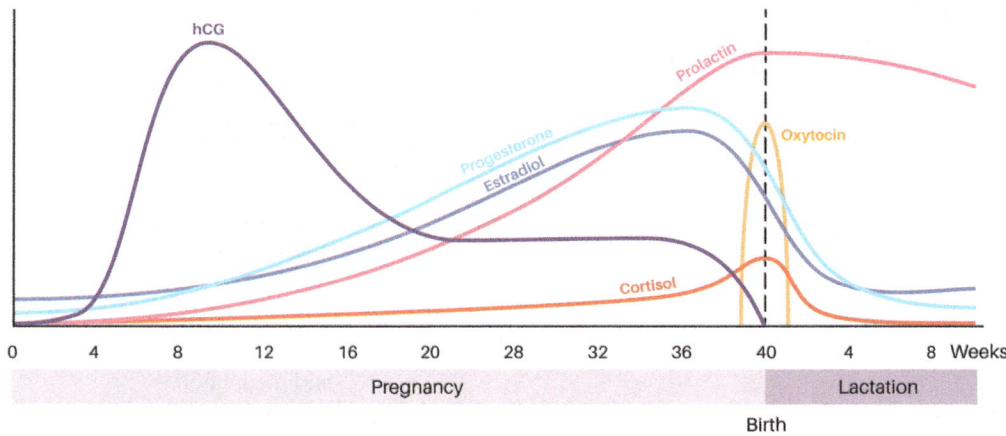

Figure 3.1 Fluctuating hormone levels throughout pregnancy.

selection of appropriate interventions and highlight the importance of avoiding certain treatments during specific trimesters or months of pregnancy due to potential contraindications. Additionally, awareness of embryological development can facilitate communication with women and their families when explaining congenital conditions or developmental anomalies of the female reproductive system. OTPs can play a role in providing education and support to individuals and families facing such challenges, helping them navigate the physical and emotional aspects of reproductive health. Table 3.2 outlines the key stages of embryological and fetal development, specific developmental processes, and their relevance to occupational therapy management practices (Figure 3.2).

Pregnancy exerts significant demands on various body systems, causing noticeable physiological shifts that impact a woman's daily life. Cardiovascular changes include increased blood volume and cardiac output to support the growing fetus. The heart has to work harder to pump the increased blood volume, which can lead to an elevated heart rate and increased cardiac output. This extra effort can make the individual feel more fatigued, especially if her body is not accustomed to the increased workload. Respiratory adjustments involve elevated diaphragm positioning, leading to reduced lung capacity and increased respiratory rates. Gastrointestinal changes often result in morning sickness, heartburn, and constipation due to hormonal and anatomical influences. Musculoskeletal adaptations, driven by the hormone relaxin, prepare the body for childbirth but can cause joint instability and back pain. The urinary system sees increased pressure on the bladder, leading to frequent urination. Integumentary changes include skin hyperpigmentation and the appearance of stretch marks. Table 3.3 outlines these physiological changes and their impact on body functions and ADLs (Figure 3.3).

Musculoskeletal changes, including forward head/neck position, may result in neck pain, tingling and numbness, pain between shoulder blades, and carpal tunnel syndrome. Forward tilting of the pelvis may result in pelvic pain, low back pain, leg pain. Hyperextension of the knees and flattening of the feet may result in knee pain, foot pain, heel pain, overworked joints. Extension of head/neck may be seen resulting in headaches and neck pain. Hyperextension of the upper back may be evident resulting in

90 Occupational Therapy and Women's Health

Table 3.2 Fetal development stages and occupational therapy considerations

Stage	Time Frame	Developmental Processes	OT Considerations for Pregnant Women (Applicable to male and female fetuses)
Fertilization and Early Cell Stages	Week 1 of gestation	Fertilization occurs, forming a zygote. The zygote undergoes several cell divisions as it travels down the fallopian tube.	Encourage rest and stress reduction to support implantation. Avoid high-impact activities and any strenuous physical exertion. Provide education on relaxation techniques, including deep breathing and meditation.
Blastocyst Formation and Implantation	Week 2 of gestation	The blastocyst forms and implants into the uterine wall. The placenta begins to develop. Possible symptoms include light spotting, mild cramping, and breast tenderness.	Continue to focus on rest and light activities. Avoid electronic muscle stimulation (E-STIM), heat modalities, and any activities that might disrupt implantation. Educate about potential symptoms like implantation bleeding and mild cramping. Offer gentle stretching and prenatal yoga.
Embryonic Disc Formation	Week 3 of gestation	The blastocyst develops into the embryonic disc, which will form the embryo. Germ layers begin to differentiate.	Emphasize gentle exercises and ergonomic adjustments. Educate on the importance of nutrition and hydration to support early development. Provide guidance on safe body mechanics for daily activities.
Early Embryonic Development	Week 4 of gestation	The neural tube forms, and the heart begins to develop. The embryo is now recognizable and starts forming basic structures.	Continue to avoid deep tissue massage near the abdomen. Support posture and ergonomic adjustments to accommodate early pregnancy changes. Introduce exercises to strengthen the core and pelvic floor.
Formation of the Gonadal Ridge	Weeks 5–6 of gestation	The presence or absence of the SRY gene on the Y chromosome determines whether the gonadal ridge develops into testes or ovaries.	Avoid high-impact activities, E-STIM, and heat modalities. Educate on gentle exercises and stress management techniques to support early pregnancy health. Introduce light resistance training and balance exercises.
Development of Müllerian and Wolffian Ducts	Weeks 6–7 of gestation	The Müllerian ducts develop into female reproductive structures (fallopian tubes, uterus, cervix, and upper vagina), while the Wolffian ducts regress in females.	Continue to avoid E-STIM and heat modalities. Focus on ergonomic adjustments and avoid heavy lifting to prevent strain on the developing uterus. Educate on body mechanics and safe lifting techniques.

(Continued)

Table 3.2 (Continued)

Stage	Time Frame	Developmental Processes	OT Considerations for Pregnant Women (Applicable to male and female fetuses)
Fusion of Müllerian Ducts	Weeks 9–12 of gestation	The Müllerian ducts fuse to form the uterovaginal primordium, which differentiates into the uterus and upper part of the vagina.	Avoid deep tissue massage near the abdomen and heavy lifting. Emphasize posture support and ergonomic adjustments. Introduce prenatal Pilates to enhance core strength.
Development of External Genitalia	Weeks 9–12 of gestation	The labioscrotal folds form the labia majora, the genital tubercle elongates into the clitoris, and the urogenital folds form the labia minora.	Continue to avoid deep tissue massage and ultrasound near the abdomen. Provide support for posture and pelvic alignment to alleviate discomfort. Introduce gentle stretching and flexibility exercises.
Finalization of Female Reproductive Anatomy	Weeks 13–20 of gestation	The female reproductive organs continue to develop and mature; the ovaries descend into the pelvis, and the external genitalia achieve their typical female appearance.	Educate on maintaining physical activity within safe limits, and emphasize the importance of hydration and nutrition. Avoid activities that involve lying flat on the back for prolonged periods. Introduce water aerobics for low-impact exercise.
Continued Development and Maturation	Weeks 20–28 of gestation	The fetus grows significantly, and organs continue to mature. Increased movement and rapid weight gain occur.	Recommend moderate physical activity, focusing on balance and core stability. Avoid activities that risk abdominal trauma. Continue to avoid E-STIM and deep tissue modalities near the abdomen. Introduce exercises to improve balance and stability.
Preparation for Birth	Weeks 29–40 of gestation	The fetus continues to grow and mature, lungs develop further, and the fetus positions itself for birth.	Educate on body mechanics and proper lifting techniques to reduce back strain. Introduce breathing exercises and relaxation techniques for labor preparation. Avoid high-impact activities, and monitor for signs of preterm labor. Use gentle techniques and avoid any interventions that increase intra-abdominal pressure. Introduce pelvic floor exercises and perineal massage.

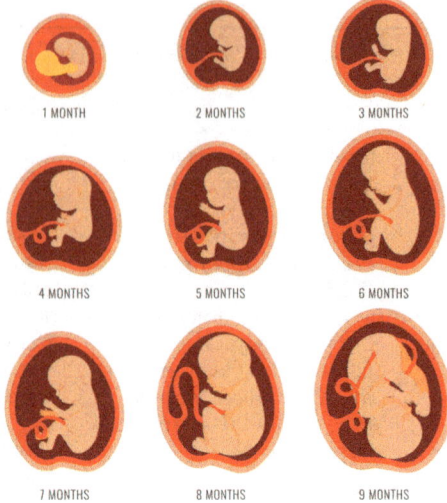

Figure 3.2 Embryo developmental stages.

rib pain and trouble breathing. Last, accentuated lumbar lordosis contributes to low back pain and tense muscles.

Neuroanatomical Differences and Changes in the Brain During Pregnancy

Understanding the neuroanatomical differences between male and female brains provides a foundation for exploring the specific changes that occur during pregnancy. The brains of men and women exhibit distinct variations in structure and function, influenced by both genetic and hormonal factors. For instance, studies have shown that women generally have a larger hippocampus relative to overall brain size, which is associated with memory and learning. Men, on the other hand, tend to have a larger amygdala, a region involved in processing emotions and fear responses. Additionally, the prefrontal cortex, responsible for decision-making and social behavior, has been found to exhibit structural differences, potentially influencing behavioural tendencies. These differences are not absolute but rather represent tendencies, with considerable overlap between male and female brains (Figures 3.4 and 3.5).

The concept of the bipotential neonatal brain highlights the brain's initial capacity to develop characteristics typically associated with either gender. Both male and female brains contain components that are traditionally linked with the opposite gender, suggesting a spectrum rather than a strict binary. For example, females can exhibit brain patterns commonly seen in males and vice versa, emphasizing the fluidity and complexity of brain development. This neuroanatomical diversity is crucial for understanding how the brain adapts to various life stages, including pregnancy.

Recent research has unveiled intriguing alterations in brain structure and function during pregnancy, particularly in the realm of white matter. White matter, composed of nerve fibers insulated with a fatty substance called myelin, plays a crucial role in communication between different regions of the brain. During pregnancy, women experience an increase in white matter volume, which is believed to enhance neural connectivity and cognitive functioning, supporting the psychological and emotional adjustments required

Table 3.3 Physiological changes during pregnancy and their impact on body functions and occupational functioning

System	Changes	Impact on Body Functions	Impact on Occupational Functioning
Cardiovascular	Blood volume increases by 40–50%, cardiac output increases	Maintains maternal blood pressure, ensures blood supply	May cause fatigue, increased need for rest. May require modifications to work schedules, energy conservation strategies, and frequent breaks during physical activities.
Respiratory	Diaphragm elevation, increased respiratory rate, decreased infra-sternal angle	Reduces lung capacity, increases breathing rate	May cause shortness of breath during physical activities. May necessitate pacing strategies, avoidance of strenuous tasks, and positioning techniques to ease breathing.
Gastrointestinal	Morning sickness, heartburn, constipation	Slowed digestion, nausea, vomiting	May affect appetite and meal routines. Requires dietary modifications, scheduling smaller and frequent meals, and strategies to manage nausea and heartburn.
Musculoskeletal	Ligament relaxation, joint instability, abdominal muscle stretching, increased anterior pelvic tilt	Supports weight of uterus, prepares for childbirth	May cause back pain, postural changes, joint discomfort. Interventions may include ergonomic adjustments, use of supportive devices like maternity belts, and exercises to strengthen core and back muscles.
Urinary	Increased bladder pressure, higher urine production	Frequent urination, increased urine flow	Increased trips to the bathroom, potential urinary tract infections (UTIs). Encourage regular bathroom breaks, hydration management, and education on recognizing UTI symptoms.
Integumentary	Skin hyperpigmentation, stretch marks, hair growth changes	Skin darkening, appearance of stretch marks	May impact self-esteem and body image. Support through body image counseling, skincare routines to manage hyperpigmentation and stretch marks, and strategies to boost self-esteem.

for motherhood. The prefrontal cortex, for instance, undergoes changes that may improve social cognition and empathy, crucial for bonding with the newborn. Additionally, the hippocampus and amygdala also exhibit structural changes, potentially influencing maternal behaviors and emotional regulation.

These changes are essential for adapting to the unique demands of pregnancy and preparing for the transition to motherhood. The following sections discuss these changes by brain lobe and their impacts on occupational engagement and daily living.

Frontal Lobe

The frontal lobe is responsible for executive functions, such as decision-making, problem-solving, and impulse control. During pregnancy, the prefrontal cortex, a part of the frontal lobe, undergoes enhanced connectivity in white matter. This enhancement may facilitate

94   *Occupational Therapy and Women's Health*

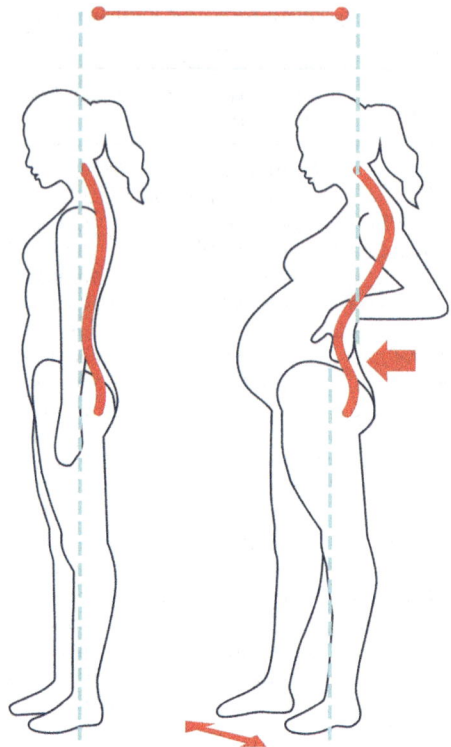

Figure 3.3 Postural changes in pregnancy.

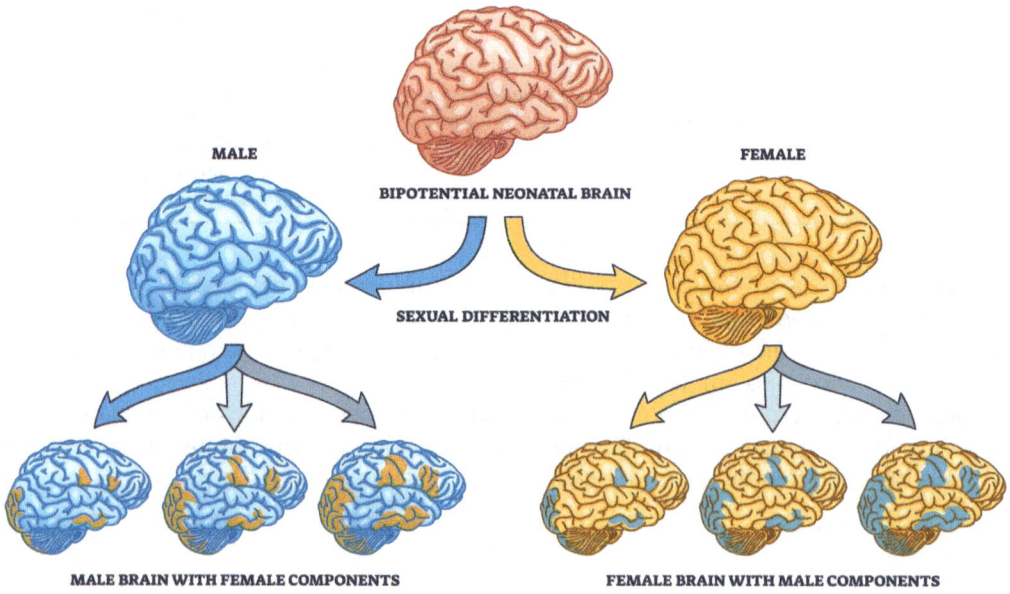

Figure 3.4 Gender differences in neuroanatomy.

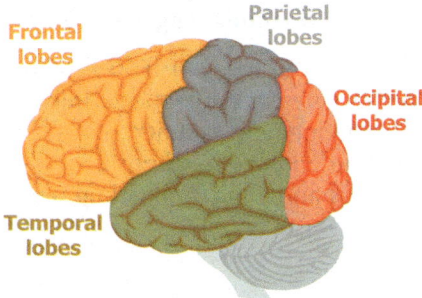

Figure 3.5 Lobes of brain.

better decision-making and impulse control, which are crucial for the upcoming responsibilities of motherhood.

Impact on Daily Activities and Occupational Engagement:

- **Benefits**: Improved decision-making and impulse control can help expectant mothers manage new responsibilities more effectively, such as planning for the baby's arrival, organizing the household, and making health-related decisions.
- **Challenges**: The increased cognitive load may lead to mental fatigue, affecting concentration and the ability to complete complex tasks. This can impact occupational performance, such as work-related duties or managing multiple household tasks simultaneously.

Parietal Lobe

The parietal lobe processes sensory information and is involved in spatial orientation. Pregnancy-related changes in this lobe may include adaptations to better process sensory inputs and manage the spatial requirements of the growing body and impending care of an infant. Enhanced white matter connectivity in this area may also support improved coordination and physical interactions.

Impact on Daily Activities and Occupational Engagement:

- **Benefits**: Improved sensory processing and spatial orientation can aid in tasks such as setting up the nursery, managing space for baby-related items, and safely navigating environments while carrying the baby.
- **Challenges**: Heightened sensory sensitivity may lead to discomfort in crowded or noisy environments, potentially limiting participation in social activities and community engagement.

Temporal Lobe

The temporal lobe is essential for processing auditory information and memory formation. During pregnancy, changes in this lobe may support the development of auditory processing skills needed to respond to a baby's cries and other sounds. Additionally, improved memory functions have been observed, potentially aiding in the management of new routines and tasks associated with motherhood.

Impact on Daily Activities and Occupational Engagement:

- **Benefits**: Enhanced auditory processing can help mothers quickly respond to their baby's needs, fostering better caregiving practices. Improved memory functions can aid in establishing and maintaining new routines.
- **Challenges**: The emotional burden of remembering numerous tasks and responsibilities can lead to increased stress and anxiety, affecting overall well-being and occupational balance.

Occipital Lobe

The occipital lobe is primarily responsible for visual processing. While there is less direct evidence of pregnancy-related changes in this lobe, it is possible that adaptations occur to enhance the mother's ability to visually monitor and care for her newborn. This might include improved visual attention and the ability to quickly recognize and respond to the baby's needs.

Impact on Daily Activities and Occupational Engagement:

- **Benefits**: Enhanced visual processing can aid in tasks such as monitoring the baby's safety, noticing changes in the baby's behavior or health, and navigating caregiving tasks.
- **Challenges**: Constant visual monitoring and heightened vigilance can lead to visual fatigue and strain, potentially impacting overall energy levels and the ability to engage in other activities.

Emotional and Cognitive Adaptations

Pregnancy is a time of emotional flux, marked by the highs of anticipation and joy, as well as the lows of anxiety and mood swings. Specific brain regions associated with emotional regulation, such as the amygdala (part of the temporal lobe) and prefrontal cortex, undergo modifications in white matter connectivity. The amygdala becomes more connected to other regions, potentially heightening emotional responses, while the prefrontal cortex's enhanced connectivity could help manage these emotions effectively.

Impact on Daily Activities and Occupational Engagement:

- **Benefits**: Enhanced emotional regulation can help mothers manage the emotional demands of pregnancy and early motherhood, improving interactions with family and healthcare providers.
- **Challenges**: Heightened emotional sensitivity can lead to mood swings and anxiety, affecting daily routines, social interactions, and overall mental health.

Preparing for Bonding

Research has indicated that white matter changes occur in brain areas associated with empathy, theory of mind (the ability to understand and interpret others' thoughts and feelings), and social cognition. The superior longitudinal fasciculus, a bundle of white matter fibers connecting different parts of the brain, is one area that experiences alterations. This change is believed to enhance a mother's ability to understand and respond to her baby's needs and emotions, fostering the mother-infant bond crucial for the baby's well-being.

Impact on Daily Activities and Occupational Engagement:

- **Benefits**: Enhanced empathy and social cognition can improve bonding and caregiving practices, fostering a strong mother-infant relationship and supporting the baby's emotional development.
- **Challenges**: The intense focus on bonding and caregiving may lead to neglect of self-care and other personal activities, potentially impacting the mother's overall health and well-being.

The brain changes during pregnancy significantly impact occupational functioning. Improved decision-making, sensory processing, and memory functions help pregnant women manage new responsibilities, respond effectively to their baby's needs, and establish new routines. However, these benefits come with challenges, including mental fatigue, heightened sensory sensitivity, emotional fluctuations, and potential neglect of self-care. These changes can affect a woman's ability to balance daily tasks, maintain social interactions, and engage in meaningful activities, highlighting the need for comprehensive support to navigate the complexities of pregnancy.

Occupational Therapy in Prenatal Care

Pregnancy is a significant phase in a woman's life that brings unique physical and emotional challenges. OTPs play a crucial role in providing comprehensive care and support to expectant mothers during this critical time. This chapter explores the multifaceted role of occupational therapy in prenatal care, addressing the physical, emotional, and environmental aspects of maternal well-being.

Comprehensive Care by OTPs

OTPs are valuable members of the healthcare team, offering specialized services to promote the health and well-being of pregnant women. Comprehensive prenatal care provided by OTPs encompasses various domains, addressing both the physical and emotional aspects of this significant journey. During pregnancy, OTPs focus on promoting wellness and health through proactive measures. They provide ergonomic recommendations and teach proper body mechanics to help expectant mothers maintain comfort and prevent discomfort as their bodies change. This includes strategies on optimal sleeping positions, safe lifting techniques, and therapeutic exercises to enhance posture and balance. Maternal well-being extends beyond physical health. OTPs also address the emotional aspects of pregnancy. They conduct psychosocial assessments to support emotional well-being and identify any signs of prenatal mood disorders like anxiety or depression. Early detection and intervention are crucial for maternal mental health, and OTPs provide coping strategies, stress management techniques, and relaxation exercises to help women navigate these emotional challenges. See Table 3.4 for prenatal interventions by OTPs.

Physical Support During Pregnancy

Supporting physical health and well-being during pregnancy is crucial for maintaining daily function and preparing for labor and delivery. OTPs can offer trimester-specific therapeutic exercises and techniques to address physical changes and challenges during

Table 3.4 Comprehensive prenatal interventions by occupational therapy practitioners

Intervention	Benefits During Pregnancy	Impact on Occupational Functioning
Adaptive ADL/IADL Techniques	Facilitates independence and safety in daily living activities.	Enhances ability to perform daily tasks with reduced strain, preventing injury and discomfort.
Diaphragmatic Breathing	Promotes relaxation, reduces stress, supports optimal oxygen exchange, strengthens pelvic floor muscles.	Enhances focus and concentration, supports pelvic floor health, and aids in managing shortness of breath.
Prenatal Affective Cognitive Training	Enhances cognitive and emotional skills to better manage the psychological demands of pregnancy.	Promotes mental resilience and emotional regulation during daily interactions, improving coping strategies.
Therapeutic Exercises	Maintains fitness, improves strength and flexibility, important for overall health during pregnancy.	Increases stamina, enhances physical capabilities for daily activities, and reduces the risk of musculoskeletal discomfort.
Therapeutic Activities	Engages expectant mothers in meaningful and purposeful activities tailored to their needs.	Promotes psychological well-being, sustains an active lifestyle, and provides a sense of accomplishment.
Pelvic Floor Exercises	Strengthens pelvic muscles, reduces risk of urinary incontinence, supports smoother delivery.	Supports bladder control, enhances comfort during daily activities, and improves postpartum recovery.
Ergonomic Recommendations	Provides posture and lifting techniques to reduce physical strain, promotes a healthier pregnancy.	Reduces pain and discomfort during activities, prevents injuries, and enhances productivity at work and home.
Psychosocial Support	Offers emotional support and coping strategies, contributes to a positive pregnancy experience.	Enhances emotional stability, improves social interactions, and reduces anxiety and depression.
Health Management	Offers guidance on balanced nutrition and understanding medication management.	Maintains energy levels, prevents fatigue, supports overall health, and improves nutritional habits.
Sleep Hygiene	Improves sleep quality, essential for mental and physical health during pregnancy.	Enhances cognitive functioning, reduces daytime fatigue, and improves mood and concentration.
Mindfulness and Stress Reduction	Teaches relaxation techniques to manage stress and improve mental well-being.	Improves mental clarity, reduces distractions, enhances participation in activities, and promotes a positive outlook.
Environmental Modifications	Recommends home and workplace adaptations for safety and comfort.	Increases safety, supports independence, enhances quality of life, and prevents falls and other injuries.
Energy Conservation	Teaches strategies to manage and conserve energy during daily tasks.	Supports sustained participation in daily and occupational activities, reduces fatigue, and improves overall efficiency.
Assistive Device Training	Educates on the use and benefits of assistive devices to enhance mobility and functionality.	Improves independence and safety in performing occupational roles, reduces physical strain, and enhances mobility.

OT in Obstetric Health Management 99

pregnancy. This section provides detailed guidance for each trimester, highlighting appropriate exercises and their impact on occupational functioning.

First Trimester (Weeks 1–12)

During the first trimester, the focus is on gentle exercises to promote relaxation and reduce early pregnancy discomfort. At this stage, it's essential to avoid high-impact exercises and heavy lifting. Gentle stretching, pelvic floor awareness, and diaphragmatic breathing are particularly beneficial. These exercises help reduce tension, strengthen pelvic muscles, and promote relaxation, setting a foundation for a healthy pregnancy. See Table 3.5 for sample exercises recommended to promote relaxation, enhance pelvic floor strength, and maintain flexibility, thereby setting a foundation for a healthy pregnancy and easing early pregnancy discomfort.

Second Trimester (Weeks 13–26)

In the second trimester, the focus shifts to strengthening and maintaining physical health as the body adapts to the growing fetus. During this period, it is crucial to avoid exercises that require lying flat on your back for extended periods and high-risk activities. Core strengthening, pelvic floor exercises, and prenatal yoga are recommended to support overall strength and stability. Table 3.6 lists therapeutic exercises with a focus on

Table 3.5 First trimester exercises to enhance maternal comfort and prepare for labor

Exercise	Description	Level	Benefits
Cat-Cow Stretch	Enhances spinal flexibility and reduces tension.	Easy	Promotes spinal flexibility and relaxation.
Seated Forward Bend	Stretches the back and hamstrings, promoting relaxation.	Easy	Enhances relaxation and reduces tension.
Child's Pose	Stretches the back, hips, and thighs while promoting relaxation.	Easy	Reduces tension and enhances relaxation.
Pelvic Floor Contractions	Strengthens pelvic muscles, preparing for increased weight.	Easy	Supports pelvic health and prepares for labor.
4-7-8 Breathing Technique	Promotes relaxation and reduces stress.	Easy	Reduces stress and promotes calmness.
Seated Marches	Strengthens the hip flexors and improves circulation.	Easy	Enhances hip strength and circulation.
Clamshells	Strengthens the hip abductors and improves stability.	Moderate	Enhances hip stability and reduces tension.
Side-Lying Leg Lifts	Strengthens the outer thigh and hip muscles.	Moderate	Improves hip stability and reduces lower body tension.
Butterfly Stretch	Stretches the inner thighs and groin area.	Easy	Enhances flexibility and reduces muscle tightness.
Standing Calf Raises	Strengthens the calf muscles and improves circulation.	Moderate	Improves lower leg strength and circulation.

Table 3.6 Second trimester strengthening and stability exercises

Exercise	Description	Level	Benefits
Standing Pelvic Tilts	Strengthens the lower back and pelvic muscles.	Easy	Supports lower back and pelvic health.
Modified Plank	Supports abdominal muscles and improves stability.	Moderate	Enhances core strength and stability.
Bridge Pose	Strengthens the glutes, hamstrings, and lower back.	Moderate	Enhances lower body strength and stability.
Bird-Dog Exercise	Improves balance and strengthens the core and back muscles.	Moderate	Enhances core stability and balance.
Glute Bridges	Strengthens the glutes and hamstrings.	Moderate	Enhances lower body strength and stability.
Seated Pelvic Tilts	Strengthens the lower back and pelvis.	Moderate	Supports lower back health and pelvic stability.
Extended Kegel Holds	Enhances endurance of pelvic muscles.	Moderate	Improves pelvic muscle endurance.
Seated Row with Resistance Band	Strengthens the upper back and shoulders.	Moderate	Improves upper body strength and posture.
Prenatal Yoga	Boosts cardiovascular health and flexibility.	Moderate	Enhances overall flexibility and cardiovascular health.
Wall Push-Ups	Strengthens the upper body muscles.	Moderate	Improves upper body strength and posture.
Side-Lying Clamshells	Strengthens the hip abductors and gluteal muscles.	Moderate	Enhances hip stability and reduces lower body tension.

strengthening core and pelvic muscles, enhancing stability, and accommodating the growing fetus, all crucial for maintaining physical health and preparing for the later stages of pregnancy.

Third Trimester (Weeks 27–40)

The third trimester focuses on preparing for labor and managing late pregnancy discomfort. It is essential to avoid exercises that involve lying flat on your back and those with a high risk of balance issues. Squats, pelvic rocking, perineal massage, and Lamaze breathing are effective in building strength, reducing pain, and preparing for childbirth. Table 3.7 lists therapeutic exercises specifically chosen for the third trimester to aid in labor preparation and alleviate late-pregnancy discomfort. It includes movements designed to strengthen the lower body, enhance pelvic flexibility, and manage pain, ensuring the mother is physically and mentally prepared for childbirth.

Supporting Women Through the Prenatal Phase

Supporting women throughout the prenatal phase is crucial for ensuring their overall well-being and optimal occupational functioning. OTPs provide comprehensive care that addresses the multifaceted needs of expectant mothers. By offering guidance and tailored interventions, OTPs help women navigate the physical and emotional changes of pregnancy, promoting health, wellness, and a positive pregnancy experience. This holistic support is essential for empowering women to manage their daily routines, prepare for parenthood, and maintain a balanced lifestyle (Table 3.8).

Table 3.7 Third trimester preparatory exercises

Exercise	Description	Level	Benefit
Squats	Strengthens the lower body and prepares for labor positions.	Moderate	Builds lower body strength and prepares for labor.
Pelvic Rocking on a Birthing Ball	Relieves back pain and enhances pelvic flexibility.	Moderate	Reduces back pain and increases pelvic flexibility.
Perineal Massage	Prepares the perineum for childbirth, reducing tearing.	Moderate	Enhances perineal flexibility and reduces tear risk.
Lamaze Breathing	Manages pain and anxiety during labor.	Moderate	Helps manage labor pain and anxiety.
Gentle Pelvic Tilts	Strengthens the lower back and relieves pelvic pressure.	Easy	Reduces pelvic pressure and enhances lower back strength.
Butterfly Stretch	Stretches the inner thighs and groin area.	Easy	Enhances flexibility and reduces muscle tightness.
Child's Pose	Stretches the back and hips, promoting relaxation.	Easy	Reduces tension and enhances relaxation.
Standing Calf Raises	Strengthens the calf muscles and improves circulation.	Easy	Reduces leg cramps and improves blood circulation.
Seated Ankle Circles	Improves ankle flexibility and reduces swelling.	Easy	Enhances lower limb mobility and reduces edema.
Deep Squats	Helps to open the pelvis and prepare for labor.	Moderate	Enhances pelvic flexibility and prepares for labor.

Table 3.8 Key areas of support by OTPs during the prenatal phase and their impact on occupational functioning

Area of Support	Description	Impact on Occupational Functioning
Promoting Independence	OTPs assess a woman's ability to perform ADLs and IADLs. They provide strategies and adaptations to enhance independence in self-care and household tasks.	Empowers expectant mothers to confidently manage their daily routines, reducing reliance on others and promoting self-sufficiency.
Training in Essential Skills	OTPs offer training in essential skills, including infant care and feeding. They address any physical limitations and adapt techniques to suit the individual needs of mothers.	Helps expectant mothers develop confidence in their roles, ensuring they are well-prepared for the demands of parenting.
Nutrition and Hydration Management	OTPs educate expectant mothers about making informed dietary choices and provide practical strategies for maintaining hydration.	Supports overall health, prevents fatigue, and ensures that both mother and baby receive essential nutrients for optimal development.
Home Environment Modifications	OTPs assess the home environment and recommend modifications and assistive devices to enhance accessibility, comfort, and convenience.	Promotes safety and independence within the home, making daily activities more manageable and reducing physical strain.
Breastfeeding/ Bottle Feeding Support	OTPs assist mothers in finding comfortable and effective positions for breastfeeding or bottle-feeding and provide ergonomic recommendations.	Reduces the risk of musculoskeletal strain, ensures comfort during feeding, and enhances the overall feeding experience for both mother and baby.
Organization and Time Management	OTPs provide strategies for time management, simplifying tasks, and balancing responsibilities.	Helps expectant mothers efficiently manage daily household tasks, prioritize self-care, and maintain a balanced lifestyle.

By addressing these key areas, OTPs ensure that expectant mothers receive the necessary support to thrive during pregnancy. This comprehensive approach not only enhances their physical and emotional well-being but also prepares them for the responsibilities of parenthood, fostering a smoother transition into this new phase of life.

Emotional and Psychological Support During Pregnancy

OTPs play a crucial role in supporting the emotional and psychological well-being of expectant mothers. Their holistic approach is pivotal in managing stress, anxiety, and prenatal mood disorders, thereby enhancing overall mental health. OTPs conduct psychosocial assessments to identify the emotional well-being of the mother and recognize any signs of prenatal mood disorders. They provide tailored counseling and coping strategies to effectively manage anxiety and stress. Additionally, OTPs offer relaxation exercises such as guided imagery and progressive muscle relaxation to promote calmness and relaxation. Furthermore, they teach mindfulness practices and meditation, which have been shown to significantly improve mental well-being. OTPs also recommend various relaxation techniques to help manage stress and enhance emotional stability throughout pregnancy. This comprehensive support ensures that expectant mothers are equipped to navigate the emotional challenges of pregnancy, leading to healthier outcomes for both the mother and the baby.

Environmental Modifications

Creating a supportive and safe home environment is essential for the well-being of expectant mothers. OTPs play a key role in assessing and recommending modifications to enhance accessibility, comfort, and safety within the home. They meticulously assess the home environment for potential hazards and recommend safety modifications, such as installing non-slip mats, ensuring adequate lighting, and fitting grab bars to prevent falls. OTPs also suggest ergonomic furniture and proper storage solutions that promote ease of movement and reduce physical strain, making daily activities safer and more comfortable for the mother-to-be.

Additionally, OTPs focus on creating a sensory-enhanced nursery that caters to the developmental needs of the newborn while also considering the comfort of the mother. They design nursery layouts that consider sensory needs, incorporating calming lighting and color schemes. OTPs recommend tactile sensory opportunities through varied textures in crib bedding and play mats, which are essential for the baby's sensory development. Furthermore, they suggest using sound machines to provide soothing auditory stimulation and toys with contrasting colors and patterns for visual stimulation, all aimed at creating an environment that supports the health and development of the child.

Musculoskeletal Dysfunction during Pregnancy: Occupational Therapy Approaches

During pregnancy, women experience substantial changes in their joints and soft tissues, particularly around the pelvic ring and lower back. These anatomical shifts, along with alterations in posture, significantly impact daily functioning and basic ADLs and IADLs. Pain and decreased mobility can make it challenging to perform essential tasks such as dressing, bathing, cooking, and maintaining a household, thereby affecting overall quality of life. The relationship between these postural changes and musculoskeletal pain is complex, as discomfort often arises before any visible changes in the lumbar spine curvature, suggesting that hormonal factors may be a significant contributor.

Interestingly, studies indicate that women with greater joint mobility during pregnancy may actually report lower instances of back pain. This finding highlights the intricate and not fully understood nature of joint and soft tissue dysfunction during this period. Clinicians must consider this complexity when discussing musculoskeletal issues with pregnant patients.

Additionally, increased fluid volume associated with pregnancy can lead to peripheral nerve entrapment or compression, resulting in conditions such as carpal tunnel syndrome, tarsal tunnel syndrome, and meralgia paresthetica. Recognizing and understanding these pathologies are essential for the effective management and treatment of MSDs in pregnant patients.

Occupational therapy plays a vital role in addressing these musculoskeletal dysfunctions, significantly impacting a woman's occupational participation and performance. Effective interventions are crucial in helping pregnant women maintain their independence and engagement in meaningful occupations. The following sections will delve into the examination of pregnant patients, providing strategies for managing these musculoskeletal challenges to support optimal occupational performance.

Occupational Therapy Evaluation and Treatment of the Pregnant Patient

Evaluating a pregnant patient requires a comprehensive and holistic approach that considers the unique physiological and anatomical changes occurring during pregnancy. The goal of the occupational therapy evaluation is to identify and address factors that may impact the patient's ability to perform daily activities and participate in meaningful occupations. It is essential to be mindful of how pregnancy impacts posture, balance, and overall body functions. Below are key components of an occupational therapy evaluation for pregnant patients.

Patient Interview and History

The patient interview and history-taking process is critical in understanding the unique needs and concerns of pregnant patients. This involves gathering detailed information about the patient's medical history, current pregnancy status, and any complications or pre-existing conditions. Additionally, the occupational profile should encompass the patient's daily routines, roles, and responsibilities, including their work environment, home life, leisure activities, and social participation. This comprehensive overview allows the therapist to identify specific challenges and tailor interventions to support the patient's occupational performance and overall well-being throughout their pregnancy. Table 3.9 lists specific additional questions that are vital in the OT evaluation of pregnant clients, compared to those typically asked of non-pregnant clients. These questions help adjust therapeutic exercises and strategies to accommodate the unique needs of pregnant patients, ensuring safety and effectiveness in treatment planning.

A thorough and empathetic evaluation process is crucial for developing an effective treatment plan that enhances the pregnant patient's occupational performance and overall quality of life. By understanding the impact of pregnancy on posture, balance, and other body functions, the occupational therapist can provide tailored interventions that

Table 3.9 Key additional questions in OT evaluation for pregnant clients

Additional Questions	Purpose	Ramifications
How far along are you in your pregnancy?	To determine the trimester and adjust interventions accordingly.	Adjust therapeutic exercises to be appropriate for the trimester; avoid exercises that may be unsafe. Modify ADL/IADL strategies to accommodate energy levels and physical capabilities.
Have you experienced any complications with this pregnancy?	To identify any medical conditions that may impact therapy	Modify exercises, monitor vitals closely, and coordinate with the healthcare team. Adapt ADL/IADL tasks to ensure safety and prevent strain or injury.
What changes have you noticed in your body since becoming pregnant?	To understand physical adaptations and their effects on function.	Tailor interventions to address specific changes and discomforts. Adjust ADL/IADL techniques to enhance comfort and efficiency.
Are you experiencing any pain or discomfort? If so, where and when?	To pinpoint specific areas of concern and tailor pain management strategies.	Develop a pain management plan and adjust activities to minimize discomfort. Recommend ergonomic modifications for ADLs/IADLs to reduce pain.
Have you noticed any changes in your ability to perform daily activities since becoming pregnant?	To assess the impact of pregnancy on ADLs and IADLs.	Implement adaptive strategies and assistive devices as needed. Educate on energy conservation techniques to maintain participation in ADLs/IADLs.
What medications were you taking before pregnancy that you have now stopped?	To identify any changes in medication that may impact health and function.	Monitor for any withdrawal symptoms or changes in health status; adapt therapy interventions as necessary.
Do you have any concerns about your posture or balance?	To address potential issues that could affect safety and function.	Focus on exercises that improve posture and balance; ensure safety precautions. Modify ADL/IADL tasks to enhance stability and prevent falls.

address these changes. This approach ensures that pregnant patients can maintain their daily activities and participate in meaningful occupations, thereby supporting their health and well-being throughout the pregnancy.

Pain Assessment

Pain assessment in pregnant patients requires a nuanced approach due to the unique physiological changes they experience. Unlike non-pregnant clients, pregnant patients may experience pain related to hormonal fluctuations, increased joint laxity, and the growing weight and shifting posture of the body. OTPs should use pain scales, such as the Visual Analog Scale (VAS) or the Numeric Rating Scale (NRS), to assess pain intensity. It is crucial to inquire about the location, frequency, and duration of the pain, as well as any activities or positions that exacerbate or relieve it.

Assess how pain affects daily living activities directly. Ask about the impact on specific tasks such as dressing, cooking, working, and caregiving. This will help prioritize interventions based on how pain limits meaningful activities. Encourage clients to keep a pain diary that tracks the activities or positions that coincide with the onset of pain. This log can be a valuable tool for identifying patterns and triggers within their daily routines and occupations. Additionally, therapists should consider pregnancy-specific conditions, which can present with distinct pain characteristics.

Functional Pain Assessment Examples

1. **Round Ligament Pain**
   - **Description**: Sharp, stabbing pain or a dull ache, typically on one or both sides of the lower abdomen or groin. It often occurs with sudden movements.
   - **Assessment**: Evaluate how actions like getting out of a car or turning over in bed affect pain levels. These activities involve sudden movements or changes in position that can stretch and stress the round ligaments.
   - **Activity and Position Log**: Track occurrences and intensity of pain during these specific movements to identify patterns and triggers.

2. **Pelvic Girdle Pain**
   - **Description**: Pain in the front or back of the pelvis, which may radiate to the hips, thighs, or lower back, often worsened by weight-bearing activities.
   - **Assessment**: Assess the impact of walking upstairs or standing on one leg (e.g., while dressing). These activities require pelvic stabilization and can exacerbate pain by stressing the pelvic joints.
   - **Activity and Position Log**: Document the specific activities that trigger pain, focusing on those that involve pelvic movement or load-bearing.

3. **Sciatica**
   - **Description**: Shooting or burning pain that starts in the lower back or buttocks and radiates down one or both legs, possibly accompanied by numbness or tingling.
   - **Assessment**: Determine how prolonged sitting or bending to pick up objects affects the pain. These activities can compress or irritate the sciatic nerve, especially if done improperly.
   - **Activity and Position Log**: Monitor and record the activities and positions that exacerbate the sciatica symptoms, particularly noting posture and duration.

4. **Symphysis Pubis Dysfunction (SPD)**
   - **Description**: Pain and tenderness in the front of the pelvis near the pubic bone, potentially radiating to adjacent areas, often described as sharp or grinding.
   - **Assessment**: Examine how movements such as getting in and out of a bathtub or turning over in bed affect the pain. These activities involve motions that can significantly strain the symphysis pubis.
   - **Activity and Position Log**: Keep a detailed log of when and during which activities the pain occurs, emphasizing those that involve leg separation or pelvic torque.

5. **Low Back Pain**
   - **Description**: Generalized aching or stiffness in the lower back, which may be exacerbated by certain postures or activities.
   - **Assessment**: Assess the impact of lifting heavy objects or prolonged standing on pain levels. These activities can increase the strain on the lower back, leading to or worsening pain.

- **Activity and Position Log**: Document tasks that lead to increased back pain, noting the specific conditions under which the pain worsens, such as during prolonged static postures or specific movements.

By understanding these specific pain descriptions and their unique triggers, OTPs can develop targeted interventions that address the particular pain-related challenges faced by pregnant patients. This tailored approach is essential for enhancing their occupational performance and overall quality of life.

Physical Examination

The physical examination of a pregnant patient requires special consideration of their physiological changes and the safety of different positioning techniques. During the first trimester, most positioning techniques, including supine and prone, are generally safe. However, as the pregnancy progresses into the second and third trimesters, lying supine can compress the inferior vena cava, leading to decreased blood flow and potential hypotension, known as supine hypotensive syndrome. Therefore, it is recommended to avoid prolonged supine positioning after the first trimester. Prone positioning is typically uncomfortable and impractical as the abdomen enlarges, so side-lying or supported semi-reclined positions are preferred for evaluations and treatments.

In conducting the physical examination, OTPs should be mindful of the patient's comfort and safety. The examination should include a thorough assessment of posture, balance, and functional mobility, considering the shift in the center of gravity and increased joint laxity. Range of motion and muscle strength tests should focus on areas commonly affected by pregnancy, such as the lower back, hips, and pelvis. Additionally, flexibility assessments should be conducted with caution to avoid overstretching, given the increased ligamentous laxity due to hormonal changes.

The physical examination of a pregnant patient differs significantly from a routine OT physical exam due to the need to accommodate the anatomical and physiological changes of pregnancy. Therapists must be particularly attentive to signs of discomfort and adjust positioning as needed to prevent adverse effects. The examination should also account for common pregnancy-related musculoskeletal dysfunctions. Table 3.10 highlights common pregnancy-related musculoskeletal dysfunctions.

Functional Mobility Assessment

Assessing functional mobility in pregnant patients is crucial to understanding how musculoskeletal issues impact their daily activities and overall occupational performance. During the functional mobility assessment, OTPs should observe the patient's gait to identify any abnormalities or compensatory movements resulting from pain, discomfort, or changes in balance and posture. Evaluating stride length, speed, and stability while walking provides insights into deviations from the norm that may indicate underlying issues. The Pregnancy Mobility Index (PMI) is a valuable tool for assessing specific mobility challenges during pregnancy, including difficulties with walking, climbing stairs, and other essential movements.

Balance and coordination are crucial areas to assess in pregnant patients, as changes in body weight and structure can significantly affect these abilities. OTPs should comprehensively evaluate both static and dynamic balance to identify potential impairments that

Table 3.10 Common musculoskeletal issues in pregnancy

Musculoskeletal Issue	Description	Clinical Presentation	Impact on Functional Activities
Thoracic and Rib Cage Dysfunction	Pain and discomfort in the thoracic spine and rib cage due to changes in posture and the expanding uterus.	Pain in the upper back and rib cage, often exacerbated by deep breathing or changes in position.	Difficulty with activities requiring upper body movement and deep breathing; impacts ADL activities involving reaching and lifting.
Lower Back Pain	The increased weight of the growing uterus places strain on the lower back, causing discomfort. Hormonal changes, such as the release of relaxin, can lead to joint instability and contribute to back pain.	Aching in the lower back, especially after prolonged periods of sitting or standing.	Difficulty with prolonged standing, sitting, and bending; may affect tasks such as cooking, cleaning, and self-care activities like dressing.
Pelvic Floor Dysfunction	Weakening or overactivity of the pelvic floor muscles, leading to issues such as urinary incontinence, pelvic pain, or pelvic organ prolapse.	Difficulty with bladder control, pelvic pain, or feeling of heaviness in the pelvic area.	Impacts toileting and sexual activity; may affect exercise routines and participation in physical activities.
Pelvic Girdle Pain (PGP)	Pain and discomfort in the pelvic area, including the pubic bone and sacroiliac joints. Hormonal changes increase joint mobility, potentially resulting in PGP.	Pain while walking, climbing stairs, or changing positions in bed.	Challenges with walking, climbing stairs, and transitioning between positions; impacts mobility-related ADLs like shopping and childcare.
Pubic Symphysis Dysfunction (PSD)	Pain and instability at the pubic symphysis, often aggravated by movements that separate the legs.	Pain in the front of the pelvis, especially when walking, climbing stairs, or turning over in bed.	Challenges with movements that involve leg separation; affects mobility and tasks such as getting in and out of bed, dressing, and walking.
Round Ligament Pain	The round ligaments, which support the uterus, stretch and relax during pregnancy.	Sharp, stabbing pain on either side of the lower abdomen, particularly when changing positions quickly or coughing.	Sudden pain can interrupt activities; may cause caution during movements like getting out of bed or standing up quickly, affecting functional mobility.
Sciatica	Sciatic nerve pain occurs when the growing uterus presses on the sciatic nerve, leading to pain radiating from the lower back down the leg.	Shooting pain, tingling, or numbness in the leg.	Difficulty with prolonged sitting, standing, or walking; may impact tasks requiring leg movement, such as driving, walking, and household chores.

(Continued)

Table 3.10 (Continued)

Musculoskeletal Issue	Description	Clinical Presentation	Impact on Functional Activities
Carpal Tunnel Syndrome (CTS)	Tingling, numbness, or pain in the wrist and hand, often due to fluid retention and swelling during pregnancy.	Challenges in gripping objects or performing fine motor tasks; numbness and pain in wrist and hand.	Difficulty with tasks requiring fine motor skills, such as writing, typing, and handling small objects; impacts ADLs like cooking and personal care.
Diastasis Recti	Separation of the abdominal muscles due to the stretching to accommodate the growing uterus.	Noticeable bulge in the abdomen; may contribute to lower back pain.	Core instability affecting posture and balance; challenges with lifting, bending, and core-related tasks like getting up from a lying position.
Swelling and Edema	Swelling in the extremities, particularly the legs and feet, due to fluid retention.	Discomfort and difficulty with mobility.	Reduced mobility and discomfort during walking and standing; affects IADLs like shopping and ADLs like dressing (especially shoes).
Postural Changes	Altered posture due to the changing center of gravity and increased weight.	Increased lumbar lordosis (inward curve of the lower spine) and anterior pelvic tilt; musculoskeletal discomfort.	Impacts balance and body mechanics; difficulties with activities requiring prolonged standing or bending; affects overall posture during daily tasks.
Osteoporosis in Pregnancy	Decrease in bone density during pregnancy, increasing the risk of fractures.	Bone pain and increased susceptibility to fractures, particularly in the spine and pelvis.	Limitations in weight-bearing activities; impacts ADLs like lifting, bending, and overall mobility.

could increase the risk of falls. Evaluations should include tasks such as standing on one leg, tandem walking, and transitioning from sitting to standing, which provide insights into balance stability.

Coordination tests, such as heel-to-toe walking or tasks that require fine motor control, are essential for pinpointing balance issues that might compromise safety. Additionally, therapists should perform postural stability assessments, observing the patient's posture while standing, sitting, and moving. It's important to note any increased lumbar lordosis, anterior pelvic tilt, or asymmetries that might indicate strain or discomfort.

Moreover, integrating these assessments into functional activities allows for a more thorough understanding of how balance and coordination affect daily living. Observing patients as they reach into cabinets, bend to pick up items from the floor, or maintain balance while carrying groceries provides valuable context. These activities help therapists gauge how well patients manage their balance and coordination during typical household tasks, ensuring that interventions are tailored to enhance safety and functional performance in everyday settings.

Transfer and transition movements are important to observe, particularly how the patient transitions between positions, such as moving from lying down to sitting up or getting in and out of bed. This helps identify any difficulties or compensatory strategies. Assessing the ease and safety of transfers is essential, especially if adaptive equipment is used. For example, observing the patient perform lower body dressing while seated on the edge of the bed can provide insights into their ability to maintain balance and coordinate movements. Similarly, evaluating the patient's ability to transfer onto a shower chair or tub bench during bathing activities can reveal challenges in mobility and stability.

Functional range of motion (ROM) assessments should focus on joint flexibility in areas most affected by pregnancy, like the hips, lower back, and pelvis. Evaluating ROM during functional tasks, such as reaching overhead to retrieve items, bending to pick up objects, or dressing, provides insights into limitations or discomfort. Strength and endurance testing in key areas, particularly the core, lower back, and lower extremities, should be included in the assessment. Evaluating muscle strength during functional tasks can help identify weaknesses that impact daily activities, such as lifting groceries or carrying a child. Endurance can be assessed by having the patient perform repetitive or sustained activities, such as walking a certain distance or standing for an extended period, to determine if fatigue affects their functional mobility.

Additionally, it is crucial to consider safe positioning during functional mobility and sleep. The American College of Obstetricians and Gynecologists (ACOG) recommends avoiding exercise in the supine position during the second and third trimesters without modifications. This recommendation also extends to the examination of pregnant patients, suggesting that therapists should not leave patients in the supine or 3/4 right side-lying position for an extended period. Therapists should use the supine position only when necessary and as expeditiously as possible. Prone lying should be avoided once the gravid uterus reaches above the pelvic brim at approximately 12 to 16 weeks' gestation. As pregnancy progresses and the abdomen enlarges, alternative positions such as using an examination table with a cut-out for the abdomen or cushioning systems should be considered. Positions such as hands-and-knees or seated may be used for examination procedures to ensure patient comfort and safety.

By incorporating these detailed assessments, OTPs can develop comprehensive treatment plans that address the specific mobility, balance, and coordination needs of pregnant patients. This approach ensures that interventions are not only effective but also enhance the patient's overall quality of life by improving their ability to safely perform daily activities and participate in meaningful occupational roles.

ADLs and IADLs Evaluation

Evaluating ADLs and IADLs in pregnant patients is essential for understanding how musculoskeletal changes impact their ability to perform routine tasks. OTPs can use a variety of assessments to gather comprehensive information on the patient's functional abilities and limitations (see Table 3.11). These assessments help identify areas where the patient may need additional support or adaptations, facilitating a client-centered approach to intervention planning. By focusing on both ADLs and IADLs, therapists can develop effective, individualized treatment plans that support the patient's daily living needs and overall well-being.

Table 3.11 Occupational therapy assessment tools for pregnant patients

Assessment Tool	Description	Focus
Canadian Occupational Performance Measure (COPM)	Identifies and prioritizes the patient's self-perceived difficulties in performing ADLs and IADLs.	ADLs and IADLs
Pregnancy-Related Pelvic Girdle Pain Questionnaire (PGQ)	Evaluates the impact of pelvic girdle pain on daily activities such as dressing, bathing, and walking.	ADLs and IADLs
Modified Barthel Index	Assesses the patient's independence in basic ADLs such as feeding, bathing, dressing, and toileting.	ADLs
Katz Index of Independence in Activities of Daily Living	Measures independence in six basic ADLs; assesses client's ability to perform basic ADLs independently, noting changes due to pregnancy.	ADLs
Assessment of Motor and Process Skills (AMPS)	Observes and analyzes the quality of performance in more complex IADLs, such as meal preparation, home maintenance, and managing finances.	IADLs
Lawton Instrumental Activities of Daily Living Scale (IADL)	Measures the patient's ability to perform more complex daily tasks such as using the telephone, shopping, and managing finances.	IADLs

Environmental and Ergonomic Assessment

An environmental and ergonomic assessment is vital for ensuring the safety and comfort of pregnant patients in their daily activities and routines. OTPs should evaluate the home and work environments to identify potential hazards and make necessary modifications. This includes assessing the arrangement of furniture and workspaces to ensure they are ergonomically sound and conducive to good posture, especially as the patient's center of gravity shifts. Recommendations may include the use of supportive chairs, adjustable desks, and proper lighting to reduce strain and fatigue. In the home, adaptive equipment such as shower chairs, grab bars, and non-slip mats can enhance safety and independence in ADLs. Additionally, therapists should educate patients on proper body mechanics and techniques for lifting, bending, and reaching to prevent injury. By addressing these environmental and ergonomic factors, OTPs can help pregnant patients maintain their functional mobility and perform daily activities with greater ease and safety.

Mental Health and Psychosocial Assessment

Assessing mental health and psychosocial well-being is crucial for pregnant patients, as pregnancy can significantly impact emotional and psychological states. OTPs should evaluate the patient's emotional health, stress levels, and coping mechanisms throughout pregnancy. This includes using tools such as the Edinburgh Postnatal Depression Scale (EPDS) to screen for symptoms of depression and anxiety, and engaging in open-ended conversations to understand the patient's feelings about their pregnancy, support system, and any fears or concerns. Understanding the patient's social context, including relationship dynamics, financial stability, and access to healthcare, is vital. Therapists should provide a safe and non-judgmental space for patients to express their emotions and concerns, fostering a therapeutic relationship built on trust and empathy. By comprehensively addressing mental health and psychosocial factors, OTPs can help pregnant patients navigate the emotional challenges of pregnancy, ultimately supporting their overall well-being and occupational performance.

Table 3.12 Mental health and psychosocial assessment tools for pregnant patients

Assessment Tool	Description	Trimester
Edinburgh Postnatal Depression Scale (EPDS)	A screening tool for identifying symptoms of depression and anxiety.	All trimesters
Prenatal Psychosocial Profile (PPP)	Assesses social support, stressors, and coping mechanisms.	First and second trimesters
Pregnancy-Related Anxiety Questionnaire (PRAQ)	Measures anxiety specifically related to pregnancy.	All trimesters
Prenatal Distress Questionnaire (PDQ)	Assesses pregnancy-specific worries and concerns.	All trimesters
Maternal Antenatal Attachment Scale (MAAS)	Evaluates the emotional bond between the mother and the unborn baby.	Second and third trimesters
Support System Inventory	Evaluates the strength and availability of the patient's support system.	All trimesters
Coping Strategies Inventory (CSI)	Assesses the patient's coping strategies and their effectiveness.	Second and third trimesters
Patient Health Questionnaire (PHQ-9)	A tool for assessing the severity of depression.	All trimesters
Generalized Anxiety Disorder 7 (GAD-7)	A tool for assessing the severity of anxiety symptoms.	All trimesters
Perceived Stress Scale (PSS)	Measures the perception of stress and how it affects the individual.	All trimesters
Role Checklist	Examines changes in roles and routines due to pregnancy.	Second and third trimesters

See Table 3.12 for a comprehensive overview of various assessment tools used by OTPs to evaluate the mental health and psychosocial well-being of pregnant patients. These tools are crucial for detecting symptoms of depression, anxiety, and stress, and for understanding the emotional bonds, coping strategies, and support systems of expectant mothers. Each tool is designed to address specific aspects of mental health across different trimesters, ensuring a holistic approach to care that supports the emotional challenges faced during pregnancy.

Pelvic Floor Assessment

Assessing the pelvic floor in pregnant patients is critical for understanding issues related to urinary and fecal incontinence, pelvic pain, and overall pelvic health. OTPs can utilize various assessments to evaluate the strength, endurance, and coordination of the pelvic floor muscles. These assessments help identify dysfunctions that may impact the patient's ability to perform daily activities and maintain a good quality of life. By addressing pelvic floor issues early, therapists can provide targeted interventions to prevent or reduce symptoms, support functional mobility, and enhance occupational performance.

It is important to note that not all women's health OTPs are trained to evaluate or treat pelvic floor dysfunction or pelvic floor health. A referral to a pelvic floor therapist is necessary if an OTP does not have training within pelvic floor rehabilitation.

Occupational therapy pelvic floor assessments typically include subjective questionnaires, physical examinations, and functional tests. These tools collectively offer a comprehensive view of the patient's pelvic health, helping to tailor individualized treatment plans. Therapists should ensure that the assessment environment is comfortable and

112 Occupational Therapy and Women's Health

Table 3.13 Assessment tools for pelvic floor health in occupational therapy

Assessment Tool	Description	Category
Pelvic Floor Distress Inventory (PFDI)	Evaluates the presence and severity of pelvic floor symptoms, including urinary and fecal incontinence, and pelvic pain.	Symptom Inventory
Pelvic Floor Impact Questionnaire (PFIQ)	Assesses the impact of pelvic floor dysfunction on daily activities and quality of life.	Quality of Life
Pelvic Organ Prolapse/Urinary Incontinence Sexual Questionnaire (PISQ-12)	Evaluates the impact of pelvic floor disorders on sexual function.	Sexual Function
International Consultation on Incontinence Questionnaire (ICIQ)	Measures the severity and impact of urinary incontinence.	Urinary Incontinence
The Brink Scale	Assesses pelvic floor muscle strength through vaginal examination.	Physical Examination
Oxford Grading Scale	Grades pelvic floor muscle strength on a scale from 0 (no contraction) to 5 (strong contraction).	Physical Examination
Modified Oxford Scale	An adaptation of the Oxford Grading Scale for clinical use, assessing muscle strength during digital examination.	Physical Examination
Visual Analog Scale for Pelvic Pain (VAS-Pelvic)	Measures the intensity of pelvic pain through patient self-report.	Pain Assessment
Incontinence Impact Questionnaire (IIQ)	Assesses the impact of urinary incontinence on physical activity, social relationships, and emotional health.	Quality of Life
Pelvic Organ Prolapse Quantification (POP-Q)	Standardized system for assessing and staging pelvic organ prolapse (POP) through physical examination.	Prolapse Assessment
Prolapse Quality of Life (QOL) Questionnaire	Assesses the impact of POP on a woman's quality of life.	Quality of Life

private, allowing patients to discuss sensitive issues openly. Understanding the patient's specific concerns and symptoms is essential for selecting the most appropriate assessments and interventions (Table 3.13).

Goal Setting and Treatment Plan

Setting goals based on assessment results is essential for creating an effective and individualized treatment plan for pregnant patients. Goals should be specific, measurable, achievable, relevant, and time-bound (SMART). They should address the unique needs identified during the assessment and prioritize improving the patient's ability to perform daily activities and maintain a good quality of life.

The treatment plan should incorporate various interventions tailored to address the physical, social, emotional, and environmental impacts of the identified musculoskeletal issues. The treatment plan must incorporate various interventions tailored to address the physical, social, emotional, and environmental impacts of the identified musculoskeletal issues. Interventions may include self-care/home management strategies, patient education, environmental modifications, therapeutic exercises, therapeutic activities, and manual therapy techniques, which are detailed in Table 3.14.

OT in Obstetric Health Management 113

Table 3.14 OT interventions for common musculoskeletal issues in pregnancy

Condition	Self-Care/Home Management	Patient Education	Environmental Modifications	Therapeutic Exercises	Therapeutic Activities	Manual Therapy Techniques
Thoracic and Rib Cage Dysfunction	ADL retraining for reaching and lifting tasks	Proper posture and body mechanics	Ergonomic adjustments for work and home	Thoracic stretches, deep breathing exercises	Upper body activities with controlled movements	Soft tissue mobilization, myofascial release
Lower Back Pain	ADL retraining for bending and lifting	Safe lifting techniques, posture education	Use of supportive seating and lumbar supports	Core strengthening, pelvic tilts	Activities to improve core stability	Massage, joint mobilizations
Pelvic Floor Dysfunction	Toileting strategies, pelvic floor exercises	Bladder training, pelvic floor health education	Installation of grab bars, raised toilet seats	Kegel exercises, pelvic floor relaxation	Functional pelvic floor strengthening activities	Internal pelvic floor muscle release techniques
Pelvic Girdle Pain (PGP)	Mobility aids, ADL retraining for mobility tasks	Pain management strategies, safe movement tips	Use of pelvic support belts, adjustable furniture	Pelvic stabilization exercises, gentle stretches	Activities to reduce pelvic strain	Manual pelvic alignment techniques
Pubic Symphysis Dysfunction (PSD)	ADL retraining for leg separation tasks	Avoiding leg separation movements, posture tips	Installation of supportive bedding	Pelvic floor strengthening, hip stabilization	Controlled leg movement activities	Soft tissue mobilization around pubic symphysis
Round Ligament Pain	Mobility aids, ADL retraining for transitional movements	Avoiding sudden movements, proper body mechanics	Use of supportive garments, ergonomic furniture	Gentle abdominal stretching	Activities focusing on smooth transitional movements	Gentle massage, myofascial release
Sciatica	ADL retraining for sitting and walking	Nerve glide techniques, posture education	Use of ergonomic chairs, supportive cushions	Sciatic nerve stretches, core strengthening	Activities to reduce nerve pressure	Soft tissue release, neural mobilization
Carpal Tunnel Syndrome (CTS)	ADL retraining for fine motor tasks	Ergonomic positioning for wrist	Ergonomic keyboards, wrist supports	Wrist stretches, nerve gliding exercises	Activities focusing on hand and wrist function	Soft tissue mobilization, joint mobilizations

(Continued)

114 Occupational Therapy and Women's Health

Table 3.14 (Continued)

Condition	Self-Care/Home Management	Patient Education	Environmental Modifications	Therapeutic Exercises	Therapeutic Activities	Manual Therapy Techniques
Diastasis Recti	ADL retraining for core-related tasks	Abdominal splinting techniques	Use of supportive garments	Core strengthening, transverse abdominis exercises	Activities to improve core stability	Gentle abdominal massage
Swelling and Edema	ADL retraining for dressing and mobility	Edema management strategies, compression techniques	Use of compression garments, adjustable furniture	Leg elevation exercises, gentle ROM	Activities to reduce fluid retention	Manual lymphatic drainage
Postural Changes	ADL retraining for standing and bending tasks	Posture education, safe movement strategies	Use of ergonomic seating and supports	Postural exercises, core strengthening	Activities to improve postural stability	Myofascial release, joint mobilizations
Osteoporosis in Pregnancy	ADL retraining for weight-bearing tasks	Bone health education, fall prevention tips	Use of non-slip mats, installation of grab bars	Weight-bearing exercises, balance training	Activities to improve bone density and strength	Gentle mobilizations, soft tissue techniques

Contraindications with Modalities

When developing a treatment plan, therapists must be aware of contraindications associated with specific therapeutic modalities to ensure the safety of both mother and child. Modalities such as electrical stimulation, ultrasound, and those that involve significant heat exposure, like hot tubs or saunas, are generally avoided. These are contraindicated because they can pose potential risks to fetal development or exacerbate existing musculoskeletal strain due to increased connective tissue extensibility in pregnant patients.

Modalities should be carefully selected to avoid any that could harm fetal development or adversely affect the mother's health. This includes avoiding transcutaneous electrical nerve stimulation (TENS) over the trunk, ultrasound therapy over the abdomen, and any form of mechanical traction. OTPs must prioritize modalities that are proven safe and effective during pregnancy, such as gentle manual therapies and approved therapeutic exercises.

Trauma-Informed Occupational Therapy Assessment and Interventions

During pregnancy, significant physiological and anatomical changes occur, and individual experiences can vary widely, particularly when influenced by past trauma or adverse life events. Understanding and addressing these unique needs through a trauma-informed care approach is vital for providing holistic care. This approach fosters a safe and supportive environment where pregnant individuals feel valued and empowered, enhancing both physical and emotional well-being.

Trauma-informed care (TIC) emphasizes creating a safe and supportive environment, fostering open communication, and tailoring assessments and interventions to respect the individual's unique needs and sensitivities. In occupational therapy, adopting a TIC approach during pregnancy involves several key elements.

1. **Building Trust and Safety**: OTPs strive to establish trust and safety by creating a nonjudgmental and empathetic atmosphere. Pregnant individuals should feel secure and comfortable sharing their concerns, experiences, and potential trauma history.
2. **Empowerment and Choice**: Empowering pregnant individuals to make informed decisions about their care is fundamental. This includes involving them in the assessment process, discussing treatment options, and respecting their choices regarding interventions.
3. **Understanding Potential Triggers**: OTPs are sensitive to potential trauma triggers that may arise during assessments or interventions. They take proactive measures to minimize triggers and provide support if a trigger does occur.
4. **Cultural Competence**: Cultural competence is vital in TIC, as cultural backgrounds can influence how individuals perceive and respond to care. OTPs respect and honor cultural differences, ensuring that care is culturally sensitive and relevant.
5. **Collaboration and Coordination**: Effective communication and collaboration with other healthcare providers involved in the individual's pregnancy care are essential. This ensures a coordinated and holistic approach to care that considers all aspects of the individual's well-being.

Principles of TIC

1. **Safety**: Prioritizing physical and emotional safety is the foundation of TIC. Pregnant individuals should feel safe and supported throughout their interactions with healthcare providers.

2. **Trustworthiness and Transparency**: Building trust through honest and transparent communication is essential. Pregnant individuals should have a clear understanding of their care and feel confident in their healthcare team.
3. **Empowerment and Choice**: Providing pregnant individuals with choices and involving them in decision-making processes empowers them to take an active role in their care.
4. **Collaboration and Mutuality**: Collaboration between healthcare providers and pregnant individuals fosters a sense of partnership and mutual respect.
5. **Cultural Sensitivity**: Recognizing and respecting cultural differences ensures that care is inclusive and responsive to the individual's cultural background.
6. **Resilience and Strength-Based**: TIC acknowledges the individual's resilience and strengths, focusing on their ability to heal and grow.

Integration of TIC into Assessment

When conducting assessments during pregnancy, OTPs integrate TIC principles by creating a safe and welcoming environment. They begin by building rapport, actively listening to the pregnant individual's concerns, and respecting their boundaries. OTPs avoid making assumptions and judgments, recognizing that everyone's journey is unique. By acknowledging the potential impact of trauma on the individual's pregnancy experience, OTPs can tailor assessments and interventions to meet their physical and emotional needs while promoting a sense of empowerment and control. This trauma-informed approach ultimately contributes to a more compassionate and supportive healthcare experience during pregnancy, enhancing overall well-being. Table 3.15 outlines trauma-informed assessment tools to guide the occupational therapy practitioner working with pregnant women to ensure a sensitive and supportive approach to care.

By integrating these assessments within a trauma-informed framework, OTPs can provide personalized care that is acutely aware of and sensitive to the woman's history and potential trauma triggers. This method involves not only using tools that directly assess trauma-related symptoms but also applying all assessment tools in a way that promotes safety, builds trust, and empowers the patient. This approach ensures that the assessments are not merely diagnostic tools but are part of a therapeutic process that enhances the woman's sense of security and validation throughout her care. Such sensitive application helps support the physical and emotional well-being of the patient during pregnancy, fostering an overall experience that enhances safety, trust, and empowerment.

Holistic Assessments

OTPs can employ various assessments with pregnant women to address their specific needs and promote their well-being. These assessments not only identify challenges but also guide the development of personalized interventions. OTPs should familiarize themselves with assessment areas and the corresponding interventions that might be initiated based on the assessment findings.

1. **Sensory Processing Assessment**
    - **Assessment**: Conduct assessments to identify sensory sensitivities or challenges using tools like the Sensory Profile Questionnaire.
    - **Interventions**: Develop a sensory diet plan tailored to the woman's needs, including activities and strategies to manage identified sensitivities.

Table 3.15 Trauma-informed assessment tools for OTPs

Category	Description	Example Assessments
Comprehensive Occupational Profile	Begins with a thorough profile considering personal history, trauma, and preferences.	- Comprehensive Occupational Performance Measure (COPM)
Perinatal Mental Health Assessment	Assesses mental health concerns, which may be exacerbated by trauma.	- Edinburgh Postnatal Depression Scale (EPDS) - Generalized Anxiety Disorder 7-item (GAD-7) scale
Pregnancy-Specific PTSD Assessment	Identifies trauma-related symptoms or triggers specific to pregnancy.	- PTSD CheckList – Civilian Version (PCL-C) - Impact of Event Scale-Revised (IES-R) adapted for pregnancy
Safety Assessment	Evaluates the physical and emotional safety of the woman's environment and routines.	- Home safety checklists - Hurt Insult Threaten Scream (HITS) Tool - Woman Abuse Screening Tool (WAST)
Coping and Resilience Assessment	Explores coping mechanisms and resilience factors.	- Coping Strategies Inventory Short Form (CSI-SF) - Resilience Assessment Questionnaire (RAQ)
Pain and Discomfort Assessment	Assesses musculoskeletal discomfort or pain, using a trauma-informed approach.	- Visual Analog Scale for Pain (VAS-Pain) - McGill Pain Questionnaire
Activity and Participation Assessment	Evaluates the ability to engage in daily activities and routines, considering trauma impacts.	- Occupational Performance History Interview (OPHI) - Canadian Occupational Performance Measure (COPM)
Social Support and Network Assessment	Assesses the quality and strength of the social support system.	- Social Support Questionnaire (SSQ) - Social Network Index
Cultural Competence Assessment	Considers the cultural background and preferences in planning and support.	- Cultural Competence Self-Assessment Checklist - Cultural Formulation Interview (CFI)
Empowerment and Goal-Setting Assessment	Sets collaborative goals, empowering the patient in care planning.	- Goal Attainment Scaling (GAS) - Patient-Specific Functional Scale (PSFS)
Communication and Consent Assessment	Establishes clear communication, emphasizing informed consent.	- Teach-back method - Informed consent verification tools
Resilience and Strength-Based Assessment	Recognizes and fosters the woman's resilience and strengths.	- Strengths and Difficulties Questionnaire (SDQ) - Resilience Scale
Progress and Outcome Monitoring	Monitors the effectiveness of interventions and adjusts as needed.	- Outcome and Assessment Information Set (OASIS) - Routine Outcome Monitoring (ROM)

2. **Cognitive Assessment**
- **Assessment**: Evaluate cognitive functions such as memory, attention, and executive functioning with tools like the Montreal Cognitive Assessment (MoCA).
- **Interventions**: Based on the findings, implement cognitive strategies or compensatory techniques to address identified challenges.

3. **Nutrition and Meal Planning Assessment**

    - **Assessment**: Assess dietary habits and nutritional needs, potentially using a dietary recall.
    - **Interventions**: Provide tailored nutrition education and meal planning guidance to align with the woman's dietary needs and restrictions.

4. **Sleep Assessment**

    - **Assessment**: Use tools like the Pittsburgh Sleep Quality Index (PSQI) to evaluate sleep patterns and quality.
    - **Interventions**: Offer recommendations for improving sleep hygiene based on the assessment findings, such as optimizing the sleep environment or establishing a bedtime routine.

5. **Medication and Health Literacy Assessment**

    - **Assessment**: Review and assess understanding of current medications and supplements, and evaluate the woman's health literacy.
    - **Interventions**: Provide education and resources to enhance understanding and safe management of health care and medication during pregnancy.

By integrating these holistic assessments and interventions, OTPs can develop a comprehensive understanding of each pregnant woman's unique needs, thereby facilitating the creation of individualized treatment plans that enhance physical and emotional well-being, support daily activity participation, and promote a positive pregnancy experience.

Strategies for Adaptation and Compensation

Navigating the physical demands of pregnancy and new parenthood requires careful attention to lifting techniques and daily activity management. Expectant and new parents must adapt their movements to accommodate the physiological changes of pregnancy, such as increased joint laxity and a shifted center of gravity. OTPs play a critical role in educating parents on these adaptations, ensuring that activities involving lifting, carrying, and daily childcare do not compromise their musculoskeletal health. Proper lifting techniques and ergonomic considerations are crucial to prevent strain and discomfort. This includes using supportive devices like baby carriers and making thoughtful modifications to daily routines to suit the changing body. For example, understanding how to correctly lift an infant from a crib, carry a toddler without exacerbating back pain, or adjust household setups for easier access can significantly enhance parental well-being.

Additionally, engaging with a child in various activities is essential for their development and bonding, but it's equally crucial for expecting mothers to make adaptations to ensure a safe and comfortable experience. These adaptations help reduce the risk of musculoskeletal strain and discomfort while participating in playtime and interactive activities. By proactively making these adaptations, pregnant women can prioritize their health and that of their growing baby, ensuring that they can fully embrace the joys of parenthood while minimizing physical strain and discomfort. Table 3.16 provides detailed guidance on specific lifting techniques and other adaptive strategies to help parents manage these challenges effectively, promoting safety and comfort during this transformative period.

Table 3.16 Adaptations for safe and comfortable playtime, childcare, and daily activities during pregnancy

Activity/Task	Technique and Description
Lifting Techniques	
Infant Car Seat	Stand close, bend knees, keep back straight, hold handle with both hands, lift using legs, and avoid twisting.
Cradling	Place one hand under baby's head and neck, slide the other hand under the body, bend at knees, and avoid stooping.
Diaper Changing	Use a changing pad for cushioning, bend at the knees, support the baby's legs with one hand, and lift their lower body gently.
Feeding	Use pillows or cushions for support, maintain good back posture, and keep the baby at breast or bottle level.
Highchair	Lower the tray or table, bend at the knees, and gently place the child in the highchair, avoiding sudden movements.
Playtime and Interactive Activities	
Floor Play	Use a cushion or bolster to support elbows and forearms, change positions frequently to prevent stiffness.
Babywearing	Use a baby carrier or sling per manufacturer's instructions, ensure snug fit and adjust straps for comfort.
Stroller Use	Bend at the knees, keep the back straight, use both hands on the stroller handles, and engage leg muscles to lift.
Lifting Child from the Floor	Bend at the knees, keep the back straight, squat down to child's level, and use both hands to lift them.
Childcare and Daily Activities	
Bathing	Use a baby bathtub or supportive bath seat or use a kneeler or cushion for knee support if using a regular tub.
Changing Table	Ensure the table is at a comfortable height, keep supplies within reach and avoid bending over the table.
Diaper Bag	Choose a bag with padded shoulder straps, use both shoulder straps, and distribute weight evenly to both shoulders.
Bedtime Routine	When putting the child to bed or lifting them in and out of a crib, keep the back straight, bend at the knees, and provide appropriate support.
Car Seat Installation	Ensure proper installation of the car seat in the vehicle and avoid twisting or straining while securing the seat.
Childproofing	Place frequently used items within easy reach and use safety gates to restrict access to potentially hazardous areas.
Holding Another Child	Hold the child in front of your body, not on the hip, to distribute their weight more evenly and maintain better alignment of your spine. Support the child with both arms to minimize lateral bending of the spine and reduce strain. See Figure 3.6b.

The position where a mom holds a baby on her hip, known as "hip carrying," can often lead to improper body mechanics. This position creates an asymmetrical load, causing uneven weight distribution and leading to a pelvic tilt where one side of the pelvis is higher than the other. Such an imbalance can result in muscle strain, particularly in the lower back and hips, and can also cause the spine to curve unnaturally, potentially leading to lower back pain and shoulder or neck strain. Over time, consistently carrying a baby on one hip may also lead to hip misalignment and discomfort.

120 Occupational Therapy and Women's Health

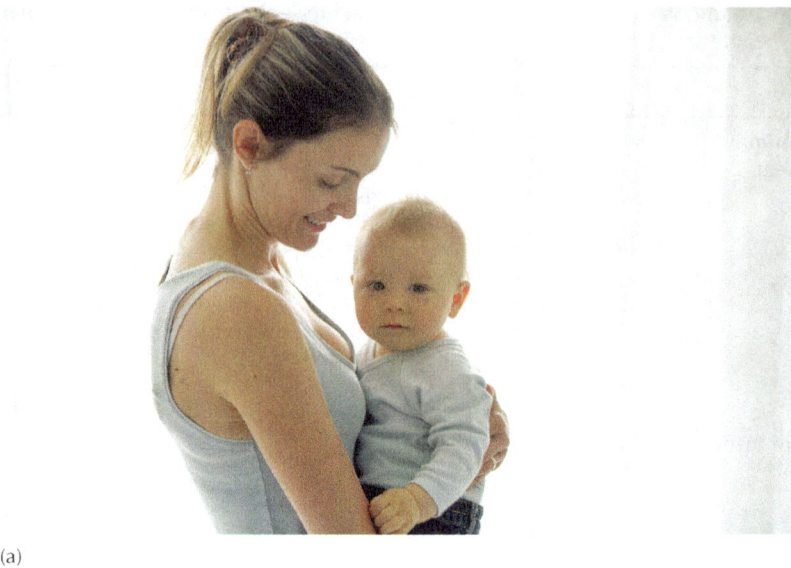

(a)

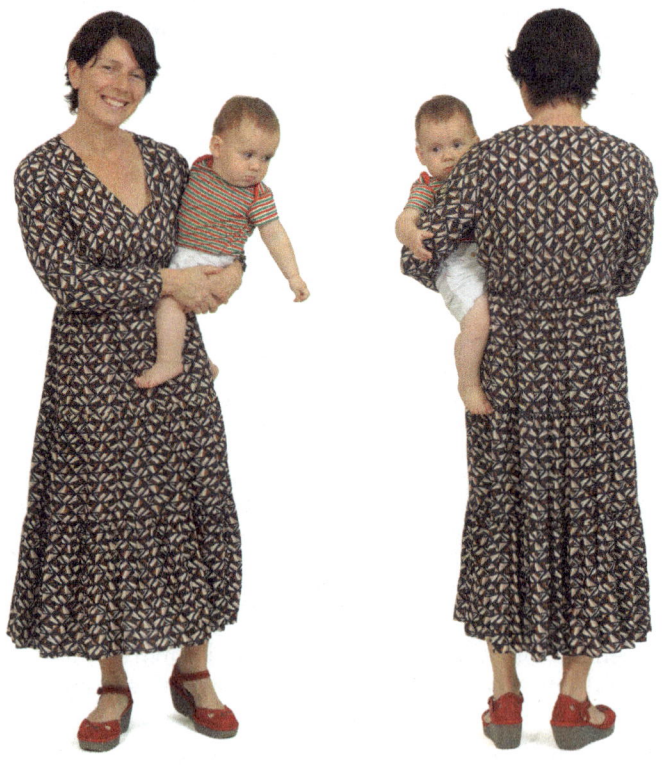

(b)

Figure 3.6 Child carrying techniques: (a) Proper spinal alignment; (b) Hip carrying position: spinal misalignment.

To avoid these issues, it is recommended to use a baby carrier or sling that distributes the baby's weight evenly across both shoulders, keeping the baby close to your chest. This promotes proper spinal alignment and reduces strain on the back and hips. If hip carrying is necessary, alternating hips regularly can help balance the load and reduce the risk of muscle imbalances. Additionally, using ergonomic baby carriers designed to support both the baby and the parent can help maintain proper posture and reduce strain. Engaging core muscles while carrying the baby can also provide additional support to the back and pelvis, promoting better overall body mechanics.

Motivational Interviewing

Motivational Interviewing (MI) is a client-centered counseling approach designed to facilitate behavior change by helping individuals explore and resolve ambivalence. This collaborative and non-confrontational method enables individuals to discover their own motivations for making healthier choices, thereby enhancing their intrinsic motivation. OTPs utilize MI to assist pregnant women in adopting positive changes in their physical activity levels during pregnancy. They apply MI principles through a series of strategic dialogues, aiming to enhance the women's engagement and empowerment in maintaining their health.

1. **Engaging**: OTPs can start by building rapport and showing empathy. For instance, they might say, "I understand that staying active during pregnancy can be challenging. Can you tell me more about your experiences and concerns?"
2. **Exploring Ambivalence**: OTPs can gently explore the woman's mixed feelings about physical activity. They might ask, "What are the pros and cons you see in incorporating exercise into your routine during pregnancy?"
3. **Reflective Listening**: Active listening is crucial. An OTP might reflect the woman's statements, saying, "I hear you're worried about overexertion. Tell me more about what's concerning you."
4. **Developing Discrepancy**: OTPs can help the woman recognize the gap between her goals and her current behavior: "You mentioned wanting a healthy pregnancy, but you're unsure about exercising. How do you think physical activity might support your goal?"
5. **Supporting Self-Efficacy**: Encourage self-belief by asking, "What strategies have worked for you in the past? How do you think you can incorporate safe physical activity into your daily life now?"
6. **Rolling with Resistance**: Avoid confrontation and respect the woman's perspective. "I see that you're concerned about time constraints. Let's explore ways to make it manageable for you."
7. **Developing a Plan**: Collaboratively create an action plan. "What small steps can you take this week to start integrating physical activity into your routine? How can I support you in this?"
8. **Strengthening Commitment**: Reinforce the woman's commitment: "You've identified several reasons for staying active. How can you remind yourself of these motivations and stay committed?"

Successfully applying MI techniques equips OTPs with the tools needed to tackle specific challenges that pregnant women face in maintaining an active lifestyle. As we delve deeper into the practical application of these techniques, it becomes crucial to address the common barriers such as unhealthy habits, roles, and routines. By focusing on these areas, OTPs can help expectant mothers overcome obstacles to physical activity, which is essential for both maternal and fetal health. Let's explore strategies that OTPs can use to identify and modify these barriers, ensuring that every intervention is tailored to support and empower women throughout their pregnancy.

Addressing Unhealthy Performance Patterns for Enhanced Well-being

OTPs play a crucial role in promoting overall well-being during pregnancy by addressing barriers such as unhealthy habits, roles, and routines. These elements can significantly influence a pregnant woman's health and are essential targets for intervention to support a more active and healthier lifestyle that respects individual circumstances and needs.

Unhealthy Habits: Research has substantiated the impact of various behaviors on pregnant women's health. Sedentary behaviors, poor dietary habits, and inadequate sleep significantly contribute to adverse outcomes. For example, a 2019 study in *BMC Public Health* found strong associations between sedentary behaviors, particularly television time, and the development of gestational diabetes mellitus (GDM) in women at high risk for GDM, with television time tripling the odds of developing GDM. Additionally, a 2020 review in the journal *Nutrients* highlighted the detrimental effects of high simple sugar intake, linking it to excessive gestational weight gain, GDM, preeclampsia, and preterm birth. Moreover, a 2022 study published in *BMJ Open* associated poor sleep quality, especially during the first and third trimesters, with high perceived stress, depression, and intimate partner violence. OTPs work with pregnant women to modify these habits by promoting healthier alternatives and activities that improve maternal and fetal health, such as interspersing screen time with short, low-impact exercises, encouraging balanced nutrition, and establishing good sleep hygiene practices.

Roles and Responsibilities: The demanding roles and responsibilities of pregnant women can significantly contribute to stress, linked to adverse pregnancy outcomes like preterm birth and preeclampsia. A 2020 study in the *American Journal of Obstetrics & Gynecology Maternal-Fetal Medicine* highlighted the link between stress and disruptions in maternal-placental-fetal endocrine and immune responses. OTPs support expectant mothers by effectively managing these stressors, such as redefining roles at work and home, delegating tasks, or setting boundaries to alleviate stress. These actions help manage the biological, social, and psychological changes during pregnancy, enhancing both maternal and fetal well-being.

Routines: Disruptions to daily routines due to pregnancy-related discomfort or fatigue often lead pregnant women towards more sedentary lifestyles. A 2022 study in the *Journal of Women's Health Reports* revealed that despite known benefits, only a small percentage of expectant mothers meet exercise guidelines, often due to poorly structured daily routines. Beyond physical activity, routines include managing time for relaxation, socializing, and pursuing hobbies, contributing to overall well-being. OTPs assist pregnant women by helping them create balanced schedules that accommodate the physical demands of pregnancy while promoting social engagement and personal time. This support ensures that pregnant women can maintain not just an active lifestyle but a holistic approach to health, crucial for their well-being and that of their developing baby.

Through collaborative goal-setting, behavioural techniques, and strategic use of MI, OTPs empower expectant mothers to embrace a more active lifestyle and overcome barriers to physical well-being. This comprehensive support helps pregnant women make positive changes, enhancing their physical and emotional health during this critical period. By addressing unhealthy habits, roles, and routines within the context of promoting overall well-being during pregnancy, OTPs foster a supportive environment for positive changes that benefit both maternal and fetal health.

Occupational Therapy in Labor and Delivery

Labor and delivery, the transition from prenatal to intrapartum care, is a critical phase in maternal healthcare. This period starts with the onset of regular contractions that lead to cervical dilation and ends with the delivery of the baby and placenta. OTPs are integral in this stage, addressing physical, emotional, sensory, and psychological factors that influence a woman's labor and delivery experience. By utilizing a holistic care approach, OTPs support women in managing their environment, emotions, and bodily sensations, contributing to a more positive labor and delivery experience.

Role of Occupational Therapy During Labor and Delivery

OTPs provide personalized care that integrates pain reduction techniques, stress management, and sensory regulation to enhance the comfort and well-being of the mother during labor. Their interventions are designed to empower expectant mothers, helping them to feel in control and supported throughout the labor process. This includes aiding women in making informed choices about their labor and delivery preferences, ensuring that each woman's unique needs and desires are respected and facilitated.

Occupational Therapy Interventions during Labor and Delivery

During labor and delivery, OTPs provide interventions aimed at reducing pain, managing stress, and enhancing the overall well-being of the mother. These interventions include physical techniques to alleviate pain, emotional support to manage stress and anxiety, and sensory regulation to create a calming environment (see Table 3.17). OTPs work closely with expectant mothers to develop personalized strategies that align with their specific labor and delivery plans, empowering them to feel in control and supported throughout the process. By helping women manage their environment, emotions, and bodily sensations, OTPs contribute to a more positive labor and delivery experience. Their expertise in holistic care allows them to support women in making informed choices about their labor preferences, ensuring that each woman's unique needs and desires are respected and facilitated.

Optimal Positioning Strategies for Labor

Understanding and utilizing various labor positions can significantly impact the labor and delivery process, particularly for managing pain, improving comfort, and facilitating labor progression. It's crucial to consider the unique needs of all women, including those with disabilities. OTPs are adept at adapting positioning strategies to accommodate limitations such as reduced range of motion, decreased strength in the lower and upper extremities, and other physical challenges. This personalized approach ensures that each woman,

Table 3.17 Comprehensive occupational therapy interventions for labor and delivery

Intervention	Description	Category	Tools/Examples	Expected Outcome
Breathing Techniques	Guided exercises to control breathing, reduce pain, and manage anxiety during labor.	Stress Management	Diaphragmatic breathing, paced breathing	Reduced anxiety, pain management
Positioning for Comfort	Assistance in finding labor positions that maximize comfort and labor progression.	Pain Relief	Birth stool, squatting bars	Enhanced comfort, reduced labor duration
Use of Birth Balls	Utilizes birth balls to support various labor positions and facilitate easier movement.	Pain Relief, Sensory Regulation	Birth balls	Decreased pain, increased mobility
Massage and Touch Therapy	Application of gentle massage to ease muscle tension and enhance emotional comfort.	Pain Relief, Emotional Regulation	Hand massage, back rubs	Muscle relaxation, emotional comfort
Visualization and Imagery	Employing mental imagery to aid relaxation, decrease stress, and distract from pain.	Stress Management	Guided visualization scripts	Enhanced relaxation, stress reduction
Sensory Modulation Techniques	Creation of a soothing environment using sensory tools to regulate sensory input.	Sensory Regulation	Dim lighting, soft music, aromatherapy	Calmer environment, sensory comfort
Hydrotherapy	Use of water immersion in a tub or shower to relieve pain and promote muscle relaxation.	Pain Relief, Sensory Regulation	Labor tub, shower	Pain relief, relaxation
Education and Advocacy	Provides comprehensive information on labor options and supports the woman's preferences.	Emotional Support, Advocacy	Informational pamphlets, birth plan discussions	Informed decisions, empowered experience

regardless of her physical capabilities, feels supported and empowered throughout her labor.

OTPs educate and assist women in finding and maintaining positions that align with their preferences and physical needs, making necessary adjustments to enhance comfort and effectiveness. Table 3.18 details several labor positions, highlighting their benefits and potential challenges, with a focus on inclusivity for women with varying physical abilities.

While various positioning strategies can significantly enhance the labor experience, it's important to acknowledge that not every birth progresses to a natural delivery. In some

Table 3.18 Labor positions and their adaptations for women with disabilities

Labor Positions	Benefits	Challenges	Adaptations for Disabilities
Upright Positions (Standing, Walking)	Uses gravity to help labor progress, can reduce pain and duration of labor.	May be tiring, requires good mobility.	Support from a partner or mobility aid; modified standing with a bar or leaning support.
Squatting	Opens pelvis, helps baby descend, uses gravity.	Can be tiring, requires leg strength.	Supported squatting with a chair or birthing stool; use of grab bars.
Hands and Knees	Reduces back pain, helps baby reposition, good for back labor.	May be tiring for arms and knees.	Use of pillows or bolsters for support under knees and arms; modified hands-and-knees position on a low bed with supports.
Side-Lying	Good for rest, reduces pressure on the perineum, helpful with epidurals.	May slow labor, less effective with gravity.	Use of pillows for support and alignment; assistance in turning and maintaining position.
Sitting (On Birth Ball or Chair)	Can be comfortable, allows for movement and rocking.	May not use gravity as effectively.	Modified sitting positions on cushioned surfaces or tailored chairs for support and stability.
Water Birth	Provides pain relief, buoyancy aids movement.	Access to water facilities required, not suitable for all women.	Support for safe entry and exit; customized support within the pool for maintaining position.

cases, circumstances may necessitate a cesarean section, for which OTPs also provide essential support.

Supporting Women's Choices and Preferences

Supporting women's choices and preferences during labor and delivery is a fundamental aspect of occupational therapy in obstetric health. OTPs work closely with expectant mothers to understand their birth plans, preferences, and any concerns they may have. By fostering a supportive and non-judgmental environment, OTPs empower women to make informed decisions about their labor and delivery. This includes discussing various labor positions, pain management options, and interventions that align with their personal and cultural values. Additionally, OTPs advocate for the woman's choices in the clinical setting, ensuring that healthcare providers respect and support her preferences. This collaborative approach helps create a positive birthing experience, where the woman feels heard, respected, and in control of her labor process.

Occupational Therapy in Postpartum Care

The postpartum period, often referred to as the "fourth trimester," spans from immediately after delivery up to six weeks, known as the acute postpartum phase. However, many experts recognize the ongoing physical and emotional changes mothers undergo, extending this period to cover the first year after birth. This comprehensive approach allows OTPs to support mothers not only immediately after delivery but also as they transition into new maternal roles.

Immediate and Extended Postpartum Support

OTPs offer tailored interventions immediately after both C-section and vaginal deliveries. For C-sections, the focus includes surgical wound care, adherence to weight lifting restrictions, and effective pain management. Vaginal deliveries often require management of birth trauma such as perineal tears or pelvic floor dysfunction. Across both delivery types, OTPs provide essential emotional and psychological support, assist with adaptations in ADLs and IADLs, and help establish a supportive home environment (see Table 3.19). These measures ensure mothers receive the comprehensive care needed to navigate both the acute and the extended postpartum periods successfully.

Table 3.19 Comparison of postpartum OT considerations for C-section and vaginal deliveries

Category	C-Section Delivery	Vaginal Delivery
Weight Lifting Restrictions	Avoid lifting objects heavier than 10–25 pounds for several weeks. Use proper body mechanics and assistive devices.	Generally fewer lifting restrictions unless there are complications. Avoid heavy lifting immediately postpartum.
Functional Mobility	Teach safe bed mobility strategies such as the log roll technique, which minimizes stress on the abdominal muscles when getting in and out of bed. This method is essential for protecting the incision site and facilitating a smoother recovery.	Support gentle mobility techniques that accommodate any soreness or perineal trauma. Encourage gradual movement and light walking as tolerated to promote healing and reduce the risk of complications like thrombosis.
Wound Care	Monitor for signs of infection (redness, swelling, increased pain, discharge). Educate on proper incision care and scar massage techniques.	Manage perineal tears and episiotomies with proper hygiene and care. Use ice packs and sitz baths for pain relief.
Pain Management	Use prescribed medications and non-pharmacological methods (breathing exercises, relaxation techniques).	Techniques for managing perineal pain and discomfort. Use pain relief medications as needed.
Emotional and Psychological Support	Provide psychosocial counseling for postpartum depression and anxiety. Encourage skin-to-skin contact and bonding activities for mother-infant dyad and family.	Provide psychosocial counseling for postpartum depression and anxiety. Encourage skin-to-skin contact and bonding activities for mother-infant dyad and family. Connect with support groups for sharing experiences and receiving peer support.
ADL/IADL Support	Train in modifying tasks to adhere to weight lifting restrictions. Assist with safe baby care techniques and ergonomic positioning.	Assist with daily routines to prevent strain. Provide training in efficient and safe baby care tasks.
Environmental Modifications	Assess home environment and recommend safety and convenience modifications.	Ensure home environment supports easy access and movement. Recommend ergonomic furniture and proper lighting.

C-Section Considerations

A Cesarean section, commonly referred to as a C-section, is a surgical procedure used to deliver a baby through incisions in the abdomen and uterus. As of 2024, the C-section is the most commonly performed surgery in the United States, highlighting its significance in obstetric care. This procedure may be planned due to medical reasons affecting the health of the mother or baby, or it may be performed as an emergency measure if complications arise during vaginal delivery. OTPs have a crucial role in preparing women for C-sections by providing comprehensive education about the procedure. They also discuss post-operative care to ensure a smooth recovery and manage potential challenges such as mobility restrictions, pain, and the emotional impact of surgery.

OTPs play a vital role in preparing women for C-sections by providing comprehensive education about the procedure. Following delivery, OTPs assist with pain management and facilitate early mobility to prevent complications such as deep vein thrombosis. They support the mother in practical aspects of newborn care, including strategies for safe movement, ergonomic positioning for breastfeeding, and adapting daily activities to manage discomfort and enhance recovery. OTPs tailor their interventions to meet the individual needs of each mother, promoting a recovery process that emphasizes safety, comfort, and maternal well-being.

Post-Cesarean Scar Management and Activity Modifications

OTPs play an essential role in the recovery process following a Cesarean section (C-section). Their expertise is critical in ensuring that new mothers manage their recovery effectively, addressing both physical and emotional challenges. The involvement of OTPs in post–C-section care helps to prevent complications, improve functional abilities, and support overall well-being during the postpartum period.

Scar Management and Infection Prevention

Managing the healing process after a Cesarean section is critical for reducing complications and enhancing recovery. Surgical site infection (SSI) is one of the most common complications following a C-section, with an incidence of 3–15%. SSIs place physical and emotional burdens on the mother and impose significant financial burdens on the healthcare system. Moreover, SSI is associated with a maternal mortality rate of up to 3%. A study published in the *International Journal of Women's Health* in 2017 highlighted the importance of recognizing the consequences and developing strategies to diagnose, prevent, and treat SSIs to reduce post-Cesarean morbidity and mortality. Effective strategies include optimizing maternal comorbidities, appropriate antibiotic prophylaxis, and evidence-based surgical techniques. OTPs play a crucial role in this process by regularly assessing the C-section scar for signs of infection, educating mothers on proper scar care techniques, and monitoring for symptoms such as fever or unusual pain. Early detection and management of infections, as emphasized by a 2022 study in *BMC Pregnancy and Childbirth*, significantly reduce maternal morbidity and mortality. This comprehensive approach underscores the importance of scar management and infection prevention in promoting a safe and healthy recovery for mothers post-Cesarean.

Activity Modifications and Energy Conservation

After a C-section, mothers may experience significant fatigue and discomfort. OTPs teach energy conservation techniques and how to modify daily activities to manage pain and avoid straining the surgical site. This includes instruction on safe bed mobility strategies like log rolling, which minimizes stress on the abdominal muscles when getting in and out of bed. Energy conservation strategies are essential for new mothers, who often struggle with balancing rest and necessary activities.

Functional Mobility and Self-Care

A 2018 study has emphasized early mobilization improves pulmonary function and tissue oxygenation, improves insulin resistance, reduces risk of thromboembolism, and shortens length of stay post C-section. OTPs provide guidance on modified dressing techniques, safe showering practices, and other personal care activities to accommodate limited mobility and pain. They also recommend ergonomic tools and adaptive equipment to facilitate independence without compromising the healing process. Ensuring that mothers can safely perform self-care tasks is vital for their physical and emotional recovery. Research has demonstrated that tailored self-care strategies and the use of adaptive equipment can significantly enhance functional independence in postpartum women recovering from C-sections.

Lifting Techniques and Childcare

Given the weight lifting restrictions following a Cesarean section, adhering to these guidelines is critical to prevent strain and facilitate proper healing. Typically, women are advised to avoid lifting anything heavier than 10–25 pounds during the initial postpartum weeks. This precaution is especially vital after a C-section to prevent complications such as incisional hernias or exacerbated post-surgical pain. OTPs play a crucial role in educating and training women on safe lifting techniques and the use of ergonomic principles. A 2021 study published in *Obstetric Medicine* highlights the importance of perinatal care in reducing complications and enhancing maternal health outcomes, reinforcing the need for OTPs to provide guidance on safe lifting practices. OTPs teach proper body mechanics, recommend assistive devices, and suggest modifications to daily tasks to help distribute weight more effectively and reduce the load on the surgical site. These strategies support women in their recovery, maintaining safety and promoting independence in caring for their newborn.

Adapting Instrumental Activities of Daily Living (IADLs)

To help mothers maintain an active role in their home and care for other children, OTPs advise on modifying household tasks. Strategies may include using a stool while cooking to reduce standing time, sliding objects along counters instead of lifting, and organizing daily tasks to match energy levels throughout the day. Adaptations for IADLs are essential for new mothers to manage their households effectively while recovering. Studies have shown that occupational therapy interventions that focus on adapting daily routines and household tasks can significantly enhance postpartum recovery and maternal satisfaction.

Weight Lifting Restrictions

Following a Cesarean section, adhering to weight lifting restrictions is critical to prevent strain and facilitate proper healing. During the initial postpartum phase, especially after a Cesarean section, it's crucial to restrict lifting to lighter weights—generally under 25 pounds—to minimize the risk of surgical complications and discomfort. Practitioners in occupational therapy are essential in offering guidance on proper lifting methods and ergonomic adjustments to ensure safe recovery and prevent strain. This training may begin during pregnancy if a C-section is anticipated, including teaching proper body mechanics, recommending assistive devices, and suggesting modifications to daily tasks to help distribute weight more effectively and reduce the load on the surgical site. These strategies support women in their recovery, maintaining safety and promoting independence in caring for their newborn.

Pelvic Floor Rehabilitation

Pelvic floor dysfunction refers to a range of issues affecting the pelvic floor muscles, including incontinence, pelvic pain, and organ prolapse. These conditions can result from weakened, tightened, or injured pelvic muscles, which are common after childbirth. Pelvic floor dysfunction can occur regardless of whether delivery was via C-section or vaginally, affecting many postpartum women. OTPs play a crucial role in addressing these issues through comprehensive pelvic floor rehabilitation. This process begins with conducting thorough assessments to identify specific pelvic floor problems and tailoring individualized intervention plans. Interventions may include exercises to strengthen, relax, and rehabilitate the pelvic floor muscles, as well as biofeedback techniques to improve muscle control. OTPs also provide education on proper posture, body mechanics, and safe lifting techniques to support the pelvic floor and prevent further complications (see Table 3.20). By addressing pelvic floor dysfunction early, OTPs help new mothers regain control, reduce discomfort, and improve their overall quality of life.

Breastfeeding and Bottle-Feeding Support

Breastfeeding and bottle feeding are crucial for the mother-infant dyad, significantly impacting both the physical health and emotional bonding between the two. Successful feeding practices ensure proper nutrition for the infant while fostering a nurturing relationship and supporting the mother's confidence and well-being. OTPs play a vital role in addressing challenges in feeding through a comprehensive, holistic approach.

Ergonomic Positioning

Proper ergonomic positioning during feeding is essential to prevent physical discomfort and strain for the mother. OTPs teach mothers how to use pillows to support the baby and their arms, as well as recommending chairs with good back support to avoid back and neck pain.

- **Example 1**: An OTP might suggest using a breastfeeding pillow to elevate the baby to breast level, reducing the need for the mother to hunch over.

Table 3.20 Common pelvic floor rehabilitation interventions used by OTPs

Intervention	Purpose	Notes
Pelvic Floor Muscle Contractions	Strengthen pelvic floor muscles.	Prescribed individually, typically as 3 sets of 10 repetitions, 3 times a day. Includes both short "flick" contractions (quick squeeze and release) and sustained contractions (hold for 5–10 seconds). Avoid overdoing; focus on quality over quantity.
Biofeedback	Improve muscle control and awareness.	Sessions often include 20–30 minutes of feedback-guided exercises.
Manual Therapy	Reduce muscle tension and improve tissue mobility.	Performed by a trained therapist; sessions usually last 30–60 minutes.
Pelvic Floor Muscle Relaxation	Alleviate muscle tightness and spasms.	Include deep breathing and relaxation techniques, practiced 5–10 minutes daily.
Bladder Training	Improve bladder control and reduce incontinence.	Scheduled voiding intervals gradually increased by 15–30 minutes, aiming for every 3–4 hours.
Electrical Stimulation	Enhance muscle contraction and strength.	Typically used for 15–20 minutes per session, 2–3 times per week.
Thermal Modalities	Use heat or cold to manage pelvic pain and inflammation.	Heat therapy can help relax and loosen tissues and stimulate blood flow to the area, while cold therapy can help reduce inflammation and numb sore tissues.
TENS (Transcutaneous Electrical Nerve Stimulation)	Reduce pain through electrical stimulation.	TENS units deliver small electrical impulses through the skin, which are thought to modify pain signals before they reach the brain.
Myofascial Release	Alleviate soft tissue restrictions to improve pain and function.	Involves applying gentle, sustained pressure into the myofascial connective tissue restrictions to eliminate pain and restore motion.
Joint Mobilization	Increase range of motion by mobilizing joint restrictions.	Techniques are applied to pelvic joints to improve mobility and decrease discomfort.
Ultrasound Therapy	Promote tissue healing and reduce pain and inflammation.	Uses sound waves to deliver deep heat to soft tissues and joints, enhancing circulation and pain relief.
Behavioural Strategies	Manage symptoms through behavior modification.	Includes bladder and bowel training strategies, dietary modifications, and stress management techniques.
Postural Education	Support pelvic floor and overall body mechanics.	Instructions on proper sitting, standing, and lifting techniques during each visit.
Education on Lifestyle Modifications	Reduce strain on the pelvic floor and prevent further issues.	Advice on weight management, proper hydration, and diet, reviewed during therapy sessions.

- **Example 2**: Conducting a home visit to assess the mother's typical feeding environment and recommending specific modifications, such as adjusting the height of the feeding chair to ensure proper alignment of the spine, or suggesting an adjustable arm support to help maintain a comfortable position during extended feeding sessions.
- **Example 3**: Demonstrating the use of a baby carrier that supports breastfeeding and bottle feeding, allowing the mother to maintain proper posture and reduce strain on her back and shoulders while feeding on the go.

Latching and Bottle-Feeding Techniques

Effective latching is crucial for successful breastfeeding, preventing nipple pain and ensuring efficient milk transfer. OTPs provide hands-on demonstrations and visual aids to help mothers understand the best positions and methods for a proper latch. For bottle feeding, OTPs teach techniques that promote comfort and bonding.

- **Example 1**: An OTP may use a doll to demonstrate various breastfeeding holds, such as the cradle hold or football hold, to find the most comfortable and effective position for both mother and baby.
- **Example 2**: Showing techniques for adjusting the baby's head position to achieve a deeper latch and reduce nipple discomfort, including the use of specific pillows or wedges to support the baby's head and neck.
- **Example 3**: Teaching mothers how to use paced bottle-feeding techniques, which mimic breastfeeding rhythms to prevent overfeeding and promote bonding.

Supportive Devices

Supportive devices can greatly assist in making feeding more comfortable and sustainable. OTPs recommend and demonstrate the use of devices like breastfeeding pillows, chairs, and specialized bottle-feeding supports.

- **Example 1**: Introducing a mother to a specially designed breastfeeding chair with armrests and lumbar support can make extended feeding sessions more comfortable.
- **Example 2**: Demonstrating the use of a breastfeeding pillow to support the baby's weight, allowing the mother to relax her arms and shoulders, and suggesting specific brands or models that offer the best support based on the mother's body type.
- **Example 3**: Recommending the use of a hands-free pumping bra for mothers who need to pump, enabling them to maintain proper posture and engage in other activities during pumping sessions. Additionally, introducing bottle-feeding aids that help parents maintain a comfortable feeding posture.

Adaptation Strategies

When mothers face persistent feeding challenges, OTPs help develop adaptation strategies to ensure successful feeding. This includes finding alternative feeding positions or transitioning between breastfeeding and bottle feeding without compromising the mother-infant bond.

- **Example 1**: If a mother has difficulty breastfeeding, an OTP might suggest paced bottle feeding, mimicking the breastfeeding rhythm to maintain a close, nurturing interaction.
- **Example 2**: Teaching side-lying breastfeeding positions for mothers recovering from a C-section to reduce strain on their incision site, and providing guidance on how to safely position pillows and the baby.
- **Example 3**: Recommending the use of nipple shields for mothers with latch difficulties, providing a temporary solution while addressing the underlying issues, and closely monitoring the mother's and baby's response to ensure continued progress. For bottle feeding, introducing slow-flow nipples to mimic the breastfeeding experience.

Education and Counseling

OTPs provide education on the physiological aspects of breastfeeding and bottle feeding, common challenges, and effective solutions. They also offer counseling to address emotional and psychological concerns, such as anxiety about milk supply or guilt over feeding choices.

- **Example 1**: An OTP can organize a support group session where mothers share their experiences and learn coping strategies for common feeding issues, fostering a supportive community and reducing feelings of isolation.
- **Example 2**: Providing individualized counseling to address specific concerns, such as low milk supply or weaning difficulties, offering evidence-based solutions and emotional support tailored to the mother's unique situation.
- **Example 3**: Educating mothers on the benefits of both breastfeeding and bottle feeding, helping them make informed choices that best suit their circumstances and preferences, and creating a personalized feeding plan that includes practical strategies and resources.

By offering tailored interventions and strategies, OTPs support mothers in overcoming feeding challenges, ensuring a positive and fulfilling feeding experience. This comprehensive support not only promotes the physical health of both mother and infant but also strengthens their emotional bond, enhancing the overall well-being of the mother-infant dyad.

Mental Health and Emotional Well-being

The postpartum period can be emotionally challenging for many new mothers, with some experiencing postpartum depression, anxiety, or significant mood swings. OTPs play a crucial role in supporting mental health and emotional well-being during this time. They conduct screenings for postpartum depression and anxiety and refer mothers to mental health professionals when necessary. OTPs provide psychosocial counseling to help postpartum mothers adjust to their new roles and transitions, focusing on enhancing performance patterns and skills needed for daily life. This counseling includes addressing changes in daily routines, managing stress, and developing coping strategies to handle the emotional demands of motherhood. OTPs also facilitate access to support groups where mothers can share their experiences and receive peer support, reducing feelings of isolation and promoting emotional healing. By providing these supports, OTPs help mothers navigate the emotional complexities of the postpartum period, fostering a sense of stability and well-being.

Infant Care Training

New mothers often need guidance on how to care for their newborns, and OTPs provide essential training and support to ensure mothers feel confident and competent in their new roles. The occupational transition to motherhood involves adapting to new routines and responsibilities, and OTPs play a crucial role in facilitating this adjustment. OTPs teach safe handling techniques to prevent injury and ensure the baby's safety, including proper methods for lifting, carrying, and positioning the baby during daily activities.

For example, OTPs might demonstrate the best way to support a newborn's head and neck when picking up or laying down the baby to prevent strain or injury. Additionally, OTPs guide mothers through the process of bathing and dressing their infants safely and efficiently, providing step-by-step demonstrations on safe bathing practices, including water temperature checks and handling a slippery baby.

This transition to the new occupation of motherhood also involves developing new routines and integrating infant care into daily life. OTPs assist mothers in establishing effective daily routines that balance the needs of the infant with the mother's self-care and household responsibilities. They provide strategies for organizing time and tasks, such as creating schedules that incorporate feeding, nap times, and play, alongside personal and household activities. By addressing the challenges of this significant occupational transition, OTPs help mothers develop the skills and confidence necessary for effective infant care, ensuring a smoother and more fulfilling adjustment to their new roles. This comprehensive support enhances the well-being of both mother and child, promoting a positive start to the parenting journey.

Return to Work and Daily Activities

Balancing the demands of motherhood with returning to work and managing daily activities can be challenging for new mothers. OTPs assist in this transition by providing practical strategies and support. They help mothers develop effective time management skills to balance childcare, self-care, and work responsibilities. This includes creating schedules and routines that accommodate the needs of both the mother and the baby.

Examples of OTP Support

Assessing Current Routine: OTPs can evaluate a mother's current daily routine to identify areas of difficulty and disruption. By understanding the existing structure, OTPs can offer tailored strategies to integrate new responsibilities and streamline activities.

Example: An OTP may work with a mother to map out her daily schedule, identifying times where she can incorporate feeding, naps, and playtime for the baby without neglecting her own needs.

Developing New Routines: OTPs assist mothers in developing new routines that balance the demands of work, home, and childcare. This includes creating schedules that incorporate work commitments, baby care, and personal time.

Example: An OTP might help a mother establish a morning routine that ensures she can prepare for work while also attending to her baby's needs, such as feeding and changing, by setting up a system of time blocks and checklists.

Time Management and Organization: OTPs provide strategies for effective time management and organization, helping mothers prioritize tasks and make the most of their time.

Example: Teaching the use of tools such as planners, apps, or calendars to organize daily tasks and set reminders for important activities, ensuring nothing is overlooked.

134   *Occupational Therapy and Women's Health*

Energy Conservation Techniques: OTPs teach energy conservation techniques to help mothers manage fatigue and maintain productivity throughout the day. This involves prioritizing tasks, taking breaks, and using efficient methods to complete daily activities.

Example: Suggesting techniques like breaking larger tasks into smaller, manageable chunks, taking short breaks between tasks, and alternating between high-energy and low-energy activities.

Ergonomic Assessments: OTPs conduct ergonomic assessments of the home and workplace to ensure environments are set up to support the mother's physical well-being. This includes advice on workstation setup, proper lifting techniques, and safe practices for daily tasks.

Example: Evaluating a mother's home office setup and suggesting ergonomic adjustments, such as chair height and monitor placement, to prevent back and neck pain while working from home.

By providing these comprehensive supports, OTPs help new mothers transition back to work and manage daily activities effectively. This promotes overall health and well-being for both mother and baby, ensuring a smoother and more fulfilling adjustment to their new roles.

Medical and Occupational Therapy Management of High-Risk Pregnancies

High-risk pregnancies significantly impact a woman's day-to-day functioning and overall well-being. These pregnancies require specialized care to manage potential complications and ensure the health of both the mother and the baby. High-risk pregnancies can affect physical, emotional, and social aspects of a woman's life, making it essential for OTPs to provide comprehensive support and interventions. By addressing the unique needs of women with high-risk pregnancies, OTPs can help optimize maternal and fetal well-being, promoting better health outcomes.

Identifying High-Risk Pregnancies and Medical Considerations

Identifying high-risk pregnancies is crucial for ensuring appropriate medical and therapeutic interventions. It is essential for women to communicate with their healthcare providers to understand any restrictions or special considerations related to their pregnancy. Healthcare providers can provide vital information about the nature of the high-risk condition, necessary precautions, and recommended activities. This information is critical for OTPs to develop safe and effective intervention plans tailored to the specific needs of the mother (see Table 3.21).

Physiological Effects of Bed Rest

Bed rest is often prescribed for high-risk pregnancies to prevent complications such as preterm labor or worsening of conditions like placenta previa. While bed rest can be beneficial, it also has several physiological effects, including muscle atrophy, decreased cardiovascular endurance, and the risk of blood clots. OTPs must address these issues through tailored interventions to maintain as much physical function as possible.

OT in Obstetric Health Management

Table 3.21 Occupational therapy considerations for high-risk pregnancies

Type of High-Risk Pregnancy	Definition	Impact on Occupational Functioning	OT Considerations
Gestational Diabetes	A form of diabetes that develops during pregnancy, affecting how cells use sugar	Fatigue, frequent medical appointments, dietary restrictions	Educate on energy conservation, meal planning, and stress management.
Pre-eclampsia	A condition characterized by high blood pressure and signs of damage to other organ systems, often the liver and kidneys	Hypertension, swelling, severe headaches	Monitor blood pressure, teach relaxation techniques, adapt activities to reduce stress.
Multiple Gestations (Twins, Triplets)	Pregnancies with more than one fetus	Increased physical strain, frequent medical monitoring	Provide ergonomic advice, assist with time management, and offer support for physical tasks.
Placenta Previa	A condition where the placenta covers the cervix, leading to bleeding	Bleeding risks, bed rest requirements	Develop modified activity plans, suggest positioning strategies, and provide mental health support.
Preterm Labor Risk	Increased likelihood of labor before 37 weeks of pregnancy	Activity limitations, frequent rest periods	Educate on recognizing signs of labor, provide gentle exercise routines, and suggest relaxation techniques.
Spinal Cord Injury	Damage to the spinal cord that can affect mobility and organ function	Mobility limitations, increased risk of complications	Adapt ADLs, provide education on skin care and positioning, recommend assistive devices.
Multiple Sclerosis (MS)	A disease where the immune system eats away at the protective covering of nerves	Fatigue, muscle weakness, mobility issues	Energy conservation techniques, adaptive equipment, home modifications, balance and coordination exercises.
Lupus	An autoimmune disease that can affect the skin, joints, kidneys, brain, and other organs	Joint pain, fatigue, risk of flares	Pain management strategies, energy conservation, education on joint protection.
Cystic Fibrosis	A genetic disorder that affects the respiratory and digestive systems	Respiratory issues, fatigue, frequent hospitalizations	Breathing exercises, energy conservation, adaptive equipment for ADLs.
Cerebral Palsy	A group of disorders affecting movement and muscle tone, often caused by damage to the developing brain	Mobility issues, muscle stiffness, coordination problems	Adapt ADLs, provide mobility aids, teach muscle relaxation techniques, and offer ergonomic advice.

Specific High-Risk Conditions and OT Considerations

Gestational diabetes, characterized by the body's inability to effectively use sugar during pregnancy, requires careful management to prevent complications. Beyond dietary management and blood sugar monitoring, OTPs can help by developing routines that integrate necessary lifestyle changes seamlessly into daily life. For example, an OTP might work with a woman to plan balanced meals and snacks that fit her schedule and energy levels, ensuring she maintains her blood sugar levels throughout the day.

Hypertensive disorders, such as pre-eclampsia, involve high blood pressure and potential organ damage. These conditions necessitate a focus on stress management and physical activity adaptations. OTPs can introduce relaxation techniques like guided imagery or progressive muscle relaxation to help manage stress. They might also suggest modifications to physical activities to ensure they remain safe and beneficial, such as recommending low-impact exercises like swimming or prenatal yoga to maintain fitness without exacerbating symptoms.

Multiple gestations increase the physical demands on the body and require frequent medical monitoring. OTPs support these mothers by advising on ergonomic setups to reduce physical strain during daily tasks, such as using supportive cushions while sitting and lifting techniques that protect the back. Additionally, OTPs can assist in creating effective time management strategies to handle multiple medical appointments and prepare for the needs of multiple infants postpartum.

Placenta previa, where the placenta covers the cervix, often leads to significant bleeding risks and bed rest requirements. OTPs develop modified activity plans that respect these limitations while maintaining engagement in meaningful activities. This might involve teaching safe positioning techniques to minimize strain and suggesting mental health strategies to cope with the isolation and anxiety that can accompany prolonged bed rest.

Women at risk of preterm labor often face strict activity limitations and frequent rest periods. OTPs educate these women on recognizing early signs of labor and provide gentle exercise routines to maintain some physical activity without risking preterm labor. Relaxation techniques are also crucial to help manage anxiety and promote calmness, which can positively impact both maternal and fetal health.

Chronic conditions, such as spinal cord injury, multiple sclerosis (MS), lupus, and cystic fibrosis, present unique challenges during pregnancy. These conditions can complicate both prenatal and postpartum periods due to their ongoing symptoms and the added physical demands of pregnancy. OTPs adapt ADLs for these women, ensuring they can manage their condition while maintaining functionality. For instance, an OTP might recommend specific assistive devices to support mobility for a woman with MS or teach energy conservation techniques to a woman with lupus to help manage fatigue effectively.

Spinal Cord Injury: Women with spinal cord injuries may experience limited mobility and increased risk of complications. During the prenatal period, OTPs can help by adapting ADLs to ensure safety and independence. For example, they may recommend assistive devices like grab bars and transfer benches for safe bathroom use, or adaptive equipment for dressing and grooming. Postpartum, OTPs can assist with safe techniques for infant care, such as modified lifting and carrying strategies to avoid strain. They can also provide education on maintaining skin integrity to prevent pressure sores and managing positioning to reduce the risk of complications.

Multiple Sclerosis (MS): Fatigue and muscle weakness are common issues for women with MS. During pregnancy, OTPs can introduce energy conservation techniques, such as planning rest periods throughout the day and prioritizing tasks to manage fatigue effectively. They might also suggest adaptive equipment, like ergonomic kitchen tools and reachers, to reduce physical strain during daily activities. Postpartum, OTPs can help with adapting infant care routines to manage fatigue and muscle weakness, ensuring that the mother can care for her baby effectively without overexerting herself.

Lupus: Joint pain, fatigue, and the risk of flares are significant concerns for pregnant women with lupus. OTPs can provide pain management strategies, including teaching joint protection techniques and recommending supportive devices like splints or braces during the prenatal period. They also offer energy conservation methods, helping women balance activity and rest to manage fatigue. Postpartum, OTPs can support the mother in managing joint pain and fatigue while caring for her newborn, offering strategies to reduce joint strain and maintain functional ability.

Cystic Fibrosis: Respiratory issues and fatigue are common in women with cystic fibrosis. During pregnancy, OTPs can teach breathing exercises to improve respiratory function and suggest energy conservation strategies to manage fatigue. They might also recommend adaptive equipment for ADLs, such as shower chairs and long-handled sponges, to reduce physical effort during self-care activities. Postpartum, OTPs can assist in planning and organizing medical equipment and supplies needed for daily treatments, ensuring the mother can balance her own health needs with infant care responsibilities.

Cerebral Palsy: Women with cerebral palsy may experience mobility issues, muscle stiffness, and coordination problems. During pregnancy, OTPs can adapt ADLs to ensure safety and independence, such as recommending mobility aids like walkers or wheelchairs. They can also teach muscle relaxation techniques to manage stiffness and provide ergonomic advice to reduce strain during daily activities. Postpartum, OTPs can help with infant care by suggesting adaptive strategies for feeding, bathing, and carrying the baby, ensuring the mother can care for her newborn effectively despite her physical limitations.

By providing tailored interventions for these chronic conditions, OTPs help women navigate the complexities of pregnancy and maintain their independence and quality of life. These interventions support both prenatal and postpartum periods, ensuring that women receive the comprehensive care they need to manage their conditions effectively while preparing for and adjusting to motherhood.

Collaborative Care Between Medical Professionals and OTPs

Collaborative care is essential for the effective management of high-risk pregnancies. OTPs work closely with obstetricians, nurses, dietitians, and other healthcare professionals to ensure a comprehensive approach to care. This multidisciplinary collaboration ensures that all aspects of a woman's health are addressed, from medical needs to functional abilities. Regular communication and coordinated efforts help in developing and implementing intervention plans that are safe and beneficial for the mother and the baby. For example, an OTP might work with a dietitian to create a balanced meal plan for a woman with gestational diabetes, ensuring her nutritional needs are met while maintaining stable blood sugar levels. Additionally, collaboration with a nurse can help in monitoring and managing pre-eclampsia by ensuring that the mother adheres to prescribed relaxation and physical activity guidelines. Such integrated care facilitates better health outcomes by providing comprehensive, cohesive support tailored to the specific needs of each high-risk pregnancy.

Strategies for Optimizing Maternal and Fetal Well-being

Optimizing maternal and fetal well-being in high-risk pregnancies involves a multifaceted approach that incorporates various therapeutic strategies tailored to each individual's unique needs. OTPs can utilize a range of strategies to support both the physical and emotional health of expectant mothers facing high-risk conditions. These strategies include comprehensive patient education, activity modification and adaptation, use of assistive devices, stress management, promoting safe physical activity, facilitating social support, ADL/IADL retraining, and consistent monitoring and follow-up (see Table 3.22). Implementing these strategies can help ensure that high-risk pregnancies are managed effectively, promoting better health outcomes for both the mother and the fetus.

By incorporating these strategies, OTPs play a crucial role in ensuring that women with high-risk pregnancies can continue to engage in meaningful daily occupations. Participation in daily activities is vital for maintaining a sense of normalcy, emotional well-being, and

Table 3.22 Strategies for high-risk pregnancies and specific occupational therapy interventions

Strategy	Description	Specific Examples
Comprehensive Patient Education	Educating mothers about their high-risk condition and self-management techniques specific to their pregnancy.	Developing customized pamphlets, patient education handouts, or videos explaining the condition and management strategies. Providing individualized sessions on understanding high-risk conditions like gestational diabetes or pre-eclampsia.
Activity Modification and Adaptation	Modifying daily activities to reduce physical strain and align with medical restrictions during high-risk pregnancies.	Suggesting safe positioning techniques and low-energy activities for mothers on bed rest. Tailoring household tasks to reduce exertion, such as using a stool for sitting while preparing meals.
Use of Assistive Devices and Ergonomics	Recommending and training on assistive devices to mitigate physical challenges and enhance comfort for high-risk pregnancy conditions.	Introducing ergonomic pillows and supports to maintain proper alignment during prolonged bed rest. Demonstrating the use of mobility aids for mothers with physical limitations due to high-risk conditions.
Stress Management and Mental Health Support	Incorporating relaxation techniques and mental health support to address emotional and psychological stresses related to high-risk pregnancies.	Conducting relaxation sessions with breathing exercises and guided imagery to alleviate anxiety related to high-risk pregnancy. Referring to mental health professionals for counseling support.
Promoting Physical Activity Within Safe Limits	Advising on safe physical activities that promote health without compromising the high-risk pregnancy.	Suggesting gentle prenatal yoga or stretching routines for mothers with high blood pressure to maintain circulation without overexertion. Providing tailored exercise plans for mothers on partial bed rest.
ADL/IADL Retraining	Helping mothers adapt their daily and instrumental activities to accommodate their high-risk pregnancy condition.	Teaching energy-saving techniques for essential activities, such as using long-handled tools to avoid bending or reaching. Demonstrating adaptive techniques for self-care tasks to reduce physical strain.
Facilitating Social Support and Community Resources	Encouraging engagement with social support networks and community resources specifically for high-risk pregnancies.	Providing information about local and online support groups for high-risk pregnancies to share experiences and advice. Connecting mothers with community resources like home health aides or nutritional counseling.
Monitoring and Follow-Up	Regularly monitoring the patient's progress and adjusting the intervention plan as needed during the high-risk pregnancy.	Scheduling frequent check-ins to assess adherence to activity modifications and overall well-being. Adjusting care plans based on changes in the mother's condition or new medical advice.

overall quality of life. High-risk pregnancies often come with restrictions that can make women feel isolated or limited in their capabilities. However, through careful planning and adaptive techniques, OTPs can help these women find ways to safely participate in their usual routines and roles, whether it's through modified household tasks, adaptive self-care practices, or safe exercise regimens. This engagement not only supports physical health but also fosters a positive mental outlook, reducing the risk of anxiety and depression. The collaborative and individualized approach of occupational therapy ensures that each woman's unique needs and preferences are respected, promoting empowerment and resilience throughout the pregnancy journey.

Impact of Spontaneous Abortion, Stillbirth, Childhood Disability

The experiences of spontaneous abortion, stillbirth, and childhood disability can have profound and long-lasting effects on families. These events not only bring significant emotional and psychological challenges but also impact daily functioning and occupational roles. OTPs play a vital role in supporting individuals and families through these difficult times, helping them navigate their grief, adjust to new circumstances, and maintain their engagement in meaningful activities.

Spontaneous Abortion (Miscarriage)

Spontaneous abortion, or miscarriage, typically involves the loss of a pregnancy before the 20th week. The suddenness of a miscarriage often leaves women grappling with shock and unresolved plans for pregnancy, which can significantly disrupt their daily life and emotional stability. Grief can profoundly disrupt occupational functioning by affecting concentration, motivation, and emotional stability, which can make it challenging for individuals to engage in daily activities and roles effectively. OTPs can educate clients on the stages of grief and provide coping mechanisms tailored to each stage, such as relaxation techniques, structured routines, and therapeutic activities, to help individuals transition through these stages and enhance participation in meaningful occupational activities (Figure 3.7).

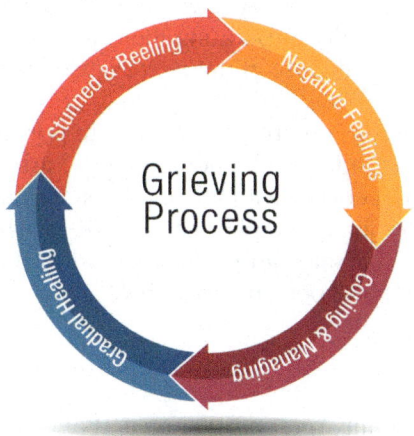

Figure 3.7 Stages of grief.

140 *Occupational Therapy and Women's Health*

OT Interventions for Miscarriage:

- **Emotional Recovery**: OTPs provide targeted counseling that focuses on coping with the shock and immediacy of loss. Techniques such as cognitive-behavioural strategies are employed to manage acute grief and mitigate feelings of guilt or blame.
- **Physical Recovery**: Guidance on physical recovery is often more straightforward due to the earlier stage of pregnancy, focusing on hormonal rebalancing and physical health restoration.
- **Routine Resumption**: OTPs assist in the gradual reintegration into normal activities, with a focus on establishing routines that acknowledge the loss but also foster a sense of future optimism, such as revisiting personal goals and hobbies that were put on hold.

For clinicians, it's crucial to provide a compassionate and responsive environment that acknowledges the loss and supports the woman's emotional and physical healing. OTPs should encourage the expression of grief in a safe setting and help integrate structured, gentle activities that aid in recovery and emotional stability. Establishing a clear plan for gradually resuming daily routines can also help the individual regain a sense of normalcy and control over their life.

Stillbirth

Stillbirth refers to the loss of a baby after the 20th week of pregnancy and is often accompanied by more intense and prolonged grief due to the advanced stage of pregnancy and the heightened anticipation of childbirth.

OT Interventions for Stillbirth:

- **Grief and Emotional Support**: The support extends to more in-depth grief counseling, possibly including family therapy, as parents navigate the profound loss of a nearly full-term pregnancy. OTPs may facilitate memorializing activities that honor the expected child, helping parents process their loss and articulate their grief.
- **Physical Recovery**: OTPs support the mother's recovery from childbirth, addressing postpartum physical care, which can be more complex due to the advanced stage of pregnancy.
- **Re-establishing Roles**: Special attention is given to helping parents redefine their roles within the family and community, supporting them in finding new meaningful roles that honor their experience while also allowing for personal growth and healing.

OTPs should focus on delivering in-depth emotional support and facilitating group or individual therapy sessions that address the complex grief associated with stillbirth. It's important to assist in physical recovery with an emphasis on managing the intense emotional aftermath that can accompany the physical healing process. Additionally, helping parents find new meaningful activities and roles can aid in adjusting to life after loss, providing pathways for healing and personal growth.

Childhood Disability

The birth of a child with a disability presents unique and ongoing challenges for families, affecting their daily routines, occupational roles, and overall quality of life. OTPs provide critical support by educating parents on the use of adaptive equipment and techniques to facilitate daily activities, making necessary home modifications for safety and accessibility, and developing structured routines that incorporate the child's needs.

OT Interventions for Childhood Disability:

- **Adaptive Equipment and Home Modifications**: OTPs might demonstrate the use of specialized equipment like feeding chairs or install home modifications such as grab bars and ramps to enhance the child's mobility and safety.
- **Routine Management**: Assisting families in creating structured schedules that balance the child's care with family activities and self-care, ensuring that all family members can continue to participate in meaningful roles.
- **Emotional and Psychological Support**: Providing counseling and facilitating support groups to help parents manage the stress and emotional impact of raising a child with a disability, fostering resilience and emotional well-being.

For OTPs, it is essential to approach each family with empathy, offering tailored interventions that address both the immediate and long-term needs. This includes not only practical support for handling daily tasks but also emotional support to help families adjust to their new reality. By fostering an environment of understanding and support, OTPs can help families of children with disabilities find balance and fulfillment.

Multidisciplinary Collaboration

Effective management of spontaneous abortion, stillbirth, and childhood disability necessitates a multidisciplinary approach. OTPs play a pivotal role, working closely with healthcare professionals such as doctors, nurses, social workers, and mental health therapists to ensure comprehensive care. This collaboration is crucial for creating tailored intervention plans that meet the unique needs of each family, enhancing overall outcomes and supporting holistic recovery.

OTPs involvement in these teams ensures that all aspects of a family's care—emotional, physical, and logistical—are addressed, facilitating a cohesive strategy for recovery and adjustment. Through this integrated approach, OTPs help families not only to cope with immediate challenges but also to build a foundation for long-term resilience and engagement in meaningful activities.

Maternal Mental Health

Maternal mental health significantly impacts both mothers and their families during pregnancy and the postpartum period. Research indicates that up to 20% of women experience mood or anxiety disorders during this time, with conditions such as postpartum depression affecting 10–15% of mothers globally. These mental health challenges can hinder a mother's ability to bond with her baby, manage daily tasks, and sustain healthy relationships, potentially leading to long-term consequences for the entire family.

OTPs are instrumental in addressing these issues, offering interventions aimed at enhancing emotional well-being, resilience, and functional independence. By facilitating early identification and intervention for maternal mental health issues, OTPs help mitigate their impact, promoting healthier family dynamics and supporting mothers in their journey towards recovery and well-being.

Common Maternal Mental Health Conditions

Understanding common maternal mental health conditions is vital for recognizing the signs and providing appropriate support.

Postpartum Depression (PPD)

- **Prevalence**: Affects approximately 10–20% of new mothers.

  Characteristics:

  - Persistent sadness and crying spells, which can disrupt daily routines and caregiving tasks.
  - Lack of interest in activities, leading to withdrawal from social interactions and hobbies.
  - Fatigue and low energy, making it difficult to perform self-care and household chores.
  - Difficulty bonding with the baby, impacting breastfeeding, and infant care routines.
  - Changes in appetite or sleep patterns, which can affect meal preparation and sleep hygiene.
  - Feelings of hopelessness or worthlessness, leading to a lack of motivation and decreased participation in daily activities.

- **Impact**: PPD can significantly interfere with a mother's ability to care for herself and her baby, leading to long-term emotional and developmental issues if untreated. The inability to engage in meaningful occupations can further exacerbate feelings of inadequacy and isolation.
- **Urgency**: Requires prompt intervention to prevent worsening symptoms and promote recovery, but typically not an immediate emergency unless there are suicidal thoughts.

Postpartum Anxiety

- **Prevalence**: Affects approximately 6–10% of new mothers.

  Characteristics:

  - Excessive worry and constant fear, which can make it challenging to leave the house or engage in social activities.
  - Restlessness and irritability, impacting interactions with family members and the ability to relax.
  - Difficulty concentrating, which can interfere with tasks requiring focus, such as managing household finances or following a schedule.
  - Physical symptoms such as heart palpitations, shortness of breath, and dizziness, making physical activities and exercise daunting.
  - Constant checking on the baby's well-being, disrupting sleep and rest periods.

- **Impact**: Postpartum anxiety can hinder a mother's ability to relax and enjoy her new role, potentially affecting her interaction with the baby and her overall quality of life. This condition can lead to overprotectiveness and avoidance of necessary activities.
- **Urgency**: Requires timely intervention to manage symptoms and prevent escalation, especially if it coexists with PPD, but not typically an immediate emergency.

Postpartum Psychosis

- **Prevalence**: A rare but severe mental health condition, occurring in approximately 1–2 out of every 1,000 deliveries.

  Characteristics:

  - Hallucinations (seeing or hearing things that are not there) can lead to confusion and dangerous behaviors.
  - Delusions (strongly held false beliefs) that can result in irrational decisions affecting safety and caregiving.
  - Extreme agitation and erratic behavior, making it difficult to engage in routine activities or care for the baby.
  - Confusion and disorientation, impacting the ability to perform basic self-care and household tasks.
  - Paranoia and disorganized thinking, leading to withdrawal from social interactions and inability to follow structured routines.

- **Impact**: Without prompt treatment, postpartum psychosis can lead to severe consequences, including hospitalization and long-term mental health issues. The inability to safely care for the baby and perform daily activities can lead to further complications.
- **Urgency**: Requires immediate medical attention due to the high risk of harm to the mother and baby. This condition is considered a psychiatric emergency and needs urgent intervention to ensure safety.

OT Interventions for Maternal Mental Health

OTPs provide a range of interventions to support maternal mental health. These interventions are tailored to the individual needs of each mother to promote emotional well-being, resilience, and functional independence.

Emotional Support and Counseling

OTPs offer emotional support and counseling to help mothers process their feelings and cope with mental health challenges. This can involve one-on-one sessions where mothers are encouraged to express their emotions and work through their grief, anxiety, or depression. For example, an OTP might use therapeutic listening techniques to help a mother who is struggling with postpartum depression articulate her feelings and develop coping strategies. Support groups facilitated by OTPs provide a platform for mothers to share their experiences with peers, fostering a sense of community and mutual support. When necessary, OTPs refer mothers to specialized mental health professionals for additional care, ensuring a comprehensive approach to mental health.

Routine and Structure

Establishing daily routines can provide a sense of normalcy and control for mothers experiencing mental health issues. OTPs assist mothers in creating structured schedules that balance caregiving responsibilities with self-care and leisure activities. For instance, an OTP might help a mother develop a daily schedule that includes time for feeding and caring for her baby, household chores, exercise, and relaxation. This structured approach can reduce feelings of overwhelm and enhance a mother's ability to manage her daily tasks effectively. By incorporating regular breaks and self-care activities, OTPs ensure that mothers have time to recharge and attend to their own needs, which is crucial for maintaining mental health.

Stress Management Techniques

Teaching stress management techniques is a key intervention for mothers dealing with anxiety and stress. OTPs introduce methods such as mindfulness, deep breathing exercises, and progressive muscle relaxation, which can be integrated into daily routines to promote relaxation and emotional well-being. For example, an OTP might guide a mother through a mindfulness meditation session to help her focus on the present moment and reduce anxious thoughts. Deep breathing exercises can be taught to help manage acute stress responses, while progressive muscle relaxation can help alleviate physical tension associated with stress. These techniques empower mothers with tools they can use independently to manage their mental health.

Activity Engagement

Encouraging engagement in meaningful activities can significantly improve mood and provide a sense of accomplishment. OTPs help mothers identify and participate in activities that they enjoy and find fulfilling, such as hobbies, social interactions, and physical exercise. For instance, an OTP might work with a mother to rediscover her passion for painting or gardening, helping her set up a space at home where she can pursue these activities. Group activities, like joining a local mom-and-baby exercise class, can provide social interaction and physical benefits. By facilitating participation in enjoyable and purposeful activities, OTPs support mothers in maintaining their mental and emotional well-being.

Social Support Networks

Facilitating connections with social support networks is crucial for maternal mental health. OTPs help mothers build and maintain support systems by connecting them with community resources, support groups, and family counseling services. For example, an OTP might introduce a mother to a local postpartum support group where she can share her experiences and receive peer support. They may also help coordinate family counseling sessions to improve communication and support within the household. Strengthening social networks ensures that mothers do not feel isolated and have access to the emotional and practical support they need.

Education and Resources

Providing education about maternal mental health conditions and available resources empowers mothers to seek help and make informed decisions about their care. OTPs can create educational materials that explain the signs and symptoms of conditions like postpartum depression and anxiety, as well as outline strategies for managing these conditions. For example, an OTP might develop a booklet that details coping strategies, self-care tips, and information on local mental health services. Guiding mothers in accessing these resources ensures they have the knowledge and tools to address their mental health proactively.

Coping Strategies

Developing effective coping strategies is essential for managing maternal mental health conditions. OTPs work with mothers to identify personalized coping mechanisms that can be used during times of stress or emotional distress. For example, an OTP might help a mother develop a "coping toolkit" that includes activities and techniques such as journaling, listening to music, or practicing yoga. These strategies are tailored to the individual's preferences and lifestyle, ensuring they are practical and sustainable. By equipping mothers with effective coping mechanisms, OTPs support their ability to manage stress and maintain emotional balance.

The Role of Multidisciplinary Collaboration

Effective management of maternal mental health requires a collaborative approach involving various healthcare professionals. OTPs work closely with obstetricians, pediatricians, mental health therapists, social workers, and community organizations to provide comprehensive care. This multidisciplinary collaboration ensures that all aspects of a mother's health are addressed, promoting holistic well-being and better outcomes for both the mother and her child.

Long-Term Support and Follow-Up

Maternal mental health needs do not end with the postpartum period. Long-term support and follow-up are essential to ensure sustained well-being. OTPs provide ongoing monitoring and adjustments to intervention plans as needed, helping mothers navigate the challenges of motherhood and maintain their mental health over time.

By addressing maternal mental health comprehensively, OTPs play a vital role in promoting the well-being of mothers and their families. Through personalized interventions, support, and collaboration, OTPs help mothers achieve emotional stability, functional independence, and a fulfilling motherhood experience.

Case Studies in Obstetric Health

CASE A: Postpartum

Background and Past Medical History: The client is a 35-year-old healthy, active woman with no significant medical history. She works as a high-school track coach, takes care of her four children, and regularly participates in marathons and half marathons. She is currently 7 weeks postpartum from the birth of her 4th child. The client has been experiencing significant challenges in her daily life due to pelvic heaviness and discomfort, impacting her ability to perform various ADLs and IADLs.

Previous Births:

- First son born vaginally via a traumatic hospital birth (12/8/2016).
- Second son delivered vaginally (04/26/2019).
- Third child delivered via traumatic Cesarean at 37 weeks due to chorioamniotic separation (01/23/2021).
- Fourth child delivered via VBAC (04/30/2022) at 41 weeks, unmedicated and without complications.

Prior Level of Function:

- Worked as a high-school track coach.
- Drove to work independently.
- Regularly participated in marathons and half marathons.
- Independent in all basic ADLs and IADLs.
- Managed household tasks independently and actively engaged in childcare for her three children.

Household Living Arrangements and Social History:

- Lives with her spouse and four children in a single-level private home.
- Strong support system with extended family nearby.
- No use of assistive equipment prior to the current postpartum period.

Change in Functional Status:

- The client reports pelvic heaviness and discomfort, impacting her ability to perform daily activities and engage in her fitness routine.
- She is experiencing challenges with managing household tasks, caring for her four children, and returning to her previous fitness level.
- Additionally, she is experiencing mild to moderate postnatal depression, affecting her emotional well-being and motivation.

Specific ADLs/IADLs that have become difficult after her recent delivery include:

- **Cooking and meal preparation**: Needs assistance with prolonged standing and bending.
- **Cleaning and maintaining the home**: Difficulty with vacuuming, mopping, and other tasks requiring bending and lifting.
- **Lifting and carrying her children**: Reports increased pelvic heaviness and discomfort.
- **Bathing and dressing herself and her children**: Difficulty with tasks requiring bending and lifting.
- **Engaging in physical exercise and fitness activities**: Unable to resume running and fitness classes due to pelvic discomfort.

OT Assessments:

- **Canadian Occupational Performance Measure (COPM)**: Identified issues in ADLs/IADLs such as managing household tasks, caring for children, and participating in fitness activities.
- **Edinburgh Postnatal Depression Scale (EPDS)**: Score of 15, indicating mild to moderate postnatal depression.
- **Pelvic Floor Impact Questionnaire (PFIQ)**: Score indicating significant impact on daily life due to pelvic floor dysfunction, with particular difficulties in physical activities and emotional well-being.

Physical Assessments:

- **Observation**: Forward shoulders, posterior translation of rib cage, posterior pelvic tilt, and reduced abdominal recruitment.
- **General Listening**: Pulling to the right posterior pelvis.
- **Energy Assessment**: Open birthing pattern.

- **Thoracic Assessment**: Wide infrasternal angle, reduced posterior-to-anterior mobility at lower thoracic segments 8–12.
- **Abdominal Assessment**: Diastasis recti with varying degrees of separation; reduced mobility at right obliques and lower abdominal fascia.
- **Bladder and Uterine Mobility**: Restrictions noted for side-to-side and rotational movements.
- **Internal Pelvic Assessment**: Perineal body, pelvic floor muscles, and urethral assessments revealed various restrictions and reduced mobility.

Occupational Therapy Plan of Care and Goals:

The client will receive skilled occupational therapy twice a week for 8 weeks to increase independence with ADLs, IADLs, and other functional activities.

Goals:

1. Client will independently manage household tasks, including cooking and cleaning, without experiencing pelvic heaviness or discomfort, as measured by the client reporting no difficulty or discomfort during these tasks within 8 weeks.
2. Client will safely and comfortably care for her four children, including lifting, bathing, and feeding, without pain or pelvic pressure, as measured by COPM performance and satisfaction scores increasing by at least 3 points within 8 weeks.
3. Client will return to running and fitness classes, achieving 20 minutes of running (10 repetitions of run 2 minutes, walk 1 minute) without pelvic heaviness or discomfort, as observed and self-reported within 12 weeks.
4. Client will demonstrate a reduction in postnatal depression symptoms, with EPDS scores decreasing to below 10 within 8 weeks.
5. Client will identify and incorporate three stress management techniques into her daily routine within 4 weeks.
6. Client will establish a consistent medication management routine, including setting reminders and tracking adherence within 4 weeks.
7. Client will report a decrease in the impact of pelvic floor dysfunction on her ability to engage in caretaking of children and household activities, as measured by a reduction in PFIQ scores by at least 50% within 8 weeks.
8. Client will improve pelvic floor muscle strength to 4/5 in all quadrants and core stabilization to enable participation in caretaking of children and household tasks without pelvic heaviness, as measured by manual muscle testing and self-reported ease of movement within 8 weeks.
9. Client will demonstrate increased mobility of the pelvic girdle and reduction in diastasis recti to less than 2 cm at all points measured to improve independence with showering and dressing, as observed and self-reported within 8 weeks.

Interventions

The following interventions will be implemented to address the client's specific needs and goals:

Manual Therapy Techniques:

- **Abdominal**: Release oblique and recti muscles, lower abdominal fascia, and scar tissue.
- **Pelvic**: Sacral correction and sheer correction, pubovesical and broad ligament release.

- **Internal Techniques**: Perineal body scar tissue release, rectal fascial release, bladder repositioning.
- **Functional Techniques**: 360 breathing, pelvic floor and transversus abdominis activation, intra-abdominal pressure management, lateral weight shifts, and yoga inversions.

Environmental Modifications:

- Adapt the home environment to facilitate safer lifting and picking up of household items and kitchen tasks, such as organizing frequently used items within easy reach.
- Use of a shower chair and long-handled sponge to relieve pressure and pain during showering.

Psychosocial Interventions:

- Referral to a mental health professional for counseling.
- Incorporation of mindfulness and stress-reduction techniques, such as deep breathing exercises and progressive muscle relaxation, practiced daily.
- Guided identification and incorporation of three stress management techniques into her daily routine.

Medication Management:

- Assist in establishing a consistent medication management routine by setting reminders and tracking adherence.

Home Program:

- 360 breathing with focus on posterior and lateral costal expansion.
- Pelvic floor and transversus abdominis activation in various positions.
- Knack technique for intra-abdominal pressure management with bending, lifting, and increased perceived exertion.
- Lateral weight shifts using adductors and abductors to balance the pelvis.
- Yoga inversions (Puppy pose) mid and late day for pressure management as needed.

Outcomes:

Post Treatment:

- Reduced pain and discomfort at rest and during activity.
- Decreased pain with intercourse.
- Reduced pelvic pressure during daily activities.
- Decreased urgency and frequency of urination.
- Improved pelvic floor strength and core stabilization.
- Increased confidence and ability to return to running with coordinated weight shifts and breathing techniques.
- Comfort and enjoyment while running up to 20 minutes total of running (10 repetitions of run 2 minutes, walk 1 minute).
- Able to care for four children without pelvic pressure present at the end of the day.
- Feeling stronger throughout her core with faster progress to return to her non-pregnancy/postpartum wardrobe 4 months sooner than with her third child.

Assessment Findings:

- Increased mobility of bony, soft tissue, and visceral structures.
- Improved mobility of abdominal and oblique fascia, particularly on the right side.
- Reduction in diastasis recti above and at the umbilicus.
- Improved bladder and uterine mobility.
- Increased sacral mobility, especially on the right side.
- Normalized position of the liver and stomach, reducing the wide infrasternal angle.
- Enhanced pelvic floor muscle strength from 2/5–3/5 to 4/5.
- Reduced urethra and bladder bulging, with alignment closer to midline.
- Improved positioning and mobility of the cervix and uterus relative to the bladder. Demonstrated increased coordination with weight shifts, breathing, and Kegel exercises, and effectively using "knack" techniques during lifting and bending tasks to minimize pressure and support pelvic floor and deep abdominal muscles.

Follow-Up Visits:

- Two additional visits for general hip girdle strengthening, core stabilization, and running progression.
- Achieved increased coordination, reduced pelvic pressure, and noticeable improvement in functional activities such as cooking, cleaning, dressing, showering, and childcare compared to previous postpartum recoveries.

The client exhibited significant improvement in pelvic floor strength, core stability, and overall function. She is now able to independently manage various ADLs and occupational activities, including cooking, cleaning, dressing, showering, and caring for her four children, without experiencing discomfort or pain. The familiarity with prior postpartum recoveries and the strong therapeutic relationship contributed to her positive outcomes. The occupational therapy approach demonstrated profound changes in her symptoms, highlighting the importance of a comprehensive, occupation-based approach in postpartum care.

CASE B: Pregnancy

Background and Past Medical History: The client is a 32-year-old woman who is currently 24 weeks pregnant with her first child. She works as a teacher and enjoys moderate physical activities such as walking and yoga. Throughout her pregnancy, she has been experiencing mild pelvic pain, occasional urinary incontinence, and sciatica, particularly when laughing or sneezing. She is concerned about maintaining her fitness levels and preparing her body for childbirth.

Prior Level of Function:

- Worked as a teacher.
- Drove to work independently.
- Regularly participated in moderate physical activities such as jogging, lifting weights, and yoga.
- Independent in all basic ADLs and IADLs.

Household Living Arrangements and Social History:

- Lives with her partner in a two-story house.
- Independent with all ADLs/IADLs.
- Driving independently.
- Has a supportive network of friends and family.
- No use of assistive equipment prior to her current pregnancy.

Change in Functional Status and Challenges:

- **Pelvic Pain**: Experiences mild pelvic pain, especially after prolonged standing or physical activity.
- **Sciatica**: Occasional shooting pain down the leg, particularly when sitting or standing for long periods.
- **Urinary Incontinence**: Occasional leakage of urine when laughing, sneezing, or coughing.
- **Fitness Maintenance**: Desire to stay active and fit during pregnancy but unsure about safe exercises.
- **Preparation for Childbirth**: Wants to ensure her pelvic floor and abdominal muscles are strong and ready for labor and delivery.

OT Assessments:

- **Pain Mapping**: Pinpointed areas of mild discomfort in the lower abdomen and pelvic region.
- **Pelvic Floor Impact Questionnaire (PFIQ)**: Scores indicated a moderate impact on her quality of life, with particular concern over urinary incontinence.

Physical Assessments:

- **Observation**: Slight anterior pelvic tilt observed, forward shoulders, and postural misalignment contributing to pelvic and sciatic pain.
- **Palpation**: Tenderness noted in the lower abdominal and pelvic areas, and along the sciatic nerve path.
- **Range of Motion (ROM)**: Limited hip external rotation and lumbar flexion.
- **Manual Muscle Testing (MMT)**: Reduced strength in hip flexors, pelvic floor muscles, and core muscles.
- **Sciatica Assessment**: Positive straight leg raise test, indicating sciatic nerve involvement.
- **Postural Assessment**: Evaluation of sitting and standing posture, noting compensatory patterns that may contribute to pelvic pain and sciatica.
- **Pelvic Floor Assessment**: Assessment of pelvic floor muscle strength, coordination, and endurance using internal and external palpation techniques.

Occupational Therapy Plan of Care and Goals: The client will receive skilled occupational therapy twice a week for 8 weeks to improve pelvic floor function, manage pelvic pain and sciatica, maintain fitness during pregnancy, and maximize participation in her teaching job.

Goals:

1. Client will report a 50% reduction in pelvic pain during daily activities within 4 weeks, as measured by self-report.

OT in Obstetric Health Management 151

2. Client will experience a 50% reduction in urinary incontinence episodes within 8 weeks, as measured by a bladder diary and pad test.
3. Client will report a 50% reduction in sciatica symptoms during daily activities within 8 weeks, as measured by self-report.
4. Client will perform a tailored prenatal exercise program safely and effectively, as observed by the therapist within 8 weeks.
5. Client will demonstrate proper activation of pelvic floor muscles during exercises, as observed and measured by the therapist within 4 weeks.
6. Client will increase hip external rotation ROM by 10 degrees within 8 weeks, as measured during physical assessments.
7. Client will be able to teach her classes with minimal discomfort, as measured by self-report and observation within 8 weeks.

Interventions

Pain Management Strategies:

- Teaching relaxation techniques such as deep breathing, progressive muscle relaxation, and guided imagery to help reduce pelvic pain and tension.
- Using modalities like heat therapy for pain relief, focusing on the lower abdomen and pelvic region.
- Ergonomic adjustments to reduce discomfort during daily activities, including proper seating and posture recommendations for work and home.

Pelvic Floor Rehabilitation:

- Conducting pelvic floor muscle exercises to strengthen the pelvic floor and reduce incontinence.
- Incorporating biofeedback to ensure proper muscle activation.
- Teaching techniques to manage pelvic pain during physical activity, such as gentle stretching and pelvic floor relaxation exercises.
- Providing education on safe body mechanics and posture to alleviate pelvic pain.

Sciatica Management:

- Teaching specific exercises to alleviate sciatic nerve pain, such as piriformis stretches and gentle nerve glides.
- Educating on proper posture and body mechanics to reduce pressure on the sciatic nerve.
- Using positional release techniques to alleviate tension in the gluteal muscles.

Therapeutic Exercises:

- Introducing low-impact exercises such as prenatal yoga and gentle stretching to maintain fitness.
- Teaching core strengthening exercises that are safe during pregnancy, such as modified planks and pelvic tilts.
- Educating on proper activation of the abdominal wall to support the pelvic floor, including exercises like single-leg rollouts and four-point kneeling exercises.

Activity Modification and Energy Conservation:

- Educating the client on how to modify activities to reduce symptom exacerbation, such as avoiding prolonged standing and taking regular rest breaks.

- Implementing energy conservation techniques, such as pacing activities and scheduling rest breaks during high-energy tasks.

Psychosocial Support:

- Offering counseling and support groups to help the client manage emotional distress related to urinary incontinence and pelvic pain.
- Teaching coping mechanisms to deal with stress and anxiety, including mindfulness practices and cognitive-behavioural techniques.

Outcomes:

Post Treatment:

- Reduced pelvic pain and improved pain management skills, with the client reporting a significant decrease in daily pain levels.
- Decreased urinary incontinence episodes, as measured by bladder diary and pad test, with fewer incidents of leakage.
- Reduced sciatica symptoms, with the client reporting fewer episodes of shooting pain down the leg.
- Improved ability to perform a tailored prenatal exercise program safely and effectively.
- Enhanced pelvic floor muscle activation, with the client demonstrating proper techniques during exercises.
- Increased hip external rotation ROM, as measured during physical assessments.
- Improved ability to teach classes with minimal discomfort, allowing her to maintain her professional responsibilities.

Follow-Up Visits:

Two additional visits will focus on reinforcing the client's progress in managing pelvic pain and urinary incontinence. During these visits, the following will be emphasized:

- **Pain Management Techniques**: Reinforcement and practice of relaxation and breathing techniques to manage pain.
- **Pelvic Floor Exercises**: Continued practice and progression of pelvic floor muscle exercises.
- **Sciatica Management**: Continued practice of exercises and techniques to alleviate sciatic nerve pain.
- **Activity Modification**: Ongoing education on modifying activities to reduce strain and discomfort.

The client exhibited significant improvement in managing her pelvic pain, sciatica, and urinary incontinence, as well as maintaining her fitness levels during pregnancy. She is now able to perform daily activities and her tailored exercise program with reduced discomfort and increased confidence. The comprehensive, occupation-based approach in managing pregnancy-related conditions demonstrates the profound impact of holistic occupational therapy care on clients' daily lives and well-being.

Further Reading

ACOG Committee Opinion No. 650: Physical activity and exercise during pregnancy and the postpartum period. (2015). *Obstetrics and Gynecology, 126*(6), e135–e142. https://doi.org/10.1097/AOG.0000000000001214

Beyers, C. N., Weaver, J. A., Huyber, C. M., Currin-McCulloch, J., & Schmid, A. A. (2024). Occupational therapists' perspectives and role with illness-induced trauma from medical conditions. *Occupational Therapy Journal of Research: Occupation, Participation and Health*, 15394492241247735. Advance online publication. https://doi.org/10.1177/15394492241247735

Chandra, M., & Paray, A. A. (2024). Natural physiological changes during pregnancy. *The Yale Journal of Biology and Medicine, 97*(1), 85–92. https://doi.org/10.59249/JTIV4138

Chauhan, A., & Potdar, J. (2022). Maternal mental health during pregnancy: A critical review. *Cureus, 14*(10), e30656. https://doi.org/10.7759/cureus.30656

Felice, E., Agius, A., Sultana, R., Felice, E. M., & Calleja-Agius, J. (2018). The effectiveness of psychosocial assessment in the detection and management of postpartum depression: A systematic review. *Minerva Ginecologica, 70*(3), 323–345. https://doi.org/10.23736/S0026-4784.17.04080-1

Franco-Antonio, C., Santano-Mogena, E., Chimento-Díaz, S., Sánchez-García, P., & Cordovilla-Guardia, S. (2022). A randomised controlled trial evaluating the effect of a brief motivational intervention to promote breastfeeding in postpartum depression. *Scientific Reports, 12*(1), 373. https://doi.org/10.1038/s41598-021-04338-w

Güngör, E., & Karakuzu Güngör, Z. (2024). Obstetric-related lower back pain: The effect of number of pregnancy on development of chronic lower back pain, worsening of lumbar disc degeneration and alteration of lumbar sagittal balance. *Journal of Orthopedic Surgery and Research, 19*(1), 174. https://doi.org/10.1186/s13018-024-04647-6

Igwe, J. N., Edikpa, E. C., Chikaodinaka, O. A., Ani, M. I., Ekeh, D. O., Eze, N. J., Nweze, B. N., Metu, I. C., Mbelede, N. G., Ezemoyih, C. M., & Ugwuanyi, C. S. (2024). Effectiveness of cognitive behavior therapy on occupational stress management among administrative, language, science and vocational education staff within open and distance learning centers: A randomized controlled trial evaluation. *Medicine, 103*(9), e37231. https://doi.org/10.1097/MD.0000000000037231

Ituk, U., & Habib, A. S. (2018). Enhanced recovery after cesarean delivery. *F1000Research, 7*, F1000 Faculty Rev-513. https://doi.org/10.12688/f1000research.13895.1

Khadivzadeh, T., Shojaeian, Z., & Sahebi, A. (2023). High risk-pregnant women's experiences of risk management: A qualitative study. *International Journal of Community-based Nursing and Midwifery, 11*(1), 57–66. https://doi.org/10.30476/IJCBNM.2022.96781.2148

Khan, S. (2023). Occupational therapy's unique role in maternal health and well-being. *OT Practice Magazine, 28*(8), 12–15.

Maman, R., Rand, D., & Avrech Bar, M. (2022). A scoping review of the maternal role at older age: Perceptions and occupations. *International Journal of Environmental Research and Public Health, 19*(1), 492. https://doi.org/10.3390/ijerph19010492

Mishra, S., & Kishore, S. (2018). Effect of physical activity during pregnancy on gestational diabetes mellitus. *Indian Journal of Endocrinology and Metabolism, 22*(5), 661–671. https://doi.org/10.4103/ijem.IJEM_618_17

Nelson, R. K., Hafner, S. M., Cook, A. C., Sterner, N. J., Butler, E. L., Jakiemiec, B. E., & Saltarelli, W. A. (2022). Exercise during pregnancy: What do OB/GYNs believe and practice? A descriptive analysis. *Women's Health Reports (New Rochelle, N.Y.), 3*(1), 274–280. https://doi.org/10.1089/whr2021.0132.

Palacio, M., & Mottola, M. F. (2023). Activity restriction and hospitalization in pregnancy: Can bedrest exercise prevent deconditioning? A narrative review. *International Journal of Environmental Research and Public Health, 20*(2), 1454. https://doi.org/10.3390/ijerph20021454

Parush, S., Lapidot, G., Edelstein, P. V., & Tamir, D. (1987). Occupational therapy in mother and child health care centers. *The American Journal of Occupational Therapy: Official Publication of the American Occupational Therapy Association, 41*(9), 601–605. https://doi.org/10.5014/ajot.41.9.601

Pitonyak, J. S. (2014). Occupational therapy and breastfeeding promotion: Our role in societal health. *The American Journal of Ocupational Therapy: Official Publication of the American Occupational Therapy Association, 68*(3), e90–e96. https://doi.org/10.5014/ajot.2014.009746

Puro, N., Kelly, R. J., Bodas, M., & Feyereisen, S. (2022). Estimating the differences in Caesarean section (C-section) rates between public and privately insured mothers in Florida: A decomposition approach. *PloS one*, *17*(4), e0266666. https://doi.org/10.1371/journal.pone.0266666

Santos-Rocha, R., Fernandes de Carvalho, M., Prior de Freitas, J., Wegrzyk, J., & Szumilewicz, A. (2022). Active pregnancy: A physical exercise program promoting fitness and health during pregnancy—Development and validation of a complex intervention. *International Journal of Environmental Research and Public Health*, *19*(8), 4902. https://doi.org/10.3390/ijerph19084902

Satone, P. D., & Tayade, S. A. (2023). Alternative birthing positions compared to the conventional position in the second stage of labor: A review. *Cureus*, *15*(4), e37943. https://doi.org/10.7759/cureus.37943

Tabatabaeichehr, M., & Mortazavi, H. (2020). The effectiveness of aromatherapy in the management of labor pain and anxiety: A systematic review. *Ethiopian Journal of Health Sciences*, *30*(3), 449–458. https://doi.org/10.4314/ejhs.v30i3.16

Takelle, G. M., Muluneh, N. Y., & Biresaw, M. S. (2022). Sleep quality and associated factors among pregnant women attending antenatal care unit at Gondar, Ethiopia: A cross-sectional study. *BMJ Open*, *12*(9), e056564. https://doi.org/10.1136/bmjopen-2021-056564

Traylor, C. S., Johnson, J. D., Kimmel, M. C., & Manuck, T. A. (2020). Effects of psychological stress on adverse pregnancy outcomes and nonpharmacologic approaches for reduction: An expert review. *American Journal of Obstetrics & Gynecology MFM*, *2*(4), 100229. https://doi.org/10.1016/j.ajogmf.2020.100229

Wagnild, J. M., Hinshaw, K., & Pollard, T. M. (2019). Associations of sedentary time and self-reported television time during pregnancy with incident gestational diabetes and plasma glucose levels in women at risk of gestational diabetes in the UK. *BMC Public Health*, *19*(1), 575. https://doi.org/10.1186/s12889-019-6928-5

Wang, S., Rexrode, K. M., Florio, A. A., Rich-Edwards, J. W., & Chavarro, J. E. (2023). Maternal mortality in the United States: Trends and opportunities for prevention. *Annual Review of Medicine*, *74*, 199–216. https://doi.org/10.1146/annurev-med-042921-123851

4 Endocrine Health

> **Chapter Objectives**
>
> Upon completion of this chapter, the reader will be able to:
>
> 1. Understand the role of hormones in women's health and the common endocrine conditions that can affect occupational performance.
> 2. Explore the occupational therapy approaches to managing endocrine conditions and hormonal imbalances, emphasizing individualized care and the importance of holistic strategies.
> 3. Discuss contraception and family planning from an occupational therapy perspective, detailing interventions that support women in integrating these aspects into their daily lives.
> 4. Address the management of perimenopausal and menopausal transitions, providing practical strategies for OTPs to support women during these significant life stages.
> 5. Highlight the use of assistive technology and community resources in managing symptoms related to hormonal changes, enhancing women's engagement in desired occupations and social participation.

Overview of Hormone Health

Hormones are critical chemical messengers produced by endocrine glands like the pituitary, thyroid, adrenal glands, pancreas, and reproductive organs. They regulate crucial functions such as growth, metabolism, reproduction, and emotional well-being. Fluctuations in hormone levels can significantly impact a woman's quality of life, influencing her ability to perform daily tasks and engage fully in life activities.

Hormonal imbalances, characterized by excess or deficiency of hormones, can lead to a range of symptoms such as weight changes, fatigue, mood swings, and altered metabolic rates. These imbalances are particularly prevalent among women, with studies indicating that up to 80% experience hormone-related symptoms at various life stages, including

156 *Occupational Therapy and Women's Health*

Table 4.1 Hormonal changes and symptoms across a woman's life

Life Stage	Hormones Impacted	Typical Changes	Potential Symptoms and Impact on Daily Life
Adolescence	Estrogen, Progesterone	Onset of menstruation; hormone levels begin to fluctuate	Mood swings, acne, initiation of menstrual pain
Reproductive Age	Estrogen, Progesterone	Hormones stabilize to support reproductive health	PMS, potential pregnancy-related hormonal shifts
Premenopause	Estrogen, Progesterone	Hormone levels decline gradually	Irregular periods, mood changes, sleep disturbances
Menopause	Estrogen, Progesterone	Significant drop in hormone levels	Hot flashes, increased risk of osteoporosis, mood swings
Post-menopause	Estrogen, Progesterone	Low levels maintained	Continued risk of osteoporosis, vaginal dryness, mood changes

premenstrual syndrome, perimenopause, and menopause. Such symptoms can severely affect daily functioning and emotional well-being.

For instance, a 2023 study published in the *Mayo Clinic Proceedings* revealed that 13.4% of women aged 45 to 60 experienced adverse work outcomes due to menopausal symptoms, with significant absenteeism costing an estimated $1.8 billion annually in lost productivity in the United States alone. This highlights the economic and personal impacts of hormonal imbalances on women's lives. To visualize how hormonal changes affect women through different life stages, Table 4.1 outlines natural hormonal transitions from adolescence through post-menopause and their implications for daily life and occupational performance.

Role of Occupational Therapy in Hormone Health Management

In line with the Occupational Therapy Practice Framework, health management involves activities that enhance health, well-being, and quality of life. This includes managing nutrition, medication routines, and lifestyle modifications. OTPs are pivotal in helping women manage the challenges posed by hormonal imbalances. Effective strategies include dietary modifications to enhance hormone production, promoting physical activity for better hormonal receptor sensitivity, and employing stress management techniques to regulate cortisol levels. Ensuring adequate sleep and managing body weight are also crucial for maintaining hormonal balance.

OTPs also educate and assist women in implementing strategies to mitigate the effects of hormonal imbalances. This holistic approach helps women maintain their roles and routines, enhancing their overall health and enabling them to engage meaningfully in occupational activities. For detailed insights into how specific hormones affect occupational activities, see Table 4.2.

Table 4.2 Key hormones in women's health, their primary functions, and considerations during occupational activities

Hormone	Source	Primary Functions	Considerations During Occupational Activities
Estrogen	Ovaries	Regulates menstrual cycle, reproductive system, and bone health	Influences mood and physical capacity; consider scheduling demanding tasks during high-energy times of the cycle; incorporate energy conservation techniques during menstruation and menopause to manage fatigue and discomfort.
Progesterone	Ovaries	Supports pregnancy, regulates menstrual cycle	Important in pregnancy management; focus on ergonomic adjustments for comfort and safety in workplace and home settings; provide education on positioning and body mechanics to reduce discomfort.
Testosterone	Ovaries and Adrenal Glands	Influences muscle mass, libido, and mood	Can affect motivation and energy; incorporate strength training exercises to enhance muscle mass and improve mood; provide strategies to boost energy levels, especially post-menopause.
Thyroid Hormones (T3 and T4)	Thyroid Gland	Regulates metabolism, energy levels, and temperature	Monitor for signs of fatigue or anxiety; tailor activity levels and work tasks to the client's energy levels; provide strategies for thermal comfort and adjustments in daily routines.
Cortisol	Adrenal Glands	Manages stress response, regulates metabolism	High levels may necessitate stress management techniques like mindfulness and relaxation exercises to prevent burnout; educate on pacing activities and incorporating regular breaks to manage stress effectively.
Insulin	Pancreas	Controls blood glucose levels	Diet and exercise interventions are crucial for energy management; provide education on meal planning, carbohydrate counting, and balancing food intake with physical activity to maintain stable blood glucose levels.
Prolactin	Pituitary Gland	Promotes milk production after childbirth	Consider scheduling flexibility for breastfeeding mothers to accommodate milk expression; provide ergonomic solutions and time management strategies to reduce stress and physical strain.
Oxytocin	Pituitary Gland	Facilitates childbirth, bonding, and lactation	Encourage social interactions and bonding activities to enhance group therapy effectiveness; support the creation of strong patient support networks to promote emotional well-being.

Table 4.3 Common endocrine conditions and associated hormonal imbalances, including associated symptoms that can affect daily functioning

Condition	Hormonal Imbalance	Symptoms
Hypothyroidism	Low thyroid hormones (T3, T4)	Fatigue, weight gain, depression, cold intolerance
Hyperthyroidism	High thyroid hormones (T3, T4)	Weight loss, anxiety, heat intolerance, palpitations
Polycystic Ovary Syndrome (PCOS)	Elevated androgens, insulin resistance	Irregular periods, weight gain, acne, hirsutism
Diabetes (Type 1 and Type 2)	Insufficient insulin production or insulin resistance	Increased thirst, frequent urination, fatigue, blurred vision
Adrenal Insufficiency	Low cortisol	Fatigue, muscle weakness, weight loss, low blood pressure
Perimenopause	Fluctuating estrogen and progesterone	Irregular periods, hot flashes, mood swings, sleep disturbances
Menopause	Decreased estrogen and progesterone	Hot flashes, mood swings, sleep disturbances, vaginal dryness

Occupational Therapy Approaches to Endocrine Conditions and Hormonal Imbalances

OTPs are essential in addressing the complex needs of women experiencing endocrine conditions and hormonal imbalances. These medical issues manifest through a spectrum of symptoms—from weight fluctuations and mood swings to more severe metabolic and physiological changes. Each symptom can profoundly impact daily living and occupational performance, necessitating specialized therapeutic interventions.

OTPs are equipped to offer customized care plans that consider the unique hormonal profiles and life circumstances of each patient. By focusing on individualized management strategies, OTPs help women navigate the challenges of hormonal imbalances, enhancing their ability to maintain personal and professional responsibilities. Table 4.3 outlines various endocrine disorders, their hormonal underpinnings, and typical symptoms, providing a foundation for OTPs to tailor their therapeutic approaches effectively.

Conditions Overview and OT Interventions

Hypothyroidism: Hypothyroidism involves low levels of thyroid hormones (T3 and T4), leading to symptoms such as fatigue, weight gain, depression, and cold intolerance. These symptoms can substantially affect daily functioning and occupational performance across a range of activities.

Impact on Daily Life:

- **ADLs**: Fatigue and muscle weakness can make it challenging to perform basic self-care tasks such as bathing, dressing, and grooming. Cold intolerance can further reduce motivation to engage in these activities.
- **IADLs**: Weight gain and low energy levels can hinder the ability to complete more complex tasks such as meal preparation, house cleaning, and managing finances. Depression can exacerbate the neglect of these responsibilities, impacting the ability to maintain an organized living environment.

- **Work**: Hypothyroidism can cause cognitive difficulties such as impaired memory and concentration, affecting job performance and productivity. The physical and mental fatigue associated with hypothyroidism further reduces work efficiency.
- **Social Participation**: The physical and emotional symptoms of hypothyroidism can reduce social engagement. Individuals may withdraw from social activities due to fatigue, low mood, or self-consciousness about weight gain.

Occupational Therapy Interventions:

- **Energy Conservation Techniques**: Instruct clients on planning and prioritizing tasks to conserve energy. Integrate rest breaks into daily routines and recommend using labor-saving devices. For instance, using a stool while cooking can minimize the strain from prolonged standing. Encouraging seated activities, like sitting while dressing or grooming, helps manage energy levels efficiently.
- **Adaptive Strategies for Cold Intolerance**: Advise on using thermal clothing and heated items such as blankets or seat warmers to maintain comfort. Recommend adjustments to the home heating system or the use of portable heaters in frequently used areas to create a warm living environment.
- **Nutrition Management**: Collaborate with dietitians to develop diet plans rich in nutrients that support thyroid function, such as iodine, selenium, and zinc. High-protein and high-fiber meals can aid in weight control and enhance energy levels.
- **Therapeutic Activities**: Promote engagement in light physical activities like walking or gentle resistance training to boost metabolism and overall energy. Tailor these activities to be indoor-friendly during colder months to accommodate cold intolerance.
- **Psychosocial Approaches**: Facilitate support groups and provide counseling to address the emotional impacts of hypothyroidism. Cognitive strategies such as using planners or smartphone reminders can help manage forgetfulness and disorganization. Encourage gradual social participation to mitigate feelings of isolation and improve emotional well-being.

Hyperthyroidism: Unlike hypothyroidism, which is characterized by low levels of thyroid hormones, hyperthyroidism involves high levels of thyroid hormones (T3 and T4). This condition presents with symptoms such as weight loss, anxiety, heat intolerance, and palpitations, which can disrupt various occupational activities including ADLs, IADLs, sleep, work, and community mobility.

Impact on Daily Life:

1. **ADLs**: Heat intolerance might make it uncomfortable for individuals to engage in warm environments or activities that raise body temperature such as taking hot showers or baths. Anxiety and restlessness can make it challenging to focus on and complete routine tasks like bathing, dressing, or grooming. Individuals may rush through these activities or avoid them due to discomfort from heat or palpitations.
2. **IADLs**: Palpitations and elevated heart rate can make sustained physical activities, such as meal preparation and household cleaning, difficult. Anxiety can also hinder the ability to concentrate on financial management or complex decision-making tasks.
3. **Work**: The symptoms of hyperthyroidism, such as difficulty concentrating and general restlessness, can diminish job performance and productivity. Anxiety and palpitations might lead to frequent breaks or absences, impacting work continuity and efficiency.

160   Occupational Therapy and Women's Health

4. **Sleep**: The increased metabolic rate and palpitations can cause insomnia and frequent awakenings, disrupting sleep patterns and leading to significant daytime fatigue that affects overall daily performance.
5. **Community Mobility**: Anxiety and palpitations may also deter individuals from engaging in community activities, fearing a public episode or inability to manage symptoms in social settings.

Occupational Therapy Interventions:

- **Adaptive Techniques for ADLs**: Recommend cooler, shorter showers and the use of lukewarm water to avoid exacerbating heat intolerance. Suggest the installation of good ventilation in bathrooms and the use of personal fans to keep the environment comfortable. For dressing, advise wearing light, breathable fabrics that do not trap heat.
- **Stress Management Techniques**: Implement mindfulness, diaphragmatic breathing, and progressive muscle relaxation to manage anxiety and reduce stress levels. Daily guided meditations can help stabilize mood and improve physiological responses to stress.
- **Therapeutic Exercises**: Encourage low-impact exercises such as yoga or swimming, which are less likely to increase body temperature excessively. These activities help maintain muscle mass and cardiovascular health while accommodating heat intolerance.
- **Environmental Adjustments**: Ensure living and work spaces are well-ventilated and cool to manage heat intolerance. This may involve using air conditioning, portable fans, and optimizing the layout of rooms for increased airflow.
- **Psychosocial Support**: Provide counseling to address anxiety and mood swings. Support groups can offer a venue for sharing coping strategies and experiences, helping clients to feel less isolated in their experiences.
- **Activity Modification**: Help clients adjust the pacing and scheduling of activities to prevent overstimulation and manage energy effectively. This might include organizing tasks to align with times when energy levels are higher and symptoms are more manageable.

Polycystic Ovary Syndrome (PCOS): PCOS is a condition characterized by elevated androgens (male hormones) and insulin resistance, which can lead to a variety of symptoms including irregular menstrual cycles, weight gain, acne, and hirsutism—the abnormal growth of hair on a woman's face and body. This condition can profoundly impact different aspects of life, including physical health, emotional well-being, and social participation.

Impact on Daily Life:

- **ADLs**: The appearance-related symptoms of PCOS, such as acne and hirsutism, can significantly affect self-esteem and body image, making routine self-care tasks like grooming and dressing emotionally challenging.
- **IADLs**: Weight gain and fatigue may hinder the ability to manage complex tasks such as meal preparation and household cleaning. Insulin resistance complicates dietary management, adding further challenges to meal planning.
- **Work**: Symptoms like fatigue and mood swings can undermine job performance and productivity. The discomfort from irregular periods can also affect physical presence and concentration at work.

- **Social Participation**: The emotional distress related to body image issues and mood fluctuations may cause individuals to withdraw from social activities, leading to decreased engagement in community events.

Occupational Therapy Interventions:

- **Lifestyle Modifications**: Develop personalized diet and exercise plans to manage weight and improve insulin sensitivity. For example, recommend a balanced diet low in processed sugars and high in fiber, along with regular physical activity such as aerobic exercises and strength training. Collaborating with a dietitian to create meal plans that fit the client's lifestyle can be beneficial.
- **Therapeutic Exercises**: Establish a structured exercise regimen including both cardiovascular and resistance training to improve overall health and address symptoms like insulin resistance and weight management.
- **Self-Management Education**: Educate clients about PCOS and assist them in monitoring symptoms and lifestyle changes effectively, using tools such as apps or journals to keep track of menstrual cycles, dietary intake, and physical activity.
- **Psychosocial Support**: Address body image issues and mood fluctuations through counseling and support groups, providing strategies to improve self-esteem and emotional resilience. Group therapy can offer a community of support and shared experiences, which is beneficial for managing the emotional aspects of PCOS.

Diabetes (type 1 and type 2): Diabetes is a chronic condition characterized by high levels of glucose in the blood due to the body's inability to produce or effectively use insulin. Type 1 diabetes is typically diagnosed in children and young adults and occurs when the body's immune system destroys insulin-producing cells in the pancreas. This type requires lifelong insulin therapy. Type 2 diabetes, which is more common, often develops in adults and is caused by insulin resistance and relative insulin deficiency. Management can involve lifestyle changes, oral medications, and sometimes insulin.

Impact on Daily Life:

- **ADLs**: Both type 1 and type 2 diabetes can cause fatigue and a general feeling of malaise, which can make it difficult to muster the energy for bathing and dressing. Additionally, neurological complications like diabetic neuropathy can decrease sensation, making it harder to handle fasteners or tie shoes, and increasing the risk of injuries from hot water during bathing. Frequent urination, a common symptom of diabetes, can disrupt routines and lead to urgency and incontinence, which affects toileting independence and may require more frequent changes of clothes or specific toileting schedules.
- **IADLs**: Managing diabetes requires careful dietary planning to control blood glucose levels, which can be time-consuming and mentally taxing. Visual impairments due to diabetic retinopathy can make it difficult to read labels or manage finances.
- **Work**: The need for regular blood glucose monitoring and potential episodes of hypo- or hyperglycemia can disrupt work tasks, necessitating breaks and potentially reducing productivity. The chronic fatigue associated with diabetes can also impair concentration and stamina.
- **Social Participation**: Dietary restrictions and the need to monitor blood sugar can complicate social dining and activities, potentially leading to isolation or reduced participation in social events.

Occupational Therapy Interventions:

- **Education and Self-Management**: Teach clients with diabetes how to effectively monitor their blood glucose levels and recognize the signs of hypo- or hyperglycemia. For type 1 diabetes, this includes insulin management education. Develop personalized meal plans in collaboration with dietitians to support blood sugar control and meet nutritional needs.
- **Therapeutic Exercises**: Recommend physical activities tailored to the client's fitness level and medical restrictions, such as low-impact exercises that are less likely to cause hypoglycemia, particularly important for those on insulin or certain diabetic medications.
- **Energy Conservation Techniques**: Provide strategies to balance activity and rest, helping clients prioritize tasks and use adaptive equipment to reduce physical strain, especially vital for those with diabetic neuropathy.
- **Stress Management Techniques**: Implement mindfulness and relaxation exercises to manage the emotional stress associated with managing a chronic condition like diabetes, enhancing overall mental well-being.

Adrenal Insufficiency: Adrenal insufficiency is a condition where the adrenal glands do not produce sufficient levels of cortisol, a hormone crucial for energy regulation, stress response, and immune function. This deficiency can lead to chronic fatigue, muscle weakness, weight loss, and low blood pressure, which profoundly affects daily life and the ability to manage stress and recover from illness.

Impact on Daily Life:

- **ADLs**: Fatigue and muscle weakness can make it exhausting to perform basic self-care, necessitating extended time or assistance. For example, the reduced stamina may make it hard to stand in the shower or manipulate buttons and zippers. Low blood pressure can lead to dizziness when standing up quickly, increasing the risk of falls during transfers to and from the toilet.
- **IADLs**: Low energy and muscle weakness can impede the ability to perform tasks that require standing or lifting, such as cooking or vacuuming. Low blood pressure may exacerbate fatigue during these activities, increasing the need for breaks. Cognitive fatigue can complicate tasks requiring concentration, such as balancing a checkbook or paying bills.
- **Work**: Muscle weakness and fatigue can drastically decrease productivity and increase the need for sick leave. Low blood pressure can lead to sudden dizziness during physical activities or stress, posing safety risks in many work environments.
- **Community Mobility**: General fatigue and muscle weakness can diminish the ability to participate in community activities, while dizziness and low stamina may discourage travel far from home, limiting social interactions and contributing to isolation.

Occupational Therapy Interventions:

- **Energy Conservation Techniques**: Educate clients on managing energy by planning and prioritizing tasks effectively, suggesting times for activities when energy levels are typically higher. Recommend using labor-saving devices like electric toothbrushes or long-handled sponges to reduce exertion.

- **Therapeutic Exercises**: Implement a tailored exercise program that includes low-impact activities such as water aerobics or stationary cycling to build endurance without overstressing the body. Strength training should be gentle but focused on maintaining muscle mass and improving stamina.
- **Nutrition Management**: Work with dietitians to ensure a nutrient-rich diet that supports energy levels and overall health. Small, frequent meals may be encouraged to manage energy better throughout the day.
- **Stress Management**: Techniques such as guided imagery, deep breathing exercises, and progressive muscle relaxation are crucial to help manage the psychological effects of living with chronic illness. These methods help reduce cortisol demand and support overall emotional resilience.
- **Environmental Modifications**: Advise on home modifications to reduce the risk of falls and make daily tasks safer and more accessible, such as installing grab bars in the bathroom and securing rugs to the floor.
- **Social and Psychological Support**: Facilitate access to counseling and support groups to address feelings of isolation or depression that may arise from living with adrenal insufficiency. Provide resources and education on the condition to empower clients and their families.

Perimenopause: Perimenopause marks the transition before menopause, characterized by fluctuating hormone levels, particularly estrogen and progesterone. This phase often brings about a range of symptoms such as irregular periods, hot flashes, mood swings, and sleep disturbances that can profoundly impact daily life.

Impact on Daily Life:

- **ADLs**: Hot flashes and night sweats can disrupt sleep, leading to significant fatigue that makes it difficult to muster the energy for bathing and dressing. Quick changes in body temperature can make these activities uncomfortable, requiring adjustments such as cooler showers or dressing in layers that are easy to modify. Mood swings can disrupt the routine and motivation needed for regular personal care, potentially leading to neglect of personal hygiene.
- **IADLs**: Fluctuations in energy and mood can complicate the planning and execution of cooking tasks. Hot flashes may make time in a warm kitchen particularly uncomfortable. Sleep disturbances and resultant fatigue can impair concentration and cognitive function, making managing finances and complex decision-making more challenging.
- **Work**: The combination of sleep disturbances, mood swings, and physical symptoms like hot flashes can significantly impair concentration, reduce productivity, and increase absenteeism. Physical discomfort during periods can further complicate maintaining a consistent work schedule.
- **Social Participation**: Mood swings and self-consciousness about menopausal symptoms can lead to withdrawal from social activities, reducing participation in community events and impacting overall social engagement.

Occupational Therapy Interventions:

- **Symptom Management**: Provide education on managing hot flashes, such as dressing in layers, staying hydrated, and using fans or cool packs. Teach sleep hygiene practices like maintaining a consistent sleep schedule and creating a restful sleep environment.

For example, recommend breathable, moisture-wicking bedding to improve comfort during sleep.
- **Therapeutic Exercises**: Recommend yoga and low-impact aerobics to manage weight, improve mood, and reduce the severity of hot flashes. These exercises can enhance flexibility, strength, and overall well-being without causing excessive strain.
- **Stress Management Techniques**: Teach mindfulness and relaxation exercises to help manage mood swings and emotional stress. Techniques such as progressive muscle relaxation and guided imagery can be integrated into daily routines to reduce stress and improve emotional regulation.
- **Psychosocial Support**: Provide counseling to address mood changes and offer support groups for sharing experiences and coping strategies. Support groups can offer a sense of community and shared understanding, which can be particularly comforting during this transitional period.
- **Activity Modification**: Adjust activities to accommodate fluctuating energy levels and ensure continued participation in meaningful activities. For instance, recommend scheduling demanding tasks during periods of higher energy and incorporating regular breaks to prevent fatigue.

Menopause: Menopause marks the end of a woman's reproductive years, characterized by the cessation of menstrual cycles due to the decline in estrogen and progesterone levels. This phase typically occurs between the ages of 45 and 55 and brings about several physiological and psychological changes. Symptoms commonly associated with menopause include hot flashes, mood swings, sleep disturbances, vaginal dryness, and a decrease in bone density. These changes can significantly affect various aspects of daily life and overall well-being.

Impact on Daily Life:
- **ADLs**: Sleep disturbances and night sweats may make it challenging to maintain personal hygiene routines. Fatigue from poor sleep can reduce the energy required for these tasks. Vaginal dryness and discomfort may also affect personal care routines, particularly those involving hygiene and comfort.
- **IADLs**: Fluctuating energy levels and mood swings can complicate tasks requiring focus and physical effort, such as cooking and home upkeep. Hot flashes may make kitchen activities uncomfortable, and decreased motivation from mood swings can affect overall task management. Cognitive changes such as reduced concentration can affect a woman's ability to manage finances and organize complex tasks effectively.
- **Work**: Menopausal symptoms like hot flashes, mood instability, and fatigue can impair focus and productivity, potentially leading to increased absenteeism and reduced work engagement.
- **Social Participation**: Physical and emotional changes may lead women to withdraw from social activities. Self-consciousness about symptoms like hot flashes or mood changes can further reduce participation in social and community events.

Occupational Therapy Interventions:
- **Symptom Management for Hot Flashes and Sleep Disturbances**: Educate on managing hot flashes through environmental control, such as adjusting the room temperature and

using fans. Recommend wearing layers of clothing that can be easily adjusted to manage body temperature changes. For sleep disturbances, advise on sleep hygiene techniques, including establishing a regular sleep schedule and creating a comfortable, cool sleeping environment.
- **Resistance Training for Bone Health**: Recommend strength training exercises to stimulate bone formation, maintain muscle mass, and reduce the risk of osteoporosis. This can include weight-bearing exercises such as walking, squats, and resistance band exercises. Strength training can help maintain bone density and muscle strength, reducing the risk of fractures.
- **Fall Prevention**: Perform home safety evaluations and recommend modifications to reduce fall risks, such as securing rugs, improving lighting, and installing grab bars in strategic areas like the bathroom.
- **Stress Management Techniques**: Implement relaxation techniques such as progressive muscle relaxation, mindfulness, and deep breathing exercises to help manage emotional stress and enhance mood stability.
- **Psychosocial Support**: Provide counseling and support groups to address emotional and psychological challenges associated with menopause. Support groups can offer a platform for sharing experiences and strategies, which is invaluable for emotional support and practical advice.
- **Diet and Nutrition Management**: Work with dietitians to ensure a diet rich in calcium, vitamin D, and other nutrients critical for bone health and overall well-being. Educate on the importance of a balanced diet that supports energy levels and health, incorporating elements like calcium-rich foods and vitamin supplements as necessary.

OTPs collaborate closely with endocrinologists and other healthcare professionals to provide holistic care that addresses the wide spectrum of symptoms associated with hormonal imbalances. Through these collaborative efforts, OTPs not only contribute their unique expertise in managing daily and occupational challenges but also ensure that interventions are well-coordinated and comprehensive, thereby significantly enhancing outcomes for women navigating these complex conditions.

Contraception and Family Planning in Women's Health

Contraception and family planning are foundational elements in women's health, offering the power of choice regarding reproductive decisions. These decisions significantly influence women's health outcomes, socioeconomic status, and opportunities for personal and career development. For OTPs, understanding and supporting effective family planning is essential as it impacts a woman's engagement in various life roles, ability to maintain balanced routines, and capacity to navigate life transitions effectively.

OTPs aid women in making informed reproductive decisions, aligning their family planning with their occupational roles and overall life goals. This support helps women manage health demands, balance work and family life, and pursue personal aspirations without the unforeseen challenges of unintended pregnancies. Effective family planning can alleviate physical and emotional stresses, fostering sustained participation in desired daily and occupational activities. OTPs are also instrumental in guiding women through the complexities of fertility treatments and postpartum contraception choices, ultimately enhancing life satisfaction and well-being (Table 4.4).

Table 4.4 Occupational therapy interventions in contraception and family planning

Intervention	Description	Examples
Education and Counseling	Providing comprehensive information about contraceptive options and family planning strategies.	Discussing hormonal methods, IUDs, barrier methods, and natural family planning techniques.
Routine and Lifestyle Management	Assisting women in integrating contraceptive routines into daily life and promoting health for pregnancy preparation.	Setting reminders for contraceptive use, advising on nutritional needs and physical activity regimens.
Support for Fertility Treatments	Offering support for physical and emotional demands associated with fertility treatments.	Stress reduction techniques, energy conservation strategies.
Postpartum Contraception Planning	Aiding new mothers in selecting and managing post-childbirth contraception methods.	Discussing options, integrating new routines, emphasizing the importance of consistent contraceptive use.
Use of Assistive Technology	Utilizing technology to enhance adherence to contraception and effective family planning.	Apps for menstrual cycle tracking, medication adherence reminders.
Addressing Barriers and Accessibility	Identifying and overcoming barriers to effective contraceptive use and accessibility.	Tailoring strategies for individuals with physical, cognitive, or emotional challenges.

OT Interventions in Contraception and Family Planning

Education and Counseling

OTPs play an important role in providing education and counseling about contraception and family planning. This includes discussing the various contraceptive options available, such as hormonal methods (pills, patches, injections), intrauterine devices (IUDs), barrier methods (condoms, diaphragms), and natural family planning techniques. OTPs can help women understand the benefits, risks, and proper use of each method, enabling them to make informed decisions that align with their health needs and personal values.

Routine and Lifestyle Management

For women planning to conceive, OTPs can offer guidance on preparing for pregnancy by promoting a healthy lifestyle. This includes nutrition management, recommending appropriate physical activity, and stress management techniques to ensure optimal health before and during pregnancy. For those not planning to conceive, OTPs can help integrate contraceptive routines into daily life, ensuring consistent and effective use. Examples include setting daily reminders for taking birth control pills or integrating contraceptive device checks into personal hygiene routines.

Support for Fertility Treatments

Women undergoing fertility treatments can benefit from the support of OTPs, who provide practical strategies for managing the intense regimen of medications and medical appointments. OTPs help clients develop relaxation techniques such as guided meditations or yoga, which can alleviate the stress associated with treatment cycles. They also offer energy conservation strategies, such as teaching how to balance rest and activity to prevent burnout. Emotional support includes facilitating discussions in therapy sessions that allow women to express their feelings and fears about the fertility process, which can be a rollercoaster of hope and disappointment.

Postpartum Contraception Planning

After childbirth, OTPs can assist new mothers in choosing and managing contraception effectively, helping integrate the use of contraceptives into their often-hectic postpartum routines. This support includes educating mothers on the various contraceptive methods that are safe during breastfeeding and helping them consider how their choice impacts their lifestyle and health. By creating reminder systems and simplifying the routine, OTPs ensure that new mothers can focus more on their recovery and less on the stress of potential subsequent pregnancies. They also provide guidance on how hormonal changes after childbirth might affect their physical and emotional health, ensuring that contraceptive choices align with their recovery.

Addressing Barriers and Accessibility

OTPs are crucial in identifying and addressing barriers to effective contraceptive use, particularly for women facing physical, cognitive, or emotional challenges. They work to adapt contraceptive methods to individual needs, such as recommending lower maintenance contraceptive options like IUDs for women who may have difficulty with daily pills due to cognitive challenges. For those with physical disabilities, OTPs might suggest devices with easier application methods or provide custom-designed aids to assist with the application of contraceptives. Additionally, they train women to use adaptive devices and modify environments to ease the use of contraceptives, ensuring that all women have the autonomy to manage their reproductive health effectively.

Use of Assistive Technology

Leveraging technology to support contraception adherence and family planning can be highly effective. OTPs evaluate the most suitable technological solutions for individual women, such as recommending smartphone apps that remind women of contraceptive doses or track fertility windows accurately. For example, they might suggest apps that sync with digital calendars to alert women of critical dates or integrate with health monitoring devices to track physiological changes. This use of technology not only supports adherence but also empowers women to take proactive roles in managing their reproductive health, providing them with data-driven insights into their bodies.

By integrating these interventions, OTPs play a pivotal role in the realm of women's health, particularly in the domains of contraception and family planning. Collaborating with endocrinologists, gynecologists, and a broader multidisciplinary team, OTPs ensure that each woman receives holistic, personalized care that supports not only her physical health but also her occupational and emotional well-being. This interprofessional approach is crucial for delivering comprehensive healthcare that aligns with the unique needs and life goals of each woman, emphasizing the critical role of occupational therapy in supporting women throughout various stages of life.

Managing Perimenopausal and Menopausal Transition

Perimenopause is the transitional period before menopause, characterized by fluctuating levels of estrogen and progesterone. This phase can last several years and includes symptoms such as irregular periods, hot flashes, night sweats, mood swings, and sleep disturbances. A woman might suspect she is in perimenopause if she experiences these symptoms and irregular menstrual cycles. Healthcare providers typically diagnose perimenopause based on a combination of symptoms, menstrual history, and sometimes hormone levels. Menopause marks the end of menstrual cycles and is diagnosed after 12 consecutive months without a period. The decrease in estrogen levels during menopause can lead to symptoms like hot flashes, mood swings, sleep disturbances, vaginal dryness, and an increased risk of osteoporosis. Table 4.5 highlights differences between perimenopause and menopause with potential impact on daily living.

Maintaining bone health during perimenopause and menopause is critically important due to the accelerated loss of bone density associated with decreased estrogen levels. This can lead to an increased risk of osteoporosis, which significantly impacts a woman's ability to engage in daily activities and maintain independence. Resistance training is especially beneficial for older adults as it helps stimulate bone formation, maintain muscle mass, and improve overall physical health. By incorporating resistance exercises, women can reduce the risk of fractures, enhance balance, and support their ability to perform daily tasks.

Table 4.5 Comparative overview of perimenopause and menopause symptoms and their impact on daily living

Aspect	Peri-menopause	Menopause
Hormonal Fluctuations	Significant fluctuations in estrogen and progesterone	Marked decrease in estrogen and progesterone
Menstrual Changes	Irregular periods, heavier or lighter menstrual flow	Absence of periods for 12 consecutive months
Hot Flashes/Night Sweats	Frequent and intense episodes affecting sleep and comfort	Persistent but may decrease in intensity over time
Mood Swings	Common, due to hormonal fluctuations	Mood may stabilize but can still experience depression or anxiety
Sleep Disturbances	Increased difficulty falling or staying asleep	Ongoing sleep issues, often due to hot flashes or night sweats
Bone Health	Beginning of bone density loss	Accelerated bone density loss, increased risk of osteoporosis
Energy Levels	Fluctuating energy, fatigue	Persistent fatigue due to hormonal changes and sleep disturbances
Cognitive Function	Memory lapses, difficulty concentrating	Potential for cognitive decline
Sexual Health	Vaginal dryness, decreased libido	Continued vaginal dryness, decreased libido
Impact on ADLs/IADLs	Disrupted daily routines due to fatigue and mood changes	Potentially decreased ability to perform daily activities due to persistent symptoms
Work Performance	Decreased productivity, increased absenteeism	Ongoing challenges with work performance and attendance
Community Mobility	May be impacted by fatigue and sleep disturbances	Continued impact due to persistent symptoms and reduced energy

Additionally, sexual health changes, such as vaginal dryness and decreased libido, are common during perimenopause and menopause. These changes can impact intimacy and overall quality of life. OTPs can provide valuable support to women experiencing these symptoms through education, lifestyle modifications, and specific therapeutic interventions.

Occupational Therapy Considerations

In the realm of women's health, OTPs play a vital role in navigating the multifaceted challenges posed by hormonal changes, particularly during menopause and other significant life transitions. As the body undergoes these changes, symptoms can arise that significantly affect daily life, requiring interventions that are not only reactive but also proactive. OTPs employ a variety of therapeutic techniques that go beyond traditional treatment, fostering holistic wellness that addresses physical symptoms, psychological well-being, and social connectivity. Such integrative approaches ensure that therapy aligns with the personal and occupational goals of the individual, promoting sustained health and a higher quality of life in a manner that respects the unique experiences of each woman.

Advanced Symptom Management

For women experiencing severe symptoms, advanced techniques such as biofeedback for managing hot flashes or cognitive-behavioural therapy (CBT) for mood disturbances can be integrated into the treatment plan. OTPs can collaborate with mental health professionals to provide comprehensive care that addresses both physical and psychological symptoms. For instance, biofeedback sessions can teach women how to modulate their physiological responses to stress, potentially lessening the frequency and severity of hot flashes. Similarly, CBT can be adapted to help women challenge unhelpful beliefs about menopause and develop healthier coping mechanisms for mood regulation.

Examples:

- **Biofeedback for Hot Flashes**: OTPs can use biofeedback techniques to help women understand and control physiological responses that trigger hot flashes. This might involve teaching clients to use breathing exercises or progressive muscle relaxation to reduce the frequency and intensity of hot flashes.
- **Cognitive-Behavioural Therapy (CBT)**: OTPs can work alongside psychologists to incorporate CBT strategies into the treatment plan. This could involve helping clients identify and change negative thought patterns related to mood swings or anxiety, improving their emotional regulation and coping skills.
- **Stress Reduction Techniques**: OTPs can teach and implement advanced stress management techniques such as guided imagery, progressive muscle relaxation, or mindfulness meditation, which can help reduce overall stress and manage symptoms more effectively.

Holistic Wellness Programs

Developing holistic wellness programs that incorporate physical, mental, and social health can be highly beneficial. These programs might include yoga classes tailored for menopausal women, mindfulness workshops, nutritional seminars, and social support groups. OTPs play a critical role in organizing and leading these initiatives, ensuring they are accessible and meet the specific needs of women at different stages of menopause. For example, yoga sessions can focus on poses that improve joint health and reduce stress, while nutritional seminars can provide strategies for managing weight and hormonal balance through diet.

Examples:

- **Yoga Classes**: OTPs can design and lead yoga classes that focus on gentle stretching, balance, and relaxation techniques specifically tailored to menopausal women. These classes can help improve flexibility, reduce stress, and enhance overall well-being.
- **Mindfulness Workshops**: OTPs can conduct workshops teaching mindfulness techniques, such as mindful breathing, body scans, and mindful movement. These workshops can help women manage stress and enhance their emotional resilience.
- **Nutritional Seminars**: Collaborating with dietitians, OTPs can organize seminars that educate women on the importance of a balanced diet rich in calcium and vitamin D to support bone health, as well as foods that can help manage menopausal symptoms.
- **Social Support Groups**: OTPs can facilitate support groups where women can share their experiences, challenges, and coping strategies related to menopause. These groups can provide emotional support and foster a sense of community.

Community Resources and Support Networks

Connecting clients with community resources and support networks is vital for providing comprehensive care. OTPs can guide clients to local and online support groups, fitness classes, and educational workshops focused on menopause and healthy aging. These resources enhance the client's support system and encourage active social engagement, which is crucial during the transition through menopause. By promoting community involvement, OTPs help clients find peer support and additional resources to manage their symptoms effectively.

Examples:

- **Local Support Groups**: OTPs can compile a list of local support groups for menopausal women and encourage clients to participate. These groups can offer peer support and a platform to discuss common challenges and solutions.
- **Fitness Classes**: Providing information on local fitness classes tailored for older adults or specifically for menopausal women, such as aqua aerobics or low-impact aerobics, can help clients stay active and healthy.
- **Educational Workshops**: OTPs can organize or recommend workshops on topics such as osteoporosis prevention, heart health, and mental well-being during menopause. These workshops can provide valuable knowledge and practical tips for managing health during this transition.

Technology Integration

Leveraging technology to support symptom management and health monitoring can significantly enhance the effectiveness of occupational therapy interventions. OTPs can introduce clients to apps for tracking menopausal symptoms, setting medication reminders, and practicing relaxation techniques. Furthermore, the use of telehealth services

Endocrine Health   171

allows for continuous support and counseling, making it easier for clients to access care when they need it. This approach not only aids in symptom management but also supports clients in maintaining independence and control over their health.

Examples:

- **Symptom Tracking Apps**: OTPs can recommend and train clients on using mobile apps that track menopausal symptoms such as hot flashes, sleep disturbances, and mood changes. These apps can help clients monitor their symptoms and identify patterns or triggers.
- **Medication Reminders**: OTPs can introduce clients to apps or smart devices that send reminders to take medications or supplements, ensuring adherence to treatment plans.
- **Relaxation Technique Apps**: Recommending apps that offer guided meditations, breathing exercises, or progressive muscle relaxation can help clients practice stress management techniques regularly.
- **Telehealth Services**: OTPs can provide virtual sessions to continue therapy, offer counseling, and monitor progress. Telehealth can be especially beneficial for clients who have difficulty attending in-person appointments due to mobility issues or other barriers.

Addressing Sexual Health Changes

Sexual health changes, such as vaginal dryness and decreased libido, are common during perimenopause and menopause and can significantly impact intimacy and quality of life. OTPs can provide critical support by educating women about safe and effective lubricants and moisturizers that alleviate discomfort. Additionally, they can teach pelvic floor exercises to enhance muscular function and reduce discomfort during sex. By addressing these changes comprehensively, OTPs help clients maintain a satisfying sexual life and enhance their overall well-being during the menopausal transition.

Examples:

- **Education on Vaginal Health**: Provide information on over-the-counter lubricants and moisturizers that can help alleviate vaginal dryness. Collaborate with healthcare providers to discuss potential prescription options if necessary.
- **Pelvic Floor Exercises**: Teach pelvic floor exercises to improve muscle tone and reduce discomfort during sexual activity.
- **Mindfulness and Stress Reduction**: Incorporate mindfulness and relaxation techniques to reduce stress and improve overall sexual health. Techniques such as guided imagery and progressive muscle relaxation can enhance relaxation and comfort.
- **Communication Strategies**: Facilitate open communication with partners about sexual health and comfort, helping clients express their needs and concerns effectively.

When suggesting lubricants for vaginal dryness, OTPs should provide information on the different types available, emphasizing options that are safe, effective, and suitable for individual preferences and needs.

1. **Water-Based Lubricants**
   - **Advantages**: These are the most common and versatile type of lubricants. They are safe to use with condoms and sex toys, easily washable, and generally well-tolerated.

- **Examples**: KY Jelly, Astroglide, and Sliquid H2O.
- **Considerations**: Some water-based lubricants may contain glycerin, which can increase the risk of yeast infections in some women. Look for glycerin-free options if this is a concern.

2. **Silicone-Based Lubricants**

    - **Advantages**: These lubricants last longer than water-based ones and do not require frequent reapplication. They are also safe to use with condoms and are hypoallergenic.
    - **Examples**: Pjur, Uberlube, and Wet Platinum.
    - **Considerations**: Silicone-based lubricants are not compatible with silicone sex toys as they can degrade the material. They are also harder to wash off and may require soap and water.

3. **Oil-Based Lubricants**

    - **Advantages**: These provide a long-lasting lubricating effect and are often preferred for their natural feel.
    - **Examples**: Coconut oil and olive oil.
    - **Considerations**: Oil-based lubricants should not be used with latex condoms as they can cause the condom to break. They can also be more difficult to wash out of fabrics and may increase the risk of vaginal infections.

4. **Moisturizers**

    - **Advantages**: Vaginal moisturizers are designed for long-term use and provide ongoing relief from dryness, unlike lubricants that are used just before sexual activity.
    - **Examples**: Replens, Hyalo Gyn, and Yes VM.
    - **Considerations**: These products can be used regularly (e.g., every few days) to maintain vaginal moisture and health.

In addressing sexual health changes during perimenopause and menopause, OTPs should take a comprehensive and personalized approach. They should begin by assessing individual needs, discussing with clients their specific symptoms, preferences, and any sensitivities or allergies in order to tailor recommendations effectively. Education on the correct application of lubricants is crucial; for instance, water-based lubricants should be applied just before sexual activity, while moisturizers might be used more regularly to alleviate symptoms of vaginal dryness. OTPs should encourage clients to experiment with different products to discover what works best for them. Additionally, collaboration with healthcare providers is essential, especially for clients experiencing persistent or severe symptoms, as they may require hormone-based treatments or other medical interventions to manage their conditions effectively. This holistic approach ensures that interventions are not only practical but also respectful of each woman's unique health journey.

Case Study in Endocrine Health

Background and Medical History: The client, a 23-year-old graduate student completing their MBA, was diagnosed with Addison's disease following an array of symptoms that progressively impaired daily functioning and occupational activities. They also manage comorbid type 1 diabetes mellitus and had an anterior cruciate ligament (ACL) repair in

2010. Recent exacerbations include unexplained fatigue, joint pain, persistent diarrhea, darkening of the skin, and a marked craving for salty foods. These symptoms, alongside decreased appetite and hyperpigmentation, suggested an advancement of their adrenal insufficiency.

Prior Level of Function:

- Worked part-time as a sales associate required to occasionally lift boxes up to 40 lbs, which has recently become challenging.
- Active graduate student facing difficulties maintaining concentration and stamina during classes.
- Previously managed all ADLs and IADLs independently.
- Independently managed commuting between home, university, and work.

Household Living Arrangements and Social History:

- Lives with their parents who provide emotional and some physical support as needed.
- Strong family ties; however, recent irritability has strained some relationships.

Change in Functional Status and Challenges:

The client reports unusual fatigue, weakness, frequent diarrhea, craving salty foods, joint pain, and prolonged hyperpigmentation, significantly impacting daily activities. Specific areas affected include:

- **ADLs**: Challenges with sustained tasks such as showering and dressing due to muscle weakness and fatigue.
- **IADLs**: Difficulty in meal preparation due to decreased appetite and managing diabetes effectively due to fluctuating glucose levels.
- **Work**: Physical tasks like lifting have become increasingly difficult, contributing to decreased work performance.
- **Social Activities**: Irritability and fatigue have led to reduced participation in social gatherings.
- **Medication Management**: Managing insulin for diabetes has become challenging due to unstable health condition.
- **Health Management**: Needs frequent monitoring and adjustment of medication due to Addison's and diabetes.
- **School**: Concentration issues and fatigue affect academic performance and attendance.

OT Assessments:

- **Barthel Index**: The client scored 40 out of 100, indicating significant assistance required for most ADLs due to muscle weakness and fatigue.
- **Modified Fatigue Impact Scale (MFIS)**: The client's score was high at 68 out of 84, reflecting severe impact of fatigue on physical, cognitive, and psychosocial functions.
- **Performance Assessment of Self-care Skills (PASS)—Meal Preparation**: The client demonstrated limited ability to prepare meals safely and efficiently, scoring 2 out of 5 on this subtest, indicative of decreased energy and manual dexterity.

- **Addison's Disease Quality of Life Questionnaire (ADQLQ)**: Scored 35 out of 100, highlighting poor quality of life, particularly in areas affecting energy levels, emotional health, and daily functioning.

Occupational Therapy Plan of Care and Goals:

The client will receive skilled occupational therapy services three times a week for 8 weeks to improve independence in ADLs, IADLs, and overall quality of life.

Goals:

1. Client will increase Barthel Index score to 75/100, reflecting improved independence in personal care tasks within 8 weeks.
2. Client will reduce MFIS score by 50%, enhancing the ability to participate in daily activities without excessive fatigue within 8 weeks.
3. Client will independently complete showering using prescribed energy conservation techniques, reducing perceived exertion by at least 50% on a self-reported fatigue scale within 8 weeks.
4. Client will prepare meals independently four times a week using adaptive strategies and assistive devices to manage decreased energy and physical limitations within 8 weeks.
5. Client will independently manage diabetes medication and adrenal supplements with 100% accuracy, as measured by a medication tracking log within 8 weeks.
6. Client will resume part-time work and MBA classes, managing tasks without significant fatigue or stress, as measured by self-report and observation within 8 weeks.

Interventions:

The following interventions will be tailored to meet the client's specific needs and address the outlined goals:

Pain and Fatigue Management Strategies:

- Employ relaxation techniques like deep breathing and progressive muscle relaxation to combat fatigue and muscle weakness.
- Utilize heat therapy to alleviate muscle and joint pain, with a focus on areas severely impacted by Addison's disease.

Activity Modification and Energy Conservation:

- Educate the client on energy conservation techniques, such as scheduling high-energy tasks at peak times and incorporating frequent rest breaks.
- Advise on modifying activities at work to manage energy, such as arranging the workspace to minimize the need to lift heavy items.

ADL Retraining and Use of Adaptive Equipment:

- Provide training on the use of adaptive equipment like reachers, long-handled sponges, and a shower chair to facilitate independent showering and dressing.
- Teach ergonomic techniques and the use of assistive devices that reduce strain during daily activities, enhancing safety and independence in ADLs.

Health and Nutrition Management:

- Collaborate with a dietitian to tailor a meal plan that supports energy management, taking into account the client's decreased appetite and diabetes.
- Educate on the importance of regular, nutritious meals that align with managing Addison's disease and diabetes effectively.

Medication Management Education:

- Instruct the client on the correct timing and dosage for diabetes and Addison's medications, emphasizing the importance of adherence to manage her conditions.

Emotional and Psychological Support:

- Offer psychosocial counseling sessions to address irritability and stress, employing cognitive-behavioural techniques to improve emotional regulation.
- Implement stress management strategies to help stabilize mood and enhance overall mental well-being.

Environmental Modifications:

- Suggest home and workplace modifications to reduce physical demands, such as reorganizing living and working spaces to ensure necessary items are within easy reach.
- Recommend adjustments in the home to facilitate easier access and mobility, especially in areas where the client performs daily routines.

Outcomes:

Post Treatment:

- **Fatigue Management**: Significant improvement in managing fatigue, evidenced by a 50% reduction in the MFIS scores, with the client reporting increased stamina and reduced daily exhaustion.
- **Health Management**: Enhanced ability to manage diabetes and Addison's disease through effective medication management and dietary adherence, demonstrated by stable blood glucose levels and proper cortisol management as documented in treatment logs.
- **ADL Independence**: Improved engagement in personal care and household tasks, with the client achieving a Barthel Index score increase from 50 to 85, reflecting increased independence and reduced need for assistance.
- **Mood Stability**: Reduction in irritability and improvement in mood stability, quantified by a 40% improvement in scores on a standardized mood assessment tool, as observed by family members and coworkers.
- **Work and Academic Engagement**: Return to part-time work and MBA classes with adapted strategies, successfully managing tasks without significant fatigue or stress.

Follow-Up Visits:

- Continuing reinforcement of energy conservation and activity modification strategies to ensure sustainability of improvements.

- Ongoing support and adjustment of the client's treatment plan based on her feedback and any changes in her condition.
- Monitoring of medication adherence and dietary management to prevent potential complications from diabetes and Addison's disease.

The client demonstrated marked improvement in managing Addison's disease and its symptoms, enhancing her overall functionality and independence. She is now capable of performing daily tasks such as cooking, cleaning, and personal care with greater efficiency and less fatigue. Additionally, her ability to manage medication for diabetes and Addison's disease has significantly stabilized her health. The strategic use of assistive devices and tailored occupational therapy interventions enabled her to resume part-time work and continue her MBA studies, effectively balancing her educational, professional, and health needs.

Further Reading

American Occupational Therapy Association. (2020). Occupational therapy practice framework: Domain and process (4th ed.). *American Journal of Occupational Therapy*, 74(Supplement_2), 7412410010. https://doi.org/10.5014/ajot.2020.74S2001

Casanova, R., Goepfert, A., Hueppchen, N. A., Weiss, P. M., & Connolly, A. (Eds.). (2023). *Beckmann and Ling's obstetrics and gynecology* (9th ed.). LWW. ISBN 978-1975180577.

Faubion, S. S., Enders, F., Hedges, M. S., Chaudhry, R., Kling, J. M., Shufelt, C. L., Saadedine, M., Mara, K., Griffin, J. M., & Kapoor, E. (2023). Impact of menopause symptoms on women in the workplace. *Mayo Clinic Proceedings*, 98(6), 833–845. https://doi.org/10.1016/j.mayocp.202302..

Feldhacker, D. R., Ikiugu, M. N., Fritz, H., Schweinle, W. E., & Wang, H. (2023). Habit formation intervention to improve type 2 diabetes self-management behaviors: A feasibility study. *The American Journal of Occupational Therapy: Official Publication of the American Occupational Therapy Association*, 77(6), 7706205100. https://doi.org/10.5014/ajot.2023.050351

Flores, V. A., Pal, L., & Manson, J. E. (2021). Hormone therapy in menopause: Concepts, controversies, and approach to treatment. *Endocrine Reviews*, 42(6), 720–752. https://doi.org/10.1210/endrev/bnab011

Geraghty, P. (2022). *Each woman's menopause: An evidence-based resource*. Springer. ISBN: 978-3-030-85483-6.

Mark, J. K. K., Samsudin, S., Looi, I., & Yuen, K. H. (2024). Vaginal dryness: A review of current understanding and management strategies. *Climacteric: The Journal of the International Menopause Society*, 27(3), 236–244. https://doi.org/10.1080/13697137.2024.2306892

Meyer, G., & Badenhoop, K. (2018). Addison-Krise – Risiko erkennen und rasch behandeln [Addisonian crisis – Risk assessment and appropriate treatment]. *Deutsche Medizinische Wochenschrift (1946)*, 143(6), 392–396. https://doi.org/10.1055/s-0043-111729

Stanikova, D., Zsido, R. G., Luck, T., Pabst, A., Enzenbach, C., Bae, Y. J., Thiery, J., Ceglarek, U., Engel, C., Wirkner, K., Stanik, J., Kratzsch, J., Villringer, A., Riedel-Heller, S. G., & Sacher, J. (2019). Testosterone imbalance may link depression and increased body weight in premenopausal women. *Translational Psychiatry*, 9(1), 160. https://doi.org/10.1038/s41398-019-0487-5

5 Autoimmune Conditions

Chapter Objectives

Upon completion of this chapter, the reader will be able to:

1. Understand the pathophysiology and prevalence of autoimmune conditions in women, including rheumatoid arthritis, systemic lupus erythematosus (SLE), Hashimoto's thyroiditis, and celiac disease.
2. Identify the unique challenges faced by women with autoimmune conditions and their impact on daily functioning, including hormonal fluctuations during menstrual cycles, pregnancy, and menopause.
3. Explore specific occupational therapy interventions tailored to the needs of women with autoimmune conditions, emphasizing holistic and individualized care.
4. Discuss the importance of energy conservation techniques, adaptive equipment, and environmental modifications in managing symptoms and improving quality of life for women with autoimmune diseases.
5. Analyze the role of occupational therapy in supporting mental and emotional well-being, addressing issues such as depression, anxiety, and cognitive difficulties associated with autoimmune conditions.
6. Highlight the significance of multidisciplinary collaboration in the management of autoimmune conditions, promoting comprehensive care and enhancing occupational performance for women.

Overview of Autoimmune Conditions in Women

Autoimmune diseases represent a significant category of chronic illnesses where the immune system erroneously attacks the body's own tissues, leading to inflammation and tissue damage. These conditions manifest a wide range of symptoms and can severely impact physical, mental, and emotional health.

Strikingly, autoimmune diseases disproportionately affect women, who account for nearly 80% of all autoimmune cases. This prevalence is thought to be influenced by a combination of factors including hormonal, genetic, and environmental elements. For instance, the X chromosome contains a high density of immune-related genes, and being typically XX, women may have an increased genetic predisposition to autoimmune conditions.

The impact of these diseases extends beyond mere physical symptoms, affecting daily activities, work, social interactions, and overall quality of life. Hormonal fluctuations during menstrual cycles, pregnancy, and menopause can significantly affect disease activity, exemplifying the need for specialized management strategies in women's health. For example, conditions like rheumatoid arthritis or multiple sclerosis may see symptom changes in intensity due to hormonal shifts during these periods.

Moreover, the intersection of chronic disease management with the roles women often hold in family and career contexts adds an additional layer of complexity. The psychological toll, including higher risks of depression and anxiety, further complicates treatment approaches. Social challenges such as isolation can emerge not only from physical limitations but also from societal misunderstandings about the invisible nature of many autoimmune symptoms.

Understanding these nuanced interactions is crucial for OTPs tasked with providing comprehensive, empathetic care that addresses both the medical and socio-emotional dimensions of autoimmune conditions in women.

OT in Rheumatoid Arthritis

Rheumatoid arthritis (RA) is a chronic inflammatory disorder in which the immune system mistakenly attacks the synovium, the lining of the membranes that surround the joints, leading to inflammation, joint damage, and pain. This disorder not only affects the joints but also has the potential to involve multiple body systems such as the skin, eyes, lungs, heart, and blood vessels. Women are up to three times more likely to develop RA than men, with hormonal influences often playing a critical role in modulating the immune system and inflammatory responses.

The progression of RA is categorized into several stages:

- **Healthy Stage**: No signs or symptoms of the disease.
- **Stage 1 (Early)**: Initial joint inflammation, mild symptoms, no visible joint damage on X-rays.
- **Stage 2 (Moderate)**: Increased inflammation and swelling, with early joint damage evident on X-rays.
- **Stage 3 (Severe)**: Advanced joint damage with significant cartilage loss and bone erosion, decreasing joint function.
- **Stage 4 (End Stage)**: Severe joint deformity and substantial loss of joint function.

As RA progresses, its impact on physical function and quality of life intensifies, often complicating daily activities and mobility. This is particularly challenging for women, who typically encounter the onset of RA during pivotal decades of their lives—spanning career peaks and active family responsibilities. The intersection of RA with pregnancy and broader hormonal changes adds complexity to managing the condition, as these factors can lead to symptom remission or flare-ups (Figure 5.1).

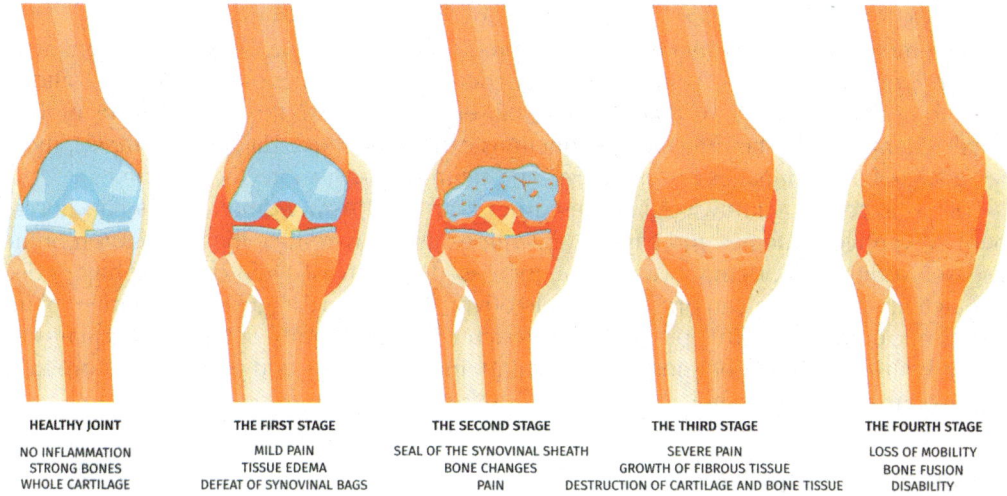

Figure 5.1 Stages of rheumatoid arthritis.

Gender-Specific Differences in Rheumatoid Arthritis

RA often presents differently in women compared to men, influenced by biological, hormonal, and possibly social factors. These gender-specific differences are crucial for understanding the unique challenges faced by women with RA and tailoring appropriate treatment strategies. Key distinctions in how RA manifests and progresses in women compared to men include:

1. **Earlier Onset**: Women are more likely to develop RA earlier in life, typically during their childbearing years, which can complicate decisions around pregnancy and family planning.
2. **More Severe Symptoms**: Women generally report more severe symptoms, including higher levels of pain and fatigue, which can significantly impact daily functioning and quality of life.
3. **Higher Disease Activity**: Clinical studies often show that women experience higher disease activity, which may require more aggressive treatment to manage symptoms and prevent joint damage.
4. **Different Response to Treatment**: Women may respond differently to certain RA medications compared to men, often requiring adjustments in drug types or dosages.
5. **Increased Risk of Comorbidities**: Women with RA are at a greater risk for developing comorbid conditions such as osteoporosis and fibromyalgia, which can further complicate disease management.
6. **Psychosocial Impact**: The disease tends to have a more pronounced psychosocial impact on women, affecting their mental health and social interactions more significantly than men.

These points highlight the need for a gender-sensitive approach in managing RA, ensuring that treatment plans are as effective and comprehensive as possible. For OTPs working with women who have RA, recognizing these gender-specific differences is crucial. It allows OTPs to design interventions that are more closely aligned with the unique needs of their female clients. Understanding these distinctions can lead to better-targeted therapies, more personalized pain management strategies, and ultimately, more effective outcomes.

For instance, by acknowledging the earlier onset of RA in women, OTPs can implement preventive strategies and early interventions that may reduce the progression of the disease. Additionally, being aware of the increased severity of symptoms and higher disease activity in women can prompt OTPs to advocate for more aggressive treatment plans and closer monitoring. This proactive approach can significantly enhance the quality of life for women with RA, helping them maintain independence and participate more fully in personal and professional activities.

Occupational Therapy Intervention

OTPs play a vital role in supporting women with RA by addressing the multifaceted impact of the condition on their daily lives. OTPs focus on enhancing physical function, managing pain, and promoting emotional well-being. Interventions include educating clients on joint protection techniques, developing individualized exercise programs, and providing adaptive strategies to maintain independence in daily activities. Additionally, OTPs offer psychosocial support through counseling and support groups, assist with workplace modifications to ensure continued employment, and recommend home adaptations to improve safety and accessibility (see Table 5.1). By considering the unique challenges faced by women with RA, OTPs can help clients maintain a balanced and fulfilling lifestyle despite the limitations imposed by the condition.

Table 5.1 Occupational therapy interventions for women with rheumatoid arthritis—Factors, interventions, descriptions, and considerations

Factor	Intervention	Description	Consideration for Women
Physical	Joint Protection Techniques	Educate clients on using assistive devices and modifying activities to reduce joint stress and prevent deformities.	Use ergonomic tools in daily activities, such as jar openers in the kitchen, to reduce strain on joints. Ensure techniques are suitable for managing joint pain during menstrual cycles, pregnancy, and childcare tasks. For example, using a baby carrier that distributes weight evenly to minimize joint stress during childcare activities.
	Therapeutic Exercises	Develop exercise programs to maintain joint flexibility, muscle strength, and overall physical fitness.	Incorporate low-impact activities like swimming or yoga that are gentle on joints but effective for maintaining fitness. Tailor exercises to consider menstrual cycles, such as gentle stretching during periods of high pain, and adapt routines for pregnancy, postpartum recovery, and menopause, like prenatal yoga or resistance training for bone health.

(Continued)

Autoimmune Conditions 181

Table 5.1 (Continued)

Factor	Intervention	Description	Consideration for Women
	Pain Management	Utilize modalities such as heat and cold therapy, ultrasound, or electrical stimulation to manage pain and inflammation.	Provide strategies for managing pain during menstrual cycles, such as using heat pads, or during pregnancy when medication use may be limited. Use non-pharmacological pain relief methods suitable for breastfeeding, such as TENS units. Offer specific pain management techniques for peri- or post-menopausal women experiencing joint pain due to hormonal changes.
Mental and Emotional	Cognitive-Behavioural Therapy (CBT)	Incorporate CBT techniques to help clients manage chronic pain, reduce stress, and improve emotional resilience.	Address gender-specific stressors, such as balancing caregiving responsibilities with self-care. Include techniques to manage stress related to hormonal fluctuations, such as mindfulness exercises during PMS or menopause.
	Counseling and Support Groups	Encourage participation in support groups where clients can share experiences and coping strategies.	Create support networks that address the unique challenges women face in managing RA alongside family and career responsibilities. Facilitate groups specifically for women, focusing on issues like pregnancy, motherhood, and hormonal changes including menopause.
Social	Workplace Modifications	Assess the client's work environment and recommend ergonomic adjustments or assistive technologies to facilitate continued employment.	Advocate for flexible work schedules or telecommuting options to accommodate flare-ups and medical appointments. Ensure modifications consider the dual roles of work and family caregiving, such as ergonomic home office setups.
	Community Participation	Facilitate engagement in community activities by identifying accessible options and providing strategies to manage fatigue and pain.	Encourage participation in community groups or activities that provide social support without exacerbating symptoms. Include recommendations for family-oriented community events that allow for socialization without overexertion.
Environmental	Home Modifications	Conduct home assessments to recommend adaptations that improve safety and accessibility.	Suggest installing grab bars in the bathroom, using non-slip mats, and rearranging furniture to create clear pathways. Consider modifications to support child-rearing activities, such as ergonomic changing tables and baby-proofing to prevent falls.

(Continued)

Table 5.1 (Continued)

Factor	Intervention	Description	Consideration for Women
	Adaptive Equipment	Recommend and train clients in the use of adaptive equipment to facilitate independence in daily activities.	Provide adaptive devices such as reachers, button hooks, and specialized kitchen tools to make daily tasks easier and reduce joint strain. Ensure devices are practical for managing household and childcare responsibilities, like using lightweight cookware for ease of handling.

A multidisciplinary approach to managing RA is essential in providing comprehensive care, as it integrates the expertise of rheumatologists, OTPs, physical therapists, and other healthcare professionals. This collaborative effort ensures that treatment plans are holistic, addressing not only the physical symptoms but also the emotional and social impacts of the disease. By leveraging the strengths of each discipline, patients can achieve improved functional outcomes, enhanced quality of life, and better disease management.

OT in Systemic Lupus Erythematosus (SLE)

Lupus is an autoimmune condition with four main types, among which systemic lupus erythematosus (SLE) is the most common and severe. SLE affects multiple organ systems, including the skin, joints, kidneys, and brain, characterized by cycles of flare-ups and remission (see Figure 5.2). Symptoms vary significantly among individuals due to a complex interplay of genetic susceptibility and environmental triggers such as infections, sunlight exposure, and certain medications. Hormonal factors also play a crucial role, contributing to the significantly higher prevalence of SLE among women compared to men.

Women are nine times more likely to develop SLE than men, typically manifesting the disease during their childbearing years, between the ages of 15 and 45. This timing poses unique challenges, as SLE often causes debilitating fatigue, joint pain, skin rashes, and organ damage, significantly impairing daily function, employment, and social engagement. Additionally, the impact of SLE extends into pregnancy, increasing the risk of complications like preeclampsia and preterm birth, which necessitate careful disease management.

Impact on Sexual Functioning

Sexual health is significantly impacted in women with SLE, correlating closely with the common occurrence of depression in approximately 40% of patients. The clinical management of SLE often includes addressing depressive states to improve sexual function, considering that impairments in mood and neuroplasticity, often exacerbated by autoimmune inflammation, can worsen sexual health. Studies indicate that women with SLE typically report lower sexual functioning compared to those with other chronic illnesses, with vaginal discomfort during intercourse being a prominent issue. The multifactorial nature of sexual dysfunction in SLE, influenced by factors such as age, relationship status, body image, and overall mental health, underscores the importance of a comprehensive approach in treatment.

Autoimmune Conditions 183

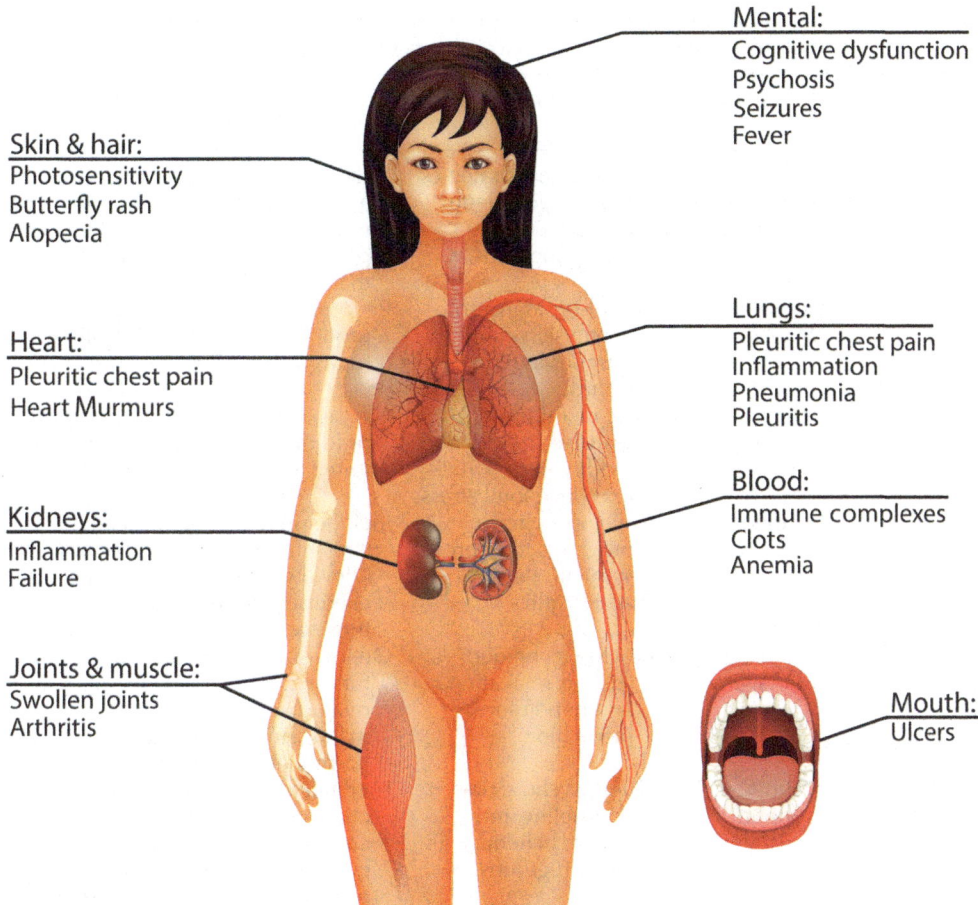

Figure 5.2 Symptoms of lupus.

OTPs are particularly positioned to address these complex needs by integrating strategies that mitigate physical discomfort and emotional stress, thereby improving overall quality of life and sexual health for women with SLE.

Occupational Therapy Interventions

OTPs play a crucial role in supporting women with SLE, addressing the physical, mental, emotional, and social impacts of the condition. Interventions focus on managing fatigue, enhancing physical function, and promoting emotional well-being. Strategies include teaching energy conservation techniques, developing individualized exercise programs, and providing support to manage both the physical and emotional symptoms of SLE. Additionally, OTPs offer psychosocial support, assist with workplace modifications, and recommend home adaptations to improve safety and accessibility. Table 5.2 specifically addresses the occupational therapy interventions needed for pregnant women with SLE, highlighting how these strategies are adapted to cater to the complexities of pregnancy.

Table 5.2 Occupational therapy interventions for women with systemic lupus erythematosus (SLE)—Factors, interventions, descriptions, and considerations

Factor	Intervention	Description	Consideration for Women During Pregnancy
Physical	Energy Conservation Techniques	Teach clients strategies to manage fatigue and use energy-saving methods.	Adapt pacing strategies to accommodate morning sickness or reduced stamina in later stages of pregnancy. Recommend rest periods that align with energy dips.
	Skin Care Management	Provide guidance on gentle skin care routines to manage rashes.	Recommend pregnancy-safe skin care products to avoid exacerbating lupus rashes.
	Joint Protection Techniques	Educate on using assistive devices and modifying activities to reduce joint stress.	Advise on the use of custom orthotics or joint supports that accommodate joint swelling during pregnancy.
	Therapeutic Exercises	Develop exercise programs to improve strength, flexibility, and health.	Include prenatal yoga and gentle stretching to maintain mobility and alleviate joint stress, ensuring exercises are modified as per trimester.
Mental and Emotional	Stress Management	Provide techniques such as relaxation and mindfulness meditation.	Offer specialized relaxation sessions focusing on reducing pregnancy-related anxiety and stress management techniques tailored to hormonal fluctuations.
	Psychological Support	Offer psychosocial counseling and connect clients with support groups.	Facilitate discussions on coping with changes in body image and concerns about pregnancy complications or postpartum recovery in support group settings.
Social	Vocational Rehabilitation	Recommend workplace accommodations and flexible schedules.	Advocate for modifications such as ergonomic seating or work-from-home arrangements during the third trimester or as prenatal visits increase.
	Social Participation	Encourage engagement in community activities that are accessible.	Organize or suggest participation in prenatal classes and motherhood preparation workshops that enhance social support and address specific SLE-related health education.
Environmental	Home Adjustments	Recommend adaptations to improve safety and reduce physical strain.	Suggest the installation of supportive aids like handrails in bathrooms and modifications to the bedroom layout to accommodate mobility aids if needed during pregnancy.
	UV Protection Strategies	Teach methods to reduce sun exposure to prevent photosensitivity reactions.	Recommend UV-protective clothing and wide-brimmed hats for outdoor activities, crucial during pregnancy to prevent lupus flares.
	Adaptive Equipment	Provide tools and devices to assist with daily activities.	Recommend ergonomic tools designed for ease of use during pregnancy, such as long-handled sponges for bathing and easy-grip utensils for kitchen tasks.

Late-Onset SLE in Women

Late-onset SLE refers to systemic lupus erythematosus diagnosed after the age of 50. While lupus typically manifests during childbearing years, approximately 10–20% of all SLE cases are diagnosed later in life. Women, even in later years, continue to be more susceptible to lupus than men, though the gender disparity in late-onset SLE is less pronounced compared to earlier onset.

The symptomatology of late-onset SLE often presents less acutely than in younger patients. Common symptoms include less severe skin manifestations and renal involvement, but more pronounced joint involvement and systemic symptoms like pulmonary and cardiac complications. The management of SLE in older adults must consider age-related changes such as decreased renal function and the presence of other chronic conditions like hypertension and diabetes, which may complicate the treatment regimen.

Occupational Therapy Considerations for Aging Adults with Lupus:

- **Mobility and Safety**: Tailoring interventions to address increased risks of falls due to joint pain and muscle weakness. OTPs may recommend assistive devices to aid mobility and modifications to the home environment to ensure safety and accessibility.
- **Pain Management**: Adapting pain management strategies to accommodate potential interactions with medications for coexisting conditions. Techniques such as thermal therapies, gentle exercise routines, and ergonomics can be especially beneficial.
- **Chronic Disease Management**: Education and support in managing multiple health conditions, focusing on simplifying medication regimens and promoting adherence to treatment plans.
- **Social and Emotional Support**: Providing strategies to combat isolation and depression, which may be exacerbated by limited mobility and chronic pain. Encouraging engagement in community activities that are accessible and fulfilling.
- **Adaptive Strategies for Reduced Physical Function**: Implementing adaptive techniques and tools to assist with daily activities, taking into account the client's reduced physical stamina and joint health. This includes ergonomic tools for household tasks and adaptive aids for personal care to maintain independence.

Working with women affected by SLE highlights the necessity of a holistic occupational therapy approach that considers both individual and gender-specific challenges. Collaborating closely with other healthcare professionals, such as rheumatologists, psychologists, and rehabilitation professionals, allows OTPs to provide integrated care tailored to the unique needs of women with SLE. This collaboration ensures that interventions are not only effective in managing symptoms but also in supporting women's roles in family, work, and society, ultimately enhancing their overall well-being and quality of life.

OT in Hashimoto's Thyroiditis

Hashimoto's thyroiditis, also known as Hashimoto's disease, is an autoimmune disorder where immune-system cells lead to the death of the thyroid's hormone-producing cells. This results in a decline in hormone production, known as hypothyroidism, which is

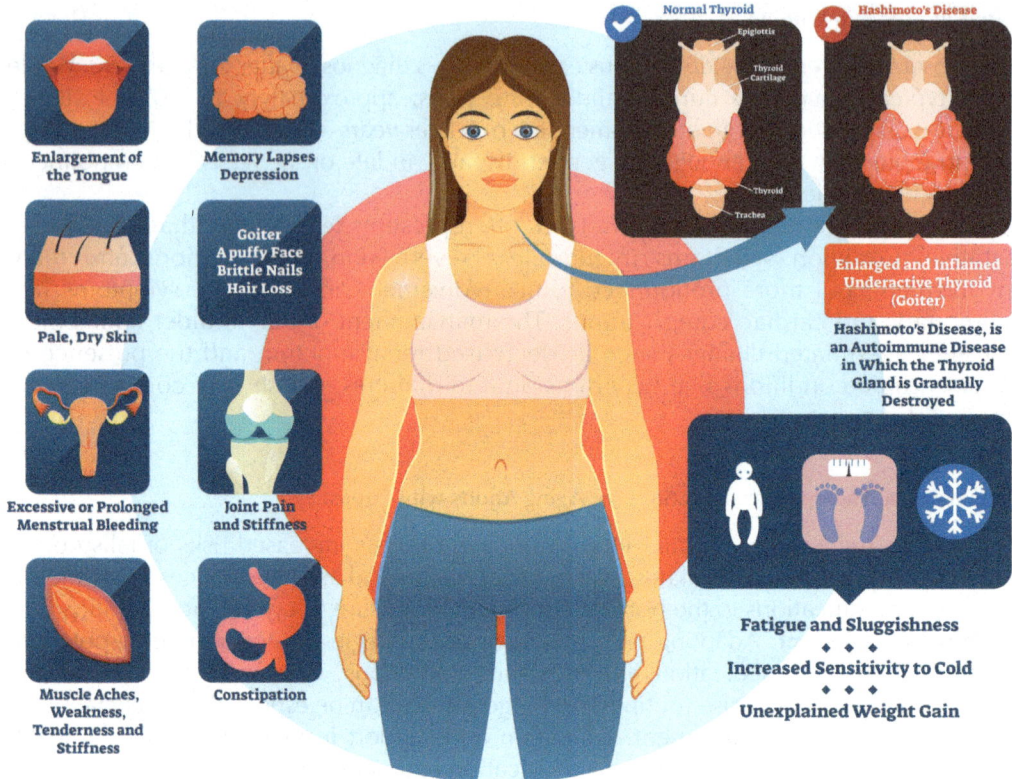

Figure 5.3 Symptoms of Hashimoto's.

particularly common among middle-aged women. Hashimoto's disease is the most prevalent cause of hypothyroidism and can lead to symptoms such as fatigue, weight gain, cold intolerance, depression, joint pain, and cognitive difficulties. These symptoms significantly impact daily life, particularly in women, affecting their ability to work, care for their family, and engage in social activities.

Hypothyroidism is treatable with medicine, but if left untreated, it can cause reproductive issues such as difficulty getting pregnant and complications during pregnancy. The management of Hashimoto's requires a nuanced approach, especially during hormonal fluctuations associated with menstrual cycles, pregnancy, and menopause, which can exacerbate symptoms or introduce new health challenges. This necessitates personalized occupational therapy interventions to manage and mitigate the effects of the disease effectively (Figure 5.3).

Occupational Therapy Intervention

OTPs play a vital role in addressing the diverse impacts of Hashimoto's thyroiditis on women. The pervasive symptoms—such as fatigue, weight gain, and cognitive difficulties—can severely limit a person's ability to perform daily tasks, work effectively, and engage socially. Occupational therapy offers targeted interventions to enhance activity and participation by teaching energy conservation techniques, cognitive strategies for managing brain fog, and physical exercises tailored to improve stamina and joint health. Additionally, OTPs provide crucial support in adapting living and work environments to better accommodate physical and cognitive limitations, ensuring that individuals can maintain independence and quality of life despite their condition. These interventions are especially critical during life stages such as pregnancy and menopause when symptoms may intensify, requiring careful management to prevent exacerbation. By focusing on tailored interventions, OTPs enhance their clients' ability to manage symptoms effectively and maintain their daily activities (see Table 5.3).

Table 5.3 Occupational therapy interventions for women with Hashimoto's thyroiditis—Factors, interventions, descriptions, and considerations

Factor	Intervention	Description	Consideration for Women
Physical	Fatigue Management	Teach energy conservation techniques and activity pacing to help clients manage fatigue and maintain productivity.	Recommend taking frequent rest breaks and prioritizing activities to conserve energy. Tailor strategies to manage energy levels during menstrual cycles, pregnancy, and menopause.
	Therapeutic Exercises	Develop exercise programs tailored to improve energy levels, manage weight, and enhance overall physical fitness.	Low-impact activities such as walking, cycling, or yoga can be beneficial. Adapt exercise routines to accommodate symptoms related to menstrual cycles and hormonal changes during menopause.
Mental and Emotional	Cognitive Strategies	Provide cognitive strategies to help clients cope with memory lapses and concentration difficulties.	Using planners, setting reminders, and organizing tasks into manageable steps can be helpful. Address cognitive challenges that may arise from hormonal fluctuations during menstrual cycles and menopause.
	Psychosocial Support	Offer counseling to address depression and anxiety, and facilitate support groups for sharing experiences and strategies.	Support groups can help women discuss reproductive health concerns and other gender-specific issues. Provide emotional support tailored to the impact of hormonal changes on mental health.
Social	Workplace Accommodations	Assess the work environment and recommend ergonomic adjustments or flexible work arrangements to support continued employment.	Advocate for flexible work schedules or telecommuting options to accommodate fatigue and cognitive difficulties. Consider the need for accommodations that address the dual roles of work and family caregiving.

(*Continued*)

Table 5.3 (Continued)

Factor	Intervention	Description	Consideration for Women
	Social Participation	Encourage engagement in social and recreational activities that align with the client's energy levels and interests.	Promote a balanced lifestyle that includes social activities without exacerbating symptoms. Develop strategies for participating in family and community events that provide support without overwhelming the client.
Environmental	Home Adjustments	Suggest home modifications to improve comfort and reduce physical strain, such as ergonomic furniture and easy-to-access storage.	Tailor modifications to accommodate family dynamics and ensure all family members are educated about the condition. Provide specific adjustments for managing household tasks and childcare activities with minimal strain.
	Adaptive Equipment	Recommend tools and devices that assist with daily activities, such as energy-efficient appliances, adaptive kitchen tools, and home automation systems to reduce physical effort.	Ensure devices are easy to use and maintain, and suitable for the client's lifestyle and preferences. Focus on tools that aid in managing household chores and family responsibilities with less physical exertion.

Hashimoto's and Exercise Intolerance

Women with Hashimoto's often experience exercise intolerance, which can significantly impact their ability to maintain physical fitness and overall health. OTPs can employ grading techniques to help clients gradually increase their activity levels without exacerbating symptoms. Key functional movements for women with Hashimoto's include pulling, pushing, squatting, lunging, hinging, anti-rotation, and carrying. If clients struggle with these movements, OTPs can introduce modifications such as floor and chair exercises, resistance bands, and isometric exercises. These strategies help clients build strength and endurance while managing fatigue and joint pain.

Exercise interventions for women with Hashimoto's

- **Floor and Chair Exercises**: These exercises are ideal for clients who experience dizziness or pain with upright activities. Examples include forearm planks, glute bridges, and chair-elevated pushups.
- **Resistance Bands**: Gentle and adaptable, resistance bands can be used in floor or seated exercises to increase strength gradually.
- **Isometric Exercises**: Exercises such as planks and wall sits help build muscle without moving joints, reducing strain on painful areas.
- **Progressive Exercise Plans**: Gradually increase the difficulty of exercises by reducing support from tools like TRX or increasing weight and repetitions as the client's strength improves.

- **Walking**: Encouraging regular walking can improve stamina and provide meditative benefits, reducing stress and promoting overall well-being.

Hashimoto's Exercise Checklist

- Start easy and slow.
- Start with low reps.
- Take long rest breaks.
- Increase fluid and salt intake.
- Adapt workouts based on stress levels and sleep quality.

Hashimoto's and Menopause

Hashimoto's thyroiditis and menopause often coincide due to overlapping age ranges, typically affecting women between the ages of 30 and 50. This convergence can exacerbate symptoms of both conditions, making diagnosis and management challenging. During menopause, fluctuating estrogen levels can trigger or worsen Hashimoto's by impacting thyroid function and increasing inflammation. Both conditions share symptoms such as fatigue, weight gain, and joint pain, which can be mistaken for normal menopausal changes. OTPs are crucial in distinguishing and managing these overlapping symptoms, providing tailored interventions that address the unique needs of middle-aged women.

Occupational therapy interventions for women in this life stage focus on optimizing thyroid function through lifestyle adjustments and managing menopausal symptoms to improve overall well-being. Effective strategies include:

1. **Thyroid and Hormone Management**
   - **Monitoring and Education**: OTPs can educate clients on the importance of regular thyroid function testing and help them understand the results. They can guide women on how to recognize and report symptoms of hormonal imbalances.
   - **Lifestyle Adjustments**: OTPs can recommend and train clients in daily routines that support hormone regulation, such as consistent sleep schedules and balanced meal planning.
   - **Coordination of Care**: Working closely with endocrinologists, OTPs can assist in developing comprehensive care plans that include medication management, monitoring for side effects, and ensuring adherence to prescribed treatments.

2. **Diet and Exercise**
   - **Nutritional Guidance**: OTPs can collaborate with dietitians to create anti-inflammatory diet plans that reduce joint pain and manage weight. They can teach clients about nutrient-dense foods that support thyroid health and overall well-being.
   - **Exercise Programs**: Developing individualized, low-impact exercise routines that improve cardiovascular health, flexibility, and muscle strength. Activities such as swimming, yoga, or tai chi are particularly beneficial.
   - **Activity Pacing**: Educating clients on pacing techniques to avoid overexertion and ensuring they can incorporate regular physical activity into their daily routines without exacerbating symptoms.

3. **Stress and Sleep Management**

   - **Relaxation Techniques**: Training clients in stress reduction methods such as deep breathing exercises, progressive muscle relaxation, and mindfulness meditation. These techniques help manage stress, which can aggravate Hashimoto's and menopausal symptoms.
   - **Sleep Hygiene**: OTPs can provide strategies for improving sleep quality, such as establishing a calming bedtime routine, optimizing the sleep environment, and using relaxation techniques before bed.
   - **Cognitive Behavioural Therapy (CBT)**: Incorporating CBT strategies to help clients manage stress and anxiety, which can impact sleep and overall health.

4. **Muscle Strength and Bone Health**

   - **Strength Training Programs**: Designing safe and effective strength training routines to counteract muscle loss and maintain bone density. OTPs can instruct clients on proper techniques to prevent injury.
   - **Weight-Bearing Exercises**: Encouraging activities that promote bone health, such as walking or resistance training. These exercises are crucial for reducing the risk of osteoporosis and fractures.
   - **Functional Activities**: Incorporating strength training into daily activities to ensure clients can maintain their independence and perform tasks efficiently.

5. **Psychosocial Support**

   - **Support Groups**: Facilitating or connecting clients with support groups where they can share experiences and strategies for managing their condition. These groups provide emotional support and reduce feelings of isolation.
   - **Counseling**: Offering individual or group counseling to address depression, anxiety, and other mental health issues related to Hashimoto's and menopause. OTPs can help clients develop coping strategies and improve their emotional resilience.
   - **Education and Advocacy**: Educating clients and their families about Hashimoto's and its impact on daily life. Advocating for clients in various settings, such as workplaces or healthcare facilities, to ensure they receive the support and accommodations they need.

OTPs play a crucial role in managing the multifaceted impact of Hashimoto's thyroiditis on women, particularly during key life stages such as pregnancy and menopause. By providing personalized interventions that address physical, cognitive, and emotional challenges, OTPs can significantly improve the quality of life for women with Hashimoto's. Collaboration with other healthcare professionals ensures comprehensive care, enabling effective management of symptoms and enhancing overall well-being.

OT in Celiac Disease

Celiac disease is an autoimmune disorder where the ingestion of gluten leads to damage in the small intestine. Gluten, a protein found in wheat, barley, and rye, triggers this immune response, resulting in a range of gastrointestinal and systemic symptoms such as diarrhea, abdominal pain, bloating, fatigue, and malnutrition. The mucosa (lining),

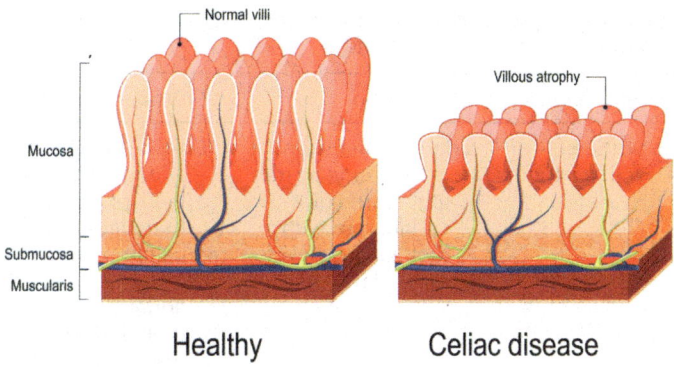

Figure 5.4 Normal villi and villi atrophy in celiac disease.

submucosa (layer beneath the lining), and muscularis (muscle layer) of the intestines are damaged in individuals with celiac disease, leading to a flattening of the villi, which are crucial for nutrient absorption. This damage severely affects nutrient absorption and overall digestive health (see Figure 5.4).

Women with celiac disease face unique challenges, including nutritional deficiencies, bone density loss, reproductive issues, and higher rates of anxiety and depression. The strict adherence to a lifelong gluten-free diet, which is the only effective treatment, can complicate social activities and affect the overall quality of life. During pregnancy and menopause, nutritional needs and hormonal changes further complicate disease management.

Occupational Therapy Intervention

OTPs can play a crucial role in supporting women with celiac disease by addressing the physical, mental, emotional, and social aspects of the condition. Interventions focus on educating clients about managing their diet, developing strategies to cope with social and emotional challenges, and ensuring they maintain an active and healthy lifestyle (see Table 5.4). OTPs work closely with clients to create personalized plans that address their unique needs and promote overall well-being.

Gastrointestinal Symptom Management in Women with Celiac Disease

Women with celiac disease must adhere to a strict gluten-free diet to manage their gastrointestinal symptoms and prevent further complications. OTPs can provide essential support in meal planning and meal preparation to ensure that clients receive adequate nutrition while avoiding gluten.

Meal Planning Strategies: OTPs can educate clients about identifying gluten-free foods, reading food labels, and understanding cross-contamination risks. This knowledge is crucial for making informed choices and maintaining a safe diet. They collaborate with dietitians to ensure meal plans are nutritionally balanced, compensating for common

Table 5.4 Occupational therapy interventions for women with celiac disease—Factors, interventions, descriptions, and considerations

Factor	Intervention	Description	Consideration for Women
Physical	Nutrition Management	Educate clients on maintaining a strict gluten-free diet and collaborate with dietitians to develop meal plans.	Collaborating with dietician, ensure adequate intake of nutrients that women may be deficient in due to malabsorption, such as calcium, iron, and vitamin D. Tailor nutritional advice to address reproductive health concerns, pregnancy, and menopause-related changes. Help client meal plan and preparation on gluten-free diet.
	Therapeutic Exercises	Develop exercise programs to improve overall physical fitness and manage symptoms such as fatigue and muscle weakness.	Focus on weight-bearing exercises to combat potential bone density loss. Recommend specific exercises that support women's health needs, such as pelvic floor exercises and activities to prevent osteoporosis.
Mental and Emotional	Cognitive Strategies	Teach clients techniques for organizing and planning meals, grocery shopping, and reading food labels to ensure adherence to a gluten-free diet.	Address potential cognitive difficulties that can arise from nutritional deficiencies and ensure strategies are practical for daily use. Offer tailored strategies for managing cognitive challenges during menstrual cycles, pregnancy, and menopause.
	Psychosocial Support	Provide counseling to manage anxiety and depression, and facilitate support groups for sharing experiences and coping strategies.	Create a supportive environment where women can discuss reproductive health concerns and other gender-specific issues. Facilitate connections with support groups specifically for women with celiac disease, focusing on unique challenges such as managing diet during pregnancy.
Social	Social Participation	Develop strategies for managing social situations, such as dining out or attending events, to maintain a gluten-free diet without feeling isolated.	Encourage participation in social activities that do not revolve around food, and teach assertiveness skills for communicating dietary needs. Provide guidance on navigating social scenarios like family gatherings, which can be particularly challenging for women managing household food preparation.

(Continued)

Table 5.4 (Continued)

Factor	Intervention	Description	Consideration for Women
	Community Resources	Connect clients with community resources and support networks, including local and online gluten-free groups.	Ensure resources are accessible and culturally appropriate, and provide information on finding gluten-free products and services. Tailor resource recommendations to address women's unique needs, such as managing gluten-free diets for their families.
Environmental	Home Environment	Assess and modify the home environment to create a safe and gluten-free kitchen, including labeling and organizing food storage areas.	Tailor modifications to accommodate family dynamics and ensure all family members are educated about celiac disease and cross-contamination. Provide specific guidance on managing a gluten-free kitchen when preparing meals for a family with mixed dietary needs.
	Assistive Devices	Recommend tools and devices that can assist with meal preparation and reduce the risk of cross-contamination.	Ensure devices are easy to use and maintain, and suitable for the client's lifestyle and preferences. Focus on tools that aid in efficient meal preparation, particularly for women balancing multiple roles and responsibilities.

deficiencies in celiac disease, such as iron, calcium, and vitamin D. OTPs help develop personalized meal plans that consider dietary preferences, lifestyle, and any additional health conditions, facilitating adherence to the gluten-free diet.

Meal Preparation Strategies: OTPs can suggest ways to organize the kitchen to minimize the risk of cross-contamination, such as having separate storage areas for gluten-free and gluten-containing products, using dedicated gluten-free cookware and utensils, and labeling items clearly. Education on safe cooking practices, such as thoroughly cleaning surfaces and cooking equipment before preparing gluten-free meals, is essential. OTPs can also introduce adaptive kitchen tools and techniques to simplify meal preparation, recommend meal prepping strategies like batch cooking and freezing meals in advance, and assist in creating weekly menus to ensure variety and efficiency.

In managing social situations involving food, OTPs can provide strategies for dining out or attending events, teaching clients how to communicate their dietary needs and choose safe options from menus. They also offer stress management techniques to handle the anxiety that often accompanies strict dietary adherence, promoting relaxation and overall well-being. By addressing these aspects, OTPs significantly enhance the ability of women with celiac disease to manage their condition and maintain an active and healthy lifestyle.

194　*Occupational Therapy and Women's Health*

Case Studies in Autoimmune Conditions

CASE A: SLE

Background and Medical History: The client, a 34-year-old woman, diagnosed with SLE at the age of 28. She experiences chronic fatigue, joint pain, skin rashes, peripheral neuropathy, and occasional cognitive difficulties. Lisa also has a history of anxiety and depression, which have been exacerbated by her diagnosis. She is married with two young children and works full-time as an accountant.

Prior Level of Function:

- Worked full time as an accountant, efficiently managing professional responsibilities.
- Actively participated in outdoor activities such as hiking and running.
- Managed all ADLs and IADLs independently.
- Independently managed commuting between home, work, and social events.

Household Living Arrangements and Social History:

- Lives with her partner and two young children.
- Strong family support.
- Active in her community and social circles before the diagnosis.

Change in Functional Status and Challenges:

The client reports unusual fatigue, weakness, frequent diarrhea, craving salty foods, joint pain, and prolonged hyperpigmentation, significantly impacting daily activities. Specific areas affected include:

ADLs:

- Peripheral neuropathy impacts her fine motor skills, making personal care tasks such as grooming and applying makeup more difficult, especially during flare-ups.
- Challenges with sustained tasks such as showering, toileting, and dressing due to muscle weakness, joint pain, and fatigue.

IADLs:

- Difficulty in meal preparation due to decreased appetite and managing diabetes effectively due to fluctuating glucose levels.
- Peripheral neuropathy further complicates tasks requiring fine motor skills, such as chopping and cooking.

Work:

- Physical tasks like lifting have become increasingly difficult, contributing to decreased work performance.
- Peripheral neuropathy impacts her ability to type and manage accounting tasks.

Social Activities:

- Irritability and fatigue have led to reduced participation in social gatherings.
- Peripheral neuropathy also affects her ability to interact with her children.

Sexual Functioning:

- Experiencing a decline in sexual health due to fatigue, joint pain, and depression, leading to decreased intimacy.

Outdoor Activities:

- Joint pain and skin rashes have limited participation in outdoor activities, which were previously a significant part of her life.
- Peripheral neuropathy further impacts her ability to engage in activities that require fine motor coordination.

Occupational Therapy Assessments

- **Canadian Occupational Performance Measure (COPM)**: Identified issues in managing self-care, productivity, and leisure activities.
- **Edinburgh Depression Scale**: High scores reflecting significant depressive symptoms.
- **Semmes–Weinstein Monofilament Test**: Assessed the extent of peripheral neuropathy, indicating reduced sensation in hands and feet.
- **Nine-Hole Peg Test**: Evaluated fine motor dexterity, revealing difficulties in tasks requiring precise hand movements.
- **Sexual Health Inventory for Women (SHIW)**: Indicated significant decline in sexual health and satisfaction due to fatigue, joint pain, and depression.
- **Modified Fatigue Impact Scale (MFIS)**: Measured the impact of fatigue on physical, cognitive, and psychosocial functioning, indicating widespread effects on daily activities.

Occupational Therapy Plan of Care and Goals:

Lisa will receive skilled occupational therapy services twice a week for 12 weeks to improve her independence in ADLs, manage fatigue, and enhance her quality of life.

Goals include:

1. Client will independently apply makeup using adaptive beauty tools, increasing independence in upper body grooming tasks as measured by a 30% improvement in COPM scores within 12 weeks.
2. Client will independently perform morning dressing routines using adapted strategies to reduce joint stress and conserve energy, aiming for a 50% reduction in perceived exertion by the end of the intervention period.
3. Client will complete bathing independently using adaptive equipment like a shower chair and long-handled sponges to reduce fatigue, with a goal of reducing perceived exertion by at least 50% on a self-reported fatigue scale within 12 weeks.
4. Client will report improved sexual functioning and reduced discomfort during intercourse by incorporating recommended therapeutic exercises and relaxation techniques, achieving at least a 30% improvement in the Sexual Functioning Questionnaire (SFQ) scores within 12 weeks.
5. Client will effectively manage symptoms of anxiety and depression, improving scores on the Edinburgh Depression Scale by 40% through targeted psychosocial interventions within 12 weeks.

6. Client will increase social participation by developing strategies for managing social situations, particularly during family gatherings and social events, without feeling isolated or overwhelmed, as measured by self-reported satisfaction and participation rates within 12 weeks.

Occupational Therapy Interventions:

The following interventions will be tailored to meet the client's specific needs and address the outlined goals:

Pain and Fatigue Management Strategies:

- Employ relaxation techniques like deep breathing and progressive muscle relaxation to combat fatigue and muscle weakness.
- Utilize heat therapy and gentle massage to alleviate muscle and joint pain, particularly in areas affected by Addison's disease.

Activity Modification and Energy Conservation:

- Educate the client on energy conservation techniques, such as scheduling high-energy tasks at peak times and incorporating frequent rest breaks.
- Advise on modifying activities at work to manage energy, such as arranging the workspace to minimize the need to lift heavy items.

ADL Retraining and Use of Adaptive Equipment:

- Provide training on the use of adaptive grooming products designed for individuals with limited mobility, such as ergonomic makeup applicators, long handled sponges, and long-handled hairbrushes.
- Teach ergonomic techniques and the use of assistive devices that reduce strain during daily activities, enhancing safety and independence in ADLs.

Health and Nutrition Management:

- Partner with a dietitian to develop a meal plan that helps maintain energy levels and supports overall health.
- Educate the client on the importance of regular, nutritious meals that are balanced and tailored to her needs, emphasizing the role of good nutrition in managing fatigue and enhancing physical function.

Emotional and Psychological Support:

- Offer psychosocial counseling sessions to address irritability and stress, employing cognitive-behavioural techniques to improve emotional regulation.
- Implement stress management strategies to help stabilize mood and enhance overall mental well-being.

Interventions for Peripheral Neuropathy:

- Introduce exercises aimed at improving nerve function and reducing discomfort, such as balance training and gentle stretching exercises.
- Recommend the use of therapeutic footwear and protective padding to alleviate discomfort during mobility and daily activities.

Environmental Modifications:

- Suggest home and workplace modifications to reduce physical demands, such as reorganizing living and working spaces to ensure necessary items are within easy reach.
- Recommend adjustments in the home to facilitate easier access and mobility, especially in areas where the client performs daily routines.

Outcomes:

Post Treatment:

- **Fatigue Management**: Significant improvement in managing fatigue, evidenced by a 50% reduction in the Modified Fatigue Impact Scale (MFIS) scores, with the client reporting increased stamina and reduced daily exhaustion.
- **ADL Independence**: Improved engagement in personal care and household tasks, with the client achieving a Barthel Index score increase from 50 to 85, reflecting increased independence and reduced need for assistance.
- **Mood Stability**: Notable improvement in mood, evidenced by a significant reduction in depressive symptoms, as observed by family members and documented in therapy sessions. The client reported feeling more positive and engaged in her daily activities and social interactions.
- **Work and Social Engagement**: Return to part-time work with adapted strategies, successfully managing tasks without significant fatigue or stress. The client effectively used occupational therapy techniques to manage her energy and physical capabilities, which improved her ability to fulfill her professional responsibilities and engage in social activities.
- **Peripheral Neuropathy Management**: Semmes–Weinstein Monofilament Test indicated improved sensation in hands and feet, with decreased severity of peripheral neuropathy symptoms.
- **Fine Motor Dexterity**: Nine-Hole Peg Test showed enhanced fine motor skills, with improved ability to perform tasks requiring precise hand movements.

Follow-Up Visits:

- Continuously reinforce energy conservation techniques and activity modifications to ensure the sustainability of the client's improvements in daily activities and work tasks.
- Provide ongoing support and adjust the client's treatment plan based on her feedback, changes in her symptoms, and any new challenges that arise in managing her lupus.

The client demonstrated marked improvement in managing her SLE and its symptoms, enhancing her overall functionality and independence. She is now capable of performing daily tasks such as cooking, cleaning, and personal care with greater efficiency and less fatigue. Additionally, her ability to manage her condition has significantly stabilized her health. The strategic use of assistive devices and tailored occupational therapy interventions enabled her to return to part-time work, effectively balancing her professional and health needs. Through the collaborative and holistic approach of occupational therapy, the client has regained a better quality of life and improved her capacity to engage in meaningful activities.

CASE B: Celiac Disease

Background and Medical History: The client is a 28-year-old woman diagnosed with celiac disease at the age of 25. She experiences chronic gastrointestinal symptoms, including abdominal pain, diarrhea, and bloating. Additionally, she struggles with fatigue, iron-deficiency anemia, and joint pain. The client works as a kindergarten teacher and enjoys baking and gardening in her free time.

Prior Level of Function:

- Worked full-time as a kindergarten teacher, managing classroom activities and engaging with young children.
- Actively participated in baking and gardening.
- Managed all ADLs and IADLs independently.
- Independently commuted between home, work, and social events.

Household Living Arrangements and Social History:

- Lives with her partner in a three-story house.
- Strong support system with family and friends.
- Active in her community and social circles before the diagnosis.

Change in Functional Status and Challenges:

The client reports increased fatigue, gastrointestinal discomfort, and joint pain, significantly impacting her daily activities. Specific areas affected include:

ADLs:

- Difficulty with grooming and personal care tasks due to fatigue and joint pain.
- Challenges with meal preparation due to dietary restrictions and fatigue.
- Increased difficulty with maintaining hygiene routines due to frequent diarrhea.

IADLs:

- Struggles with meal planning and preparation, requiring adherence to a strict gluten-free diet.
- Difficulty managing household chores such as cleaning and gardening due to joint pain and fatigue.

Work:

- Physical tasks like standing for long periods and managing classroom activities have become challenging.
- Difficulty with meal planning and eating at work due to dietary restrictions and frequent bathroom breaks.

Social Activities:

- Reduced participation in social gatherings due to anxiety about dietary restrictions and gastrointestinal symptoms.
- Difficulty enjoying hobbies like baking and gardening due to fatigue and joint pain.

Sexual Functioning:
- Experiencing a decline in sexual health due to fatigue and joint pain, leading to decreased intimacy.

Occupational Therapy Assessments:
- **Canadian Occupational Performance Measure (COPM):** Identified issues in managing self-care, productivity, and leisure activities.
- **Beck Depression Inventory (BDI):** Scores reflecting significant depressive symptoms.
- **Meal Planning Assessment:** Evaluated the client's ability to plan and prepare gluten-free meals, highlighting challenges in maintaining a strict diet.
- **Bristol Stool Form Scale:** Used to track and log the frequency and consistency of bowel movements, assessing the impact of diarrhea and constipation on daily life.
- **Sexual Health Inventory for Women (SHIW):** Indicated a significant decline in sexual health and satisfaction due to fatigue and joint pain.
- **Modified Fatigue Impact Scale (MFIS):** Measured the impact of fatigue on physical, cognitive, and psychosocial functioning, indicating widespread effects on daily activities.

Occupational Therapy Plan of Care and Goals:

The client will receive skilled occupational therapy services twice a week for 12 weeks to improve her independence in ADLs, manage fatigue, and enhance her quality of life.

Goals:

1. Client will independently prepare gluten-free meals using adaptive kitchen tools, improving her ability to manage dietary restrictions as measured by a 30% improvement in COPM scores within 12 weeks.
2. Client will independently perform morning dressing routines using adapted strategies to reduce joint stress and conserve energy, aiming for a 50% reduction in perceived exertion by the end of the intervention period.
3. Client will complete bathing independently using adaptive equipment like a shower chair and long-handled sponges to reduce fatigue, with a goal of reducing perceived exertion by at least 50% on a self-reported fatigue scale within 12 weeks.
4. Client will report improved sexual functioning and reduced discomfort during intercourse by incorporating recommended therapeutic exercises and relaxation techniques, achieving at least a 30% improvement in the Sexual Functioning Questionnaire (SFQ) scores within 12 weeks.
5. Client will effectively manage symptoms of anxiety and depression, improving scores on the Beck Depression Inventory by 40% through targeted psychosocial interventions within 12 weeks.
6. Client will increase social participation by developing strategies for managing social situations, particularly during family gatherings and social events, without feeling isolated or overwhelmed, as measured by self-reported satisfaction and participation rates within 12 weeks.
7. Client will improve bowel function management, reducing the frequency and impact of diarrhea and constipation by 50% through toileting interventions and dietary modifications, as measured by the Bristol Stool Form Scale and a bathroom visit log within 12 weeks.

Occupational Therapy Interventions:

The following interventions will be tailored to meet the client's specific needs and address the outlined goals:

Pain and Fatigue Management Strategies:
- Employ relaxation techniques like deep breathing and progressive muscle relaxation to combat fatigue and muscle weakness.
- Utilize heat therapy and gentle massage to alleviate muscle and joint pain, particularly in areas affected by celiac disease.

Activity Modification and Energy Conservation:
- Educate the client on energy conservation techniques, such as scheduling high-energy tasks at peak times and incorporating frequent rest breaks.
- Advise on modifying activities at work to manage energy, such as arranging the workspace to minimize the need to lift heavy items.

ADL Retraining and Use of Adaptive Equipment:
- Provide training on the use of adaptive kitchen tools designed for individuals with limited mobility, such as ergonomic knives and long-handled cooking utensils.
- Teach ergonomic techniques and the use of assistive devices that reduce strain during daily activities, enhancing safety and independence in ADLs.

Health and Nutrition Management:
- Partner with a dietitian to develop a meal plan that helps maintain energy levels and supports overall health.
- Educate the client on the importance of regular, nutritious meals that are balanced and tailored to her needs, emphasizing the role of good nutrition in managing fatigue and enhancing physical function.

Emotional and Psychological Support:
- Offer psychosocial counseling sessions to address irritability and stress, employing cognitive-behavioural techniques to improve emotional regulation.
- Implement stress management strategies to help stabilize mood and enhance overall mental well-being.

Interventions for Peripheral Neuropathy:
- Introduce exercises aimed at improving nerve function and reducing discomfort, such as balance training and gentle stretching exercises.
- Recommend the use of therapeutic footwear and protective padding to alleviate discomfort during mobility and daily activities.

Bowel Function Management:
- Teach toileting interventions, such as using a stool to elevate knees above hips and bending over to facilitate bowel movements.
- Develop a bathroom visit log to track the frequency and consistency of bowel movements, using the Bristol Stool Form Scale to monitor progress.
- Provide dietary recommendations to manage constipation and diarrhea, focusing on high-fiber and gluten-free foods.

Environmental Modifications:
- Suggest home and workplace modifications to reduce physical demands, such as reorganizing living and working spaces to ensure necessary items are within easy reach.
- Recommend adjustments in the home to facilitate easier access and mobility, especially in areas where the client performs daily routines.

Outcomes:

Post Treatment:

- **Fatigue Management**: Significant improvement in managing fatigue, evidenced by a 50% reduction in the Modified Fatigue Impact Scale (MFIS) scores, with the client reporting increased stamina and reduced daily exhaustion.
- **ADL Independence**: Improved engagement in personal care and household tasks, with the client achieving a Barthel Index score increase from 50 to 85, reflecting increased independence and reduced need for assistance.
- **Mood Stability**: Notable improvement in mood, evidenced by a significant reduction in depressive symptoms, as observed by family members and documented in therapy sessions. The client reported feeling more positive and engaged in her daily activities and social interactions.
- **Work and Social Engagement**: Return to part-time work with adapted strategies, successfully managing tasks without significant fatigue or stress. The client effectively used occupational therapy techniques to manage her energy and physical capabilities, which improved her ability to fulfill her professional responsibilities and engage in social activities.
- **Peripheral Neuropathy Management**: Semmes–Weinstein Monofilament Test indicated improved sensation in hands and feet, with decreased severity of peripheral neuropathy symptoms.
- **Bowel Function Management**: Reduced frequency and impact of diarrhea and constipation, with improved bowel movements as monitored by the Bristol Stool Form Scale and bathroom visit log.

Follow-Up Visits:

- Continuously reinforce energy conservation techniques and activity modifications to ensure the sustainability of the client's improvements in daily activities and work tasks.
- Provide ongoing support and adjust the client's treatment plan based on her feedback, changes in her symptoms, and any new challenges that arise in managing her celiac disease.

The client demonstrated marked improvement in managing her celiac disease and its symptoms, enhancing her overall functionality and independence. She is now capable of performing daily tasks such as cooking, cleaning, and personal care with greater efficiency and less fatigue. Additionally, her ability to manage her condition has significantly stabilized her health. The strategic use of assistive devices and tailored occupational therapy interventions enabled her to return to part-time work, effectively balancing her professional and health needs. Through the collaborative and holistic approach of occupational therapy, the client has regained a better quality of life and improved her capacity to engage in meaningful activities.

Further Reading

American Occupational Therapy Association. (2020). Occupational therapy practice framework: Domain and process (4th ed.). *American Journal of Occupational Therapy, 74*(Suppl. 2), 7412410010. https://doi.org/10.5014/ajot.2020.74S2001

Cerasola, D., Argano, C., Chiovaro, V., Trivic, T., Scepanovic, T., Drid, P., & Corrao, S. (2023). Physical exercise and occupational therapy at home to improve the quality of life in subjects affected by rheumatoid arthritis: A randomized controlled trial. *Healthcare (Basel, Switzerland), 11*(15), 2123. https://doi.org/10.3390/healthcare11152123

Gavin, J. P., Rossiter, L., Fenerty, V., Leese, J., Adams, J., Hammond, A., Davidson, E., & Backman, C. L. (2024). The impact of occupational therapy on the self-management of rheumatoid arthritis: A mixed methods systematic review. *ACR Open Rheumatology, 6*(4), 214–249. https://doi.org/10.1002/acr2.11650

George, P., Jagun, O., Liu, Q., Wentworth, C., Napatalung, L., Wolk, R., Anway, S., & Zwillich, S. H. (2023). Prevalence of autoimmune and inflammatory diseases and mental health conditions among an alopecia areata cohort from a US administrative claims database. *The Journal of Dermatology, 50*(9), 1121–1128. https://doi.org/10.1111/1346-8138.16839

Mälstam, E., Bensing, S., & Asaba, E. (2018). Everyday managing and living with autoimmune Addison's disease: Exploring experiences using photovoice methods. *Scandinavian Journal of Occupational Therapy, 25*(5), 358–370. https://doi.org/10.1080/11038128.2018.1502351

Mincer, D. L., & Jialal, I. (2023). Hashimoto thyroiditis. In *StatPearls*. StatPearls Publishing.

Posner, E. B., & Haseeb, M. (2023). Celiac disease. In *StatPearls*. StatPearls Publishing.

Yin, R., Xu, B., Li, L., Fu, T., Zhang, L., Zhang, Q., Li, X., & Shen, B. (2017). The impact of systemic lupus erythematosus on women's sexual functioning: A systematic review and meta-analysis. *Medicine, 96*(27), e7162. https://doi.org/10.1097/MD.0000000000007162

6 Non-Cisgender Health in the Context of Women's Health

Chapter Objectives

Upon completion of this chapter, the reader will be able to:

1. Understand the unique health needs of non-cisgender individuals assigned female at birth and the impact of gender dysphoria, hormone therapy, and surgical interventions on occupational performance.
2. Explore occupational therapy approaches to managing healthcare disparities and barriers faced by non-cisgender individuals, emphasizing inclusive and client-centered care.
3. Discuss strategies for promoting mental health and well-being among non-cisgender individuals, including stress management, resilience building, and access to supportive resources.
4. Address the role of occupational therapy in navigating gender-affirming care, including preoperative and postoperative support, hormone therapy management, and legal and administrative assistance.
5. Highlight the importance of social support and community engagement in enhancing the quality of life for non-cisgender individuals, and the occupational therapy interventions that facilitate social participation and advocacy.

Understanding Unique Health Needs of Non-Cisgender Individuals Assigned Female at Birth

Non-cisgender individuals assigned female at birth (AFAB) include transgender men, non-binary individuals, and genderqueer individuals, among others. Their health needs often differ significantly from those of cisgender women due to the complexities of gender dysphoria, hormone therapy, surgical interventions, and the psychosocial challenges associated with navigating a society that may not fully accept their gender identity. Understanding these unique needs through an occupational lens allows OTPs to provide comprehensive, client-centered care that enhances the quality of life for these individuals. See Table 6.1 for common terms related to gender diversity.

Hormone therapy, particularly testosterone for those seeking masculinization, plays a crucial role in aligning an individual's physical appearance with their gender identity. Testosterone therapy can induce physical changes such as increased muscle mass, deepening of the voice, redistribution of body fat, and cessation of menstruation. These changes can significantly impact an individual's self-esteem and mental health but also come with potential side effects such as fluctuations in energy levels, mood changes, and impacts on bone density and cardiovascular health. Initial phases of hormone therapy can cause fatigue, which may impact one's ability to engage fully in daily tasks or work responsibilities.

Occupational Therapy Interventions

OTPs can support clients in managing these changes by developing personalized energy conservation strategies, pacing techniques, and adaptive routines that accommodate fluctuations in energy and mood. Additionally, OTPs can provide education on the potential physical changes and how to safely engage in functional activities that align with their gender identity goals.

Surgical Interventions

Gender-affirming surgeries, such as chest masculinization (top surgery), hysterectomy, and other procedures, are often pursued by non-cisgender AFAB individuals to achieve physical characteristics that are congruent with their gender identity. These surgeries can greatly enhance psychological well-being and reduce gender dysphoria. However, they require significant postoperative care and rehabilitation, which can impact an individual's ability to perform daily activities, work, and engage in social participation.

Impact on Daily Living

Gender-affirming surgeries such as chest masculinization (top surgery) or hysterectomy require significant postoperative care and rehabilitation. These surgeries can affect functional mobility, self-care routines, and participation in daily activities.

Table 6.1 Key terminology related to gender diversity

Term	Definition
Cisgender	Describes a person whose gender identity aligns with their sex assigned at birth.
Gender diverse or expansive	An umbrella term for a person with a gender identity and/or expression broader than the male or female binary.
Gender dysphoria	Clinically significant distress that a person may feel when sex or gender assigned at birth is not the same as their identity.
Gender identity	One's internal sense of self as man, woman, both, or neither.
Nonbinary	Describes a person who does not identify with the man or woman gender binary.
Transgender	Describes a person whose gender identity and/or expression is different from their sex assigned at birth, and societal and cultural expectations around sex.

OT Interventions

OTPs can facilitate recovery through interventions focused on mobility, pain management, and scar care. This includes teaching clients how to safely perform ADLs and IADLs during the recovery period, as well as providing ergonomic recommendations to prevent strain on surgical sites. Furthermore, OTPs can develop tailored exercise programs to aid in the recovery process and improve physical strength and flexibility.

Example Intervention: Post-Top Surgery Recovery Plan

1. **Mobility and Pain Management**
   - **Education on Safe Movement**: Educate the client on how to safely get in and out of bed, perform transfers, and engage in light activities without putting undue strain on the surgical site.
   - **Pain Management Techniques**: Teach relaxation techniques, such as deep breathing exercises, and recommend appropriate use of pain relief modalities, such as ice packs and prescribed pain medications.

2. **Scar Care**
   - **Scar Massage**: Educate the client on scar massage techniques to prevent adhesions and improve scar mobility once the incision sites have healed sufficiently.
   - **Use of Silicone Gel Sheets**: Recommend silicone gel sheets or ointments to reduce scar formation and improve the appearance of scars.

3. **ADLs and IADLs**
   - **Adaptive Equipment**: Provide adaptive equipment, such as long-handled reachers and dressing aids, to help the client perform self-care tasks independently.
   - **Ergonomic Recommendations**: Offer ergonomic advice to help the client avoid postural strain during activities such as working at a desk or engaging in household chores.

4. **Exercise Programs**
   - **Gentle Stretching**: Develop a gentle stretching program to maintain shoulder and upper body mobility without stressing the surgical site.
   - **Strengthening Exercises**: Gradually introduce strengthening exercises to improve overall physical strength and endurance, tailored to the client's recovery stage and physical capabilities.

5. **Pacing and Energy Conservation**
   - **Pacing Techniques**: Teach the client how to pace activities, alternating periods of rest with activity to manage fatigue.
   - **Energy Conservation Strategies**: Develop energy conservation strategies to help the client prioritize tasks and reduce unnecessary exertion.

6. **Psychosocial Support**
   - **Support Groups**: Facilitate connections with support groups or peer networks for emotional support during recovery.

- **Stress Management**: Implement stress management techniques, such as mindfulness and cognitive-behavioural strategies, to help the client cope with any emotional challenges related to the recovery process.

By incorporating these interventions, OTPs can provide comprehensive support to non-cisgender AFAB individuals undergoing gender-affirming surgeries, enhancing their recovery and improving their overall quality of life.

Mental Health

Mental health challenges are prevalent among non-cisgender AFAB individuals, with higher rates of anxiety, depression, and suicidal ideation compared to their cisgender peers. These challenges are often exacerbated by societal stigma, discrimination, and a lack of acceptance. The emotional burden of navigating gender dysphoria and the physical and social changes associated with transition can significantly impact mental health.

Impact on Occupational Engagement

High rates of anxiety, depression, and suicidal ideation are prevalent among non-cisgender AFAB individuals due to societal stigma and discrimination. These mental health challenges can significantly impact engagement in meaningful occupations.

OT Interventions

OTPs can incorporate stress management techniques, mindfulness practices, and cognitive-behavioural strategies into therapy to help clients manage anxiety and depression. Creating a safe and supportive environment in therapy sessions where clients feel respected and understood is crucial. OTPs can also offer psychoeducation on gender identity and the impact of societal stigma, and facilitate access to gender-affirming mental health services.

Social Support

Social support is a critical component of overall well-being for non-cisgender AFAB individuals. Acceptance and support from family, friends, and the community can significantly impact mental health and quality of life. Conversely, lack of support and social isolation can exacerbate mental health issues and hinder the transition process.

Impact on Social Participation

Social support is critical for the well-being of non-cisgender AFAB individuals. Lack of acceptance from family, peers, and community can lead to social isolation and reduced participation in social activities.

OT Interventions

OTPs can help clients build and maintain social support networks by facilitating connections with supportive community resources, organizing peer support groups, and encouraging participation in inclusive social activities. Educating families and communities about gender diversity can also foster a more supportive environment. OTPs can also develop social skills training programs to help clients navigate social interactions and build confidence in their identity.

Addressing Specific Occupational Needs

Addressing the specific occupational needs of non-cisgender AFAB individuals is crucial in women's health, as these needs significantly impact their daily lives, social roles, and overall well-being. OTPs play a vital role in helping clients navigate the complexities of identity and role transitions, self-care and health management, and community and social participation. Understanding and addressing these needs through an occupational lens ensures that interventions are tailored to support the unique challenges faced by this population

Identity and Role Transitions

Identity and role transitions are significant for non-cisgender AFAB individuals, impacting their social roles, work identity, and self-perception. These transitions can create challenges in maintaining existing occupational roles and developing new ones that align with their gender identity. Non-cisgender AFAB individuals often undergo significant identity and role transitions, which can impact their occupational roles and routines. This includes changes in social roles, work identity, and self-perception.

OT Interventions: OTPs can support clients through these transitions by helping them explore and establish new roles and routines that align with their gender identity. This might involve career counseling, developing new leisure interests, and supporting identity exploration through meaningful activities. OTPs can also facilitate life skills training to help clients effectively adapt to their new roles and responsibilities.

Self-Care and Health Management

Managing hormone therapy, surgical recovery, and mental health requires effective self-care and health management skills. Non-cisgender AFAB individuals may face unique challenges in maintaining these routines due to barriers in accessing knowledgeable healthcare providers and supportive resources. Managing hormone therapy, surgical recovery, and mental health requires effective self-care and health management skills. Non-cisgender AFAB individuals may face unique challenges in maintaining these routines due to barriers in accessing knowledgeable healthcare providers and supportive resources.

OT Interventions: OTPs can provide education on self-care practices, including medication management, nutrition, and physical activity. They can also assist in developing health management routines that are sustainable and integrate seamlessly into clients' daily lives. OTPs can offer specialized training in safe binding practices for transgender men and non-binary individuals, and provide resources on safe tucking techniques for those who need them.

Community and Social Participation

Engaging in community and social activities is essential for overall well-being, but non-cisgender AFAB individuals often face barriers due to discrimination and lack of inclusive spaces.

OT Interventions: OTPs can help clients identify and access inclusive community resources and social groups. They can also work with community organizations to develop more inclusive programming and environments. OTPs can facilitate community integration programs that promote social participation and advocacy for gender diversity.

By adopting an occupational lens, OTPs can better understand and address the unique health needs of non-cisgender AFAB individuals. This holistic approach ensures that therapy interventions are tailored to enhance clients' participation in meaningful activities, promote overall well-being, and support their journey toward living authentically and comfortably in their gender identity.

Addressing Healthcare Disparities and Barriers

Non-cisgender AFAB individuals face significant healthcare disparities and barriers, which can negatively impact their access to quality care and overall health outcomes. According to a 2015 U.S. Transgender Survey, 33% of transgender individuals reported having at least one negative experience with a healthcare provider in the past year, such as verbal harassment, refusal of treatment, or having to teach the provider about transgender care. These barriers include discrimination, lack of knowledgeable healthcare providers, limited access to gender-affirming care, and financial constraints. OTPs can play a crucial role in mitigating these disparities and improving the healthcare experience for non-cisgender individuals.

Discrimination in Healthcare Settings

Discrimination and bias in healthcare settings are common challenges for non-cisgender individuals. They may encounter providers who lack understanding or exhibit prejudiced attitudes, leading to distrust and avoidance of medical care. Discrimination can manifest in various ways, such as misgendering, refusal to provide care, or inadequate treatment.

OT Interventions:

1. **Creating Inclusive Environments**: OTPs can ensure their practices are inclusive by using gender-neutral language, displaying inclusive signage, and implementing non-discrimination policies. Simple steps such as asking for and consistently using a client's chosen name and pronouns can create a more welcoming environment. OTPs can also develop inclusive intake forms and assessments that allow clients to self-identify their gender and pronouns.
2. **Education and Training**: OTPs should participate in ongoing cultural competency training to better understand the unique experiences and needs of non-cisgender individuals. This training can include topics such as gender identity, the impact of discrimination, and best practices for providing gender-affirming care. OTPs can advocate for these training sessions to be incorporated into staff development programs within their workplaces.
3. **Advocacy**: OTPs can advocate for systemic changes within healthcare institutions to promote inclusivity and reduce discrimination. This may involve working with administration to develop and enforce inclusive policies and advocating for the inclusion of LGBTQ+ health topics in professional education curricula. OTPs can also collaborate

with interdisciplinary teams to ensure that all staff members are trained in providing respectful and inclusive care.

Lack of Knowledgeable Providers

Many healthcare providers lack adequate knowledge about the health needs of non-cisgender individuals, leading to gaps in care. This can result in misdiagnosis, inappropriate treatment, or neglect of important aspects of health related to gender transition.

OTP Interventions:

1. **Self-Education**: OTPs should actively seek out resources and training opportunities to increase their knowledge of non-cisgender health issues. This includes understanding the effects of hormone therapy, surgical options, and the psychosocial challenges associated with gender transition. OTPs can engage in continuing education courses, attend conferences, and participate in professional networks focused on LGBTQ+ health.
2. **Collaborative Care**: OTPs can collaborate with other healthcare professionals, such as endocrinologists, surgeons, and mental health providers, to ensure comprehensive and coordinated care for non-cisgender clients. Building a network of knowledgeable providers can enhance the quality of care. OTPs can also facilitate interdisciplinary team meetings to discuss complex cases and ensure that all aspects of a client's health are addressed.
3. **Resource Sharing**: Sharing educational materials and resources with colleagues can help improve overall provider knowledge within a healthcare setting. OTPs can also develop informational brochures or resource lists for clients to help them find knowledgeable providers. OTPs can organize and lead workshops or in-service training sessions for healthcare staff to disseminate knowledge on best practices in caring for non-cisgender individuals.

Limited Access to Gender-Affirming Care

Accessing gender-affirming care can be challenging due to geographical barriers, limited availability of specialized providers, and restrictive insurance policies. These barriers can delay or prevent necessary treatments, leading to negative health outcomes.

OTP Interventions:

1. **Resource Navigation**: OTPs can assist clients in navigating the healthcare system to access gender-affirming care. This includes helping clients find local or telehealth providers, understand their insurance coverage, and apply for financial assistance programs. OTPs can create detailed guides or resource maps that outline steps for accessing care and available financial resources.
2. **Telehealth Services**: Telehealth can be a valuable tool for providing access to gender-affirming care, especially for clients in rural or underserved areas. OTPs can offer telehealth services for follow-up care, consultations, and ongoing support. Telehealth can also be used to conduct virtual support groups and workshops that provide education and peer support for non-cisgender individuals.

3. **Community Outreach**: OTPs can work with community organizations to increase awareness and availability of gender-affirming services. Partnering with LGBTQ+ organizations can help bridge the gap between clients and providers. OTPs can participate in community events, health fairs, and advocacy campaigns to raise awareness about the importance of gender-affirming care and the resources available.

Financial Barriers

The cost of healthcare, including gender-affirming surgeries and hormone therapy, can be prohibitive for many non-cisgender individuals. Financial constraints can lead to delayed or forgone care, exacerbating health disparities.

OTP Interventions:

1. **Financial Counseling**: OTPs can provide financial counseling to help clients understand their insurance benefits, navigate coverage for gender-affirming care, and explore options for financial assistance. This includes connecting clients with programs that offer grants or subsidies for medical expenses. OTPs can collaborate with social workers or financial counselors to provide comprehensive support.
2. **Assistance with Applications**: Helping clients complete applications for financial assistance programs, charity care, or sliding-scale clinics can reduce the financial burden of care. OTPs can also assist with appeals processes if insurance claims are denied. Providing templates and checklists for applications can streamline the process for clients.
3. **Cost-Effective Care Strategies**: Developing cost-effective care strategies, such as recommending affordable adaptive equipment or home modifications, can help clients manage their health within their financial means. OTPs can also educate clients on DIY adaptations and low-cost solutions for home modifications.

Creating Inclusive Healthcare Environments

Fostering an inclusive and welcoming healthcare environment is essential for improving the healthcare experience of non-cisgender individuals. OTPs can take active steps to ensure their practice is inclusive and affirming.

OTP Interventions:

1. **Inclusive Language**: Consistently use gender-inclusive language in all communications, including intake forms, medical records, and verbal interactions. Avoid making assumptions about gender identity or pronouns. OTPs can develop training materials and workshops to educate staff on the importance of inclusive language.
2. **Visible Inclusivity**: Display symbols of inclusivity, such as LGBTQ+ pride flags or inclusive posters, in the therapy space to signal that it is a safe and welcoming environment. OTPs can also create inclusive waiting areas by providing diverse reading materials and ensuring that educational resources reflect the experiences of non-cisgender individuals.
3. **Non-Discrimination Policies**: Implement and enforce non-discrimination policies that explicitly include gender identity and expression. Ensure that all staff members are trained on these policies and understand their importance. OTPs can advocate for the inclusion of these policies in their workplace and monitor their implementation.

4. **Client Feedback**: Regularly seek feedback from clients about their experiences and use this feedback to make improvements. Creating an open dialogue can help identify areas for improvement and ensure that the practice remains inclusive and responsive to client needs. OTPs can use surveys, suggestion boxes, and focus groups to gather feedback and implement changes based on client input.

Side Effects of Hormone Replacement Therapy

Hormone replacement therapy is a crucial component for many non-cisgender individuals seeking to align their physical appearance with their gender identity. While HRT can have profound positive effects on mental health and self-esteem, it is also important to be aware of the potential side effects and health risks associated with this treatment. Understanding these side effects allows OTPs to provide comprehensive and informed care. See Table 6.2 for a comparison of the physical changes, potential side effects, and health risks associated with hormone replacement therapy for transgender men and women.

Understanding the side effects of HRT is essential for OTPs when developing and implementing intervention plans. By considering these potential side effects, OTPs can tailor their approaches to address specific challenges and enhance the overall well-being of their clients. For example:

- **Activity Modification**: Clients experiencing fatigue or mood swings may benefit from energy conservation techniques and stress management strategies integrated into their daily routines.

Table 6.2 Effects and potential risks of hormone replacement therapy for transgender individuals

HRT for Transgender Men (Testosterone Therapy)	HRT for Transgender Women (Estrogen Therapy)
Physical Changes:	Physical Changes:
- Increased muscle mass and body hair growth - Deepening of the voice - Cessation of menstruation - Redistribution of body fat	- Development of breast tissue - Redistribution of body fat to hips and thighs - Reduced muscle mass - Decreased body hair growth
Potential Side Effects: Cardiovascular Issues:	Potential Side Effects: Cardiovascular Issues:
- Increased risk of high blood pressure - Elevated cholesterol levels	- Increased risk of blood clots and stroke - Elevated triglycerides
Emotional and Psychological Effects:	Emotional and Psychological Effects:
- Mood swings and irritability - Increased aggression or anxiety	- Mood fluctuations - Risk of depression or anxiety
Other Health Risks:	Other Health Risks:
- Acne and skin oiliness - Risk of liver dysfunction - Changes in libido	- Risk of liver dysfunction - Increased risk of certain cancers (e.g., breast cancer) - Reduced libido

- **Health Management**: OTPs can work with clients to monitor and manage cardiovascular health, including promoting physical activity and healthy eating habits.
- **Psychosocial Support**: Providing emotional support and resources for mental health services can help clients navigate mood changes and psychological impacts.
- **Education and Advocacy**: Educating clients about potential side effects and encouraging regular medical check-ups can ensure early detection and management of health risks.

By addressing these healthcare disparities and barriers, OTPs can significantly improve the health outcomes and quality of life for non-cisgender AFAB individuals. Providing inclusive, knowledgeable, and supportive care is essential for fostering a healthcare environment where all clients feel respected and valued.

Inclusive Approaches in Occupational Therapy for Diverse Women's Health

Inclusive approaches in occupational therapy are essential for effectively addressing the diverse health needs of non-cisgender individuals within the context of women's health. These approaches ensure that all clients feel respected, understood, and supported. By adopting a client-centered approach, OTPs can create tailored interventions that recognize and honor the unique experiences of non-cisgender clients.

Using inclusive language is crucial for creating a welcoming environment. This involves consistently using clients' chosen names and pronouns, avoiding assumptions about gender identity, and integrating gender-neutral language into all communications. OTPs can modify intake forms and medical records to include options for gender identity and preferred pronouns. For example, when discussing daily routines, an OTP might say, "Can you describe your morning routine?" instead of assuming gender-specific tasks.

Client-centered care involves engaging clients in shared decision-making, respecting their preferences, and developing individualized care plans that align with their goals and values. OTPs can use the Canadian Occupational Performance Measure (COPM) to identify and prioritize clients' goals and concerns, ensuring interventions are tailored to their unique needs. For example, an OTP working with a transgender man recovering from top surgery might focus on activities that support both physical recovery and the client's personal goals, such as returning to work or resuming physical fitness routines.

Safe and affirming environments are essential for effective therapy. This includes both the physical space and the interpersonal interactions within it. OTPs can create safe spaces by displaying inclusive materials, ensuring confidentiality, and fostering an atmosphere of respect and understanding. Providing private changing areas and inclusive restrooms can help non-cisgender clients feel more comfortable during therapy sessions. Table 6.3 lists specific considerations and examples of safe inclusive spaces.

Continuous cultural competency training helps OTPs understand the unique experiences and needs of non-cisgender individuals, improving the quality of care provided. OTPs can attend workshops, seminars, and online courses focused on LGBTQ+ health and cultural competency. They can also join professional networks and organizations that offer resources and support. For example, participating in a workshop on the impact of minority stress on non-cisgender individuals can enhance an OTP's ability to provide empathetic and informed care.

Adapting traditional women's health interventions to be inclusive involves recognizing and addressing the specific needs of non-cisgender individuals. OTPs can modify interventions to accommodate the unique experiences of non-cisgender clients, such as

Table 6.3 Strategies for creating safe and inclusive environments in rehabilitation for non-cisgender clients

	Specific Examples	*Implementation Tips*
Physical Environment	- Provide gender-neutral restrooms and changing areas with clear signage. - Display LGBTQ+ inclusive symbols, such as pride flags, rainbow decals, or inclusive posters in common areas and therapy rooms. - Create private spaces for changing and personal care that are easily accessible.	- Conduct regular environmental audits to identify areas for improvement. - Involve LGBTQ+ staff or consultants in the design and layout of facilities. - Ensure privacy curtains and partitions are available in shared therapy spaces.
Intake and Documentation	- Use intake forms that include options for gender identity (e.g., "man," "woman," "non-binary," "transgender," "prefer to self-describe") and preferred pronouns. - Include sections for chosen name and sex assigned at birth. - Avoid using "Mr." or "Ms." unless specifically requested by the client.	- Regularly review and update forms to ensure they remain inclusive. - Train administrative staff on the importance of inclusive documentation and how to discuss these forms with clients. - Use electronic health records that allow for customization of gender identity fields.
Communication	- Consistently use clients' chosen names and pronouns during all interactions. - Include gender-neutral language in all verbal and written communications, such as "partner" instead of "husband" or "wife." - Avoid gendered terms like "ladies and gentlemen" and use inclusive alternatives like "everyone."	- Incorporate inclusive language training into staff development programs. - Create a culture of respect and inclusivity in all interactions. - Encourage staff to practice using inclusive language in team meetings and role-playing scenarios.
Staff Training	- Conduct ongoing cultural competency training focused on LGBTQ+ health, including modules on non-cisgender health needs. - Include training on specific health disparities faced by non-cisgender clients and the impact of minority stress. - Provide workshops on the use of inclusive language and the importance of pronouns.	- Schedule regular refresher courses and include guest speakers from the LGBTQ+ community. - Evaluate training effectiveness through staff feedback and client satisfaction surveys. - Encourage participation in external LGBTQ+ health conferences and seminars.
Client-Centered Care	- Engage clients in shared decision-making regarding their care plans by asking about their goals, preferences, and concerns. - Use tools like the COPM to identify and prioritize individual goals related to occupational performance. - Customize care plans to include gender-affirming practices, such as recognizing the impact of hormone therapy on physical and emotional health.	- Foster open communication and ensure clients feel comfortable expressing their needs and preferences. - Document and respect clients' care preferences consistently. - Schedule regular check-ins with clients to reassess goals and adjust care plans as needed.

(Continued)

Table 6.3 (Contiuned)

	Specific Examples	Implementation Tips
Support Services	- Facilitate connections with LGBTQ+ support groups and community resources, such as LGBTQ+ centers, peer support networks, and online forums. - Offer peer support programs within the rehabilitation setting where clients can share experiences and strategies.	- Maintain an updated list of local and online resources, including mental health professionals experienced in gender-affirming care. - Encourage clients to participate in support groups and peer programs. - Organize social events and workshops that promote community building and peer support.
Privacy and Confidentiality	- Ensure private consultation and therapy rooms for discussions about sensitive topics. - Maintain strict confidentiality regarding clients' gender identities and medical histories by using secure data storage and communication methods. - Clearly communicate privacy policies to clients and ensure they understand their rights.	- Develop clear policies on privacy and confidentiality. - Train all staff members on these policies and regularly monitor compliance. - Use electronic health records with privacy settings that limit access to sensitive information.
Advocacy and Policy Development	- Advocate for inclusive policies within the healthcare setting, such as non-discrimination policies that explicitly include gender identity and expression. - Develop and implement policies that support the use of chosen names and pronouns in all interactions and documentation. - Work with healthcare administrators to ensure inclusive practices are part of the organizational culture.	- Work with administration to develop policies and ensure they are communicated to all staff. - Involve clients in policy development to ensure their needs are met. - Participate in or form diversity and inclusion committees to continually assess and improve policies.
Holistic Care Approaches	- Integrate physical, mental, and social health interventions into care plans by collaborating with multidisciplinary teams. - Address both medical and psychosocial needs of clients through comprehensive assessments and individualized care plans. - Incorporate gender-affirming practices into all aspects of care, such as hormone therapy support and gender-affirming surgery preparation and recovery.	- Use interdisciplinary teams to provide comprehensive care. - Regularly review and adjust care plans to reflect clients' evolving needs and goals. - Provide ongoing education to clients about holistic health practices and self-care strategies.

adapting pelvic floor therapy for transgender men or non-binary individuals. For example, when providing pelvic floor therapy, an OTP might offer specific exercises and education on pelvic health that align with the client's anatomy and gender identity.

Promoting Mental Health and Well-being

Promoting mental health and well-being is crucial for non-cisgender individuals, given the high prevalence of mental health challenges in this population. OTPs play a key role in supporting mental health through targeted interventions and supportive care. By addressing both the psychological and social aspects of health, OTPs can help clients build resilience, improve coping skills, and enhance their overall quality of life.

Non-cisgender individuals often face higher rates of anxiety, depression, and suicidal ideation due to societal stigma, discrimination, and the stress associated with gender dysphoria. Addressing these challenges is essential for promoting overall well-being. OTPs can use the Kawa Model to understand clients' life flow and identify barriers and supports affecting their mental health. For example, an OTP might use the Kawa Model to explore a client's experiences with gender dysphoria and societal stigma, identifying strategies to enhance resilience and support.

Access to counseling and peer support groups that affirm gender identity can provide essential emotional support and community connection. OTPs can facilitate referrals to gender-affirming mental health professionals and local support groups, and can also create and lead support groups within their practice. Creating a peer support group for non-cisgender individuals can provide a safe space for sharing experiences and coping strategies.

Stress management techniques such as mindfulness, progressive muscle relaxation, and cognitive-behavioural strategies can help manage anxiety and stress. OTPs can integrate stress management techniques into therapy sessions, teaching clients how to incorporate these practices into their daily routines. For example, an OTP might teach a client mindfulness meditation techniques to reduce anxiety and improve focus during daily activities.

Fostering resilience involves helping clients identify and build on their strengths and coping strategies, enhancing their ability to navigate challenges. OTPs can use strengths-based approaches to help clients recognize their capabilities and develop new skills for managing stress and adversity. For example, using the strengths-based approach, an OTP might help a client identify personal strengths, such as creativity or problem-solving, and apply these strengths to overcome challenges.

Providing crisis intervention support is essential for clients experiencing acute mental health crises, ensuring their safety and well-being. OTPs can develop safety plans with clients, connect them with emergency mental health services, and provide immediate support during crises. For example, developing a crisis plan that includes emergency contacts, coping strategies, and steps to take in case of a mental health emergency. See Table 6.4 for specific mental health and well-being interventions for non-cisgender clients.

Following the implementation of these mental health and well-being interventions, it is crucial for OTPs to continuously evaluate and adjust the care plans to meet the evolving needs of their clients. Regular follow-ups and feedback sessions can ensure that the interventions remain effective and relevant. Additionally, creating a supportive and inclusive

Table 6.4 Mental health and well-being interventions for non-cisgender clients

Intervention Area	Specific Strategies	Examples for Practice
Cognitive-Behavioural Therapy (CBT)	Use CBT techniques to address negative thought patterns and emotional regulation.	Work with clients to identify and challenge negative thoughts related to gender dysphoria and replace them with positive affirmations. Integrate these techniques into everyday activities like journaling or during routines to create a more structured day.
Dialectical Behavior Therapy (DBT)	Incorporate DBT strategies to help clients manage intense emotions and improve interpersonal effectiveness.	Teach clients DBT skills such as distress tolerance, emotional regulation, and mindfulness to cope with gender dysphoria and societal stressors. Practice these skills in sessions through role-playing social situations or during relaxation activities. **(Note: Requires specialized training)**
Acceptance and Commitment Therapy (ACT)	Utilize ACT to help clients accept their thoughts and feelings while committing to behavior changes aligned with their values.	Guide clients in identifying their core values and developing actions that align with these values despite the presence of distressing thoughts. Apply ACT principles during daily decision-making processes and during goal-setting activities. **(Note: Requires specialized training)**
Expressive Arts Therapy	Utilize creative arts such as painting, music, and dance to help clients express emotions and process experiences.	Organize weekly art therapy sessions where clients can use various art forms to explore and express their feelings about their gender identity. Encourage clients to integrate these practices into their leisure activities at home.
Mindfulness and Relaxation Techniques	Teach mindfulness meditation, progressive muscle relaxation, and guided imagery.	Conduct a series of mindfulness workshops that include guided meditation and practical tips for incorporating mindfulness into daily routines. Practice mindfulness during everyday tasks such as eating or walking.
Stress Management	Provide training in stress management techniques, such as deep breathing exercises and progressive muscle relaxation.	Develop personalized stress management plans that include daily relaxation exercises and strategies for managing stress triggers. Practice these techniques during sessions and create stress-relief kits for clients to use at home.
Social Skills Training	Teach and practice social skills to improve communication and social interactions.	Role-play social scenarios where clients may face misgendering or discrimination, and provide strategies to manage these situations effectively. Implement these skills in social outings or community engagement activities.
Peer Support and Networking	Facilitate connections with peer support groups and community resources.	Organize peer support groups within the therapy setting for sharing experiences and coping strategies. Provide information about local LGBTQ+ organizations and online forums for additional support. Encourage participation in group activities that reinforce these connections.

(Continued)

Table 6.4 (Contiuned)

Intervention Area	Specific Strategies	Examples for Practice
Resilience Building	Use strengths-based approaches to help clients build resilience and coping strategies.	Help clients develop a personal strengths inventory and explore ways to apply these strengths in managing daily stress. Integrate resilience-building activities into daily routines, such as through goal-setting and reflecting on achievements.
Crisis Intervention	Develop safety plans, connect clients with emergency mental health services, and provide immediate support during crises.	Create a crisis intervention protocol that includes step-by-step instructions for clients and contacts for immediate support. Role-play crisis scenarios to help clients prepare and feel more confident in using their plans.
Trauma-Informed Care	Implement trauma-informed care practices to address past trauma and its impact on current functioning.	Provide a safe and supportive environment, recognizing the impact of trauma on mental health, and offer tailored interventions that acknowledge past experiences. Use trauma-informed approaches during routine therapy activities and when introducing new interventions.
Family and Caregiver Support	Educate and support families on understanding and affirming their non-cisgender loved one's identity.	Facilitate family therapy sessions where families can discuss challenges, learn about gender diversity, and enhance communication and support. Offer caregiver group sessions to educate parents and caregivers on gender-affirming practices and provide a supportive space for sharing experiences and strategies.

Note: Some of the approaches listed, such as Dialectical Behavior Therapy (DBT) and Acceptance and Commitment Therapy (ACT), may require additional specialized training for OTPs.

environment within therapy sessions encourages clients to express their needs and concerns openly, fostering a collaborative approach to care. By integrating these comprehensive strategies, OTPs can significantly enhance the mental health and well-being of non-cisgender clients, empowering them to lead fulfilling and balanced lives.

Navigating Gender-Affirming Care

Navigating gender-affirming care involves coordinating multiple aspects of healthcare to align outward physical traits with clients' gender identities and support their transition process. OTPs play a crucial role in facilitating access to and management of gender-affirming treatments and surgeries, addressing the comprehensive physical, mental, and social health needs of clients. See Table 6.5 for a description of gender affirming care.

Comprehensive care before and after gender-affirming surgeries is vital for successful outcomes and overall well-being. OTPs can provide preoperative education on surgical procedures and expected outcomes, develop postoperative care plans, and assist with pain management and mobility. For example, an OTP might create a postoperative care plan for a client undergoing top surgery, including exercises to prevent lymphedema, pain management strategies, and guidance on scar care.

Table 6.5 Gender affirming care examples

Affirming Care	Description	When is it used?	Reversible or not
Social Affirmation	Adopting gender-affirming hairstyles, clothing, name, gender pronouns, restrooms and other facilities	At any age or stage	Reversible
Puberty Blockers	Using certain types of hormones to pause pubertal development	During puberty	Reversible
Hormone Therapy	Testosterone hormones for those who were assigned female at birth Estrogen hormones for those who were assigned male at birth	Early adolescence onward	Partially reversible
Gender-Affirming Surgeries	"Top" surgery—to create male-typical chest shape or enhance breasts "Bottom" surgery—surgery on genitals or reproductive organs Facial feminization or other procedures	Typically used in adulthood or case-by-case in adolescence	Not reversible

Assisting clients in navigating legal and administrative processes related to gender transition, such as changing names and gender markers on identification documents, is another critical aspect of gender-affirming care. Connecting clients with community resources that offer gender-affirming services and support is crucial for holistic care. OTPs can identify and provide information about local and online support groups, LGBTQ+ health clinics, and advocacy organizations.

A holistic approach to gender-affirming care addresses physical, mental, and social health, ensuring comprehensive support for clients. OTPs can develop care plans that integrate physical rehabilitation, mental health support, and community engagement activities (see Table 6.6).

Following the implementation of these gender-affirming care interventions, it is essential for OTPs to maintain a client-centered approach that respects and validates the individual experiences and identities of their clients. Continuous collaboration with clients ensures that their evolving needs and goals are met. OTPs should engage in ongoing education and training on gender-affirming practices to stay informed about best practices and emerging trends in transgender healthcare.

Moreover, OTPs can advocate for systemic changes within healthcare institutions to promote inclusivity and accessibility for non-cisgender individuals. This might include developing educational materials for healthcare providers, participating in policy development, and fostering an environment that supports diversity and inclusion. By advocating for these changes, OTPs not only improve individual client outcomes but also contribute to broader societal shifts toward acceptance and equality.

In practice, incorporating occupation-based interventions tailored to the unique needs of non-cisgender clients can significantly enhance their daily functioning and overall quality of life. For instance, assisting clients in developing routines that incorporate self-care, social participation, and community engagement can foster a sense of belonging and identity affirmation. Additionally, supporting clients in navigating healthcare and legal systems ensures they have access to necessary resources and services, further empowering them to live authentically and confidently.

Table 6.6 Gender-affirming care interventions for non-cisgender clients

Intervention Area	Specific Strategies	Examples for Practice
Preoperative and Postoperative Care	- Provide preoperative education and develop postoperative care plans. - Assist with pain management and mobility post-surgery.	Develop a detailed postoperative care plan for a client undergoing top surgery, including exercises to prevent lymphedema, pain management strategies, and guidance on scar care. Integrate these strategies into daily routines and occupational activities, such as dressing, bathing, and house chores, to ensure safe recovery.
Hormone Therapy Management	- Monitor physical changes, manage side effects, and promote overall health.	Work with a client to create an exercise plan that addresses weight changes and muscle mass increases due to hormone therapy. Incorporate these exercises into daily routines, such as using resistance bands while preparing meals or doing household tasks.
Legal and Administrative Support	- Assist with legal processes for changing names and gender markers. - Provide resources and referrals for legal assistance.	Help a client complete and file paperwork to change their name and gender marker, providing step-by-step guidance. Schedule these tasks into their weekly routine to ensure timely completion and reduce stress.
Community Resources	- Identify and connect clients with local and online support groups and health clinics.	Create a resource guide with contact information for local LGBTQ+ organizations and healthcare providers. Encourage clients to participate in community activities and support groups to build a strong social network.

By integrating these comprehensive strategies and maintaining a commitment to advocacy and education, OTPs can play a pivotal role in the well-being of non-cisgender individuals, facilitating their journey toward a healthier and more fulfilling life.

Case Study in Non-Cisgender Individuals Health

Background and Medical History: The client is a 27-year-old non-binary individual who is being seen for mental health reasons associated with their gender transition. They are currently navigating significant psychological distress related to their gender identity exploration and societal acceptance challenges. The client has a history of gender dysphoria and has recently begun hormone replacement therapy (HRT) to align their physical appearance with their gender identity. Prior to starting HRT, they experienced heightened anxiety, depression, and social isolation due to gender dysphoria, impacting their occupational and social functioning.

Prior Level of Function:

- Functioned independently across all areas of occupation.
- Engaged in a career in graphic design, working part-time from home and freelancing.
- Actively participated in LGBTQ+ advocacy events, demonstrating leadership and organizational skills.
- Managed daily living tasks and maintained social connections within the LGBTQ+ community.

Household Living Arrangements and Social History:

- Lives alone in an urban apartment with supportive friendships within the LGBTQ+ community.
- Receives emotional support from distant parents via phone and video calls.
- Strained relationships with friends due to social anxiety and feelings of isolation related to gender dysphoria.

Change in Functional Status and Challenges:

The client's mental health concerns, primarily associated with their gender transition journey, have significantly impacted their ability to engage in daily activities across various domains of life:

- **ADLs**: Anxiety and depression have led to decreased frequency of showering and difficulty maintaining personal hygiene routines independently.
- **Work**: Challenges with concentration and motivation have affected productivity in graphic design work and freelancing projects.
- **Social Activities**: Increased anxiety and difficulty adjusting in social settings have led to decreased participation in LGBTQ+ advocacy events and community gatherings.
- **Health Management**: Struggles with managing medication adherence have emerged, impacting the client's ability to maintain stable mental health and physical well-being.

OT Assessments:

- **Barthel Index**: The client scored 40 out of 100, indicating significant assistance required for most ADLs due to challenges related to depression and anxiety.
- **Patient Health Questionnaire-9 (PHQ-9)**: The client scored 18, indicating moderate to severe depression symptoms affecting daily life and overall mood.
- **Generalized Anxiety Disorder-7 (GAD-7)**: The client scored 15, indicating moderate anxiety symptoms impacting daily functioning and social interactions.
- **Body Image Assessment**: The client scored 25 on the Body Image Disturbance Questionnaire, reflecting dissatisfaction and distress related to body image changes during their gender transition.

Occupational Therapy Plan of Care and Goals:

The client will receive skilled occupational therapy services two times a week for 8 weeks to improve independence in ADLs, IADLs, and overall quality of life.

Goals:

1. Increase Barthel Index score to 65/100, demonstrating improved independence in personal care tasks within 8 weeks.
2. Utilize coping skills to independently complete showering three times per week, employing cognitive-behavioural techniques to reduce anxiety and improve consistency in personal hygiene routines within 8 weeks.
3. Reduce PHQ-9 score to 10, indicating a reduction in depressive symptoms and improved mood within 8 weeks.
4. Reduce GAD-7 score to 8, indicating decreased anxiety symptoms and improved ability to manage social interactions within 8 weeks.

5. Improve body image perception and satisfaction, as evidenced by a 30% decrease in the Body Image Disturbance Questionnaire score within 8 weeks.
6. Develop assertive communication skills to effectively express needs and preferences in social and professional settings, demonstrated by increased participation in community events and advocacy activities to 2 events/month.

Interventions:

The following interventions will be tailored to meet the client's specific needs and address the outlined goals:

Coping Skills and Anxiety Management:

- Implement cognitive-behavioural techniques to address anxiety related to gender dysphoria and social interactions.
- Teach mindfulness and relaxation exercises to reduce stress and improve coping mechanisms during gender transition.

Activity Modification and Energy Conservation:

- Educate the client on using energy conservation techniques during daily activities, adapting schedules to optimize energy levels.
- Provide guidance on modifying personal care routines and household tasks to minimize fatigue and increase efficiency.

Body Image and Self-Perception:

- Facilitate discussions and activities to explore and enhance body image perception and self-acceptance during gender transition.
- Incorporate strategies to promote self-confidence and positive self-talk regarding physical changes associated with hormone replacement therapy.

Communication and Assertiveness Skills:

- Develop assertive communication skills to express needs and preferences confidently in social and professional settings.
- Role-play scenarios to practice assertiveness and effective communication strategies with peers and healthcare providers.

Health and Wellness Support:

- Collaborate with healthcare providers to monitor hormone replacement therapy effects and manage associated physical health needs.
- Educate on nutrition and healthy lifestyle choices that support hormone therapy and overall well-being.

Outcomes:

Post Treatment:

- **Anxiety and Coping Skills**: Demonstrated improvement in anxiety symptoms, reflected by a 40% reduction in GAD-7 scores, indicating enhanced ability to manage social interactions and stress.

- **Body Image and Self-Perception**: Increased satisfaction and comfort with body image changes, evidenced by a 30% improvement in Body Image Disturbance Questionnaire scores.
- **ADL Independence**: Achieved increased independence in personal care tasks, as indicated by a Barthel Index score improvement from 40 to 80.
- **Social Participation**: Enhanced engagement in community events and advocacy activities, demonstrating improved social integration and confidence.
- **Academic and Vocational Engagement**: Successfully resumed graphic design work and freelance projects with adapted strategies, managing tasks effectively without significant stress or fatigue.

Follow-Up Visits:

- Continued reinforcement of coping skills and communication techniques to sustain progress in managing anxiety and enhancing social interactions.
- Ongoing support in navigating gender transition challenges and adjusting therapy goals as the client's needs evolve.
- Regular monitoring of mental health indicators and adaptation of interventions to promote long-term emotional well-being and functional independence.

At the conclusion of therapy, the client demonstrated marked improvements across various domains, showcasing enhanced resilience and adaptive skills in managing the complexities of their gender transition journey. Significant progress was noted in anxiety management, with a notable reduction in symptoms and increased confidence in social interactions. The client also showed substantial gains in self-perception and body image satisfaction, reflecting a positive adjustment to physical changes facilitated by hormone replacement therapy. Improved independence in daily activities, including personal care and vocational pursuits, underscored their strengthened ability to navigate professional responsibilities and engage actively in community advocacy. The client's commitment to therapy and the collaborative efforts with the occupational therapy team resulted in sustainable improvements in mental well-being, highlighting their capacity for growth and resilience in the face of personal challenges.

Further Reading

Brown, C., Porta, C. M., Eisenberg, M. E., McMorris, B. J., & Sieving, R. E. (2020). Family relationships and the health and well-being of transgender and gender-diverse youth: A critical review. *LGBT Health*, *7*, 407–419. https://doi.org/10.1089/lgbt.2019.0200

Hughto, J. M. W., Gunn, H. A., Rood, B. A., & Pantalone, D. W. (2020). Social and medical gender affirmation experiences are inversely associated with mental health problems in a U.S. non-probability sample of transgender adults. *Archives of Sexual Behavior*, *49*(7), 2635–2647. https://doi.org/10.1007/s10508-020-01655-5

Karaba Bäckström, M., Luiz Moura de Castro, A., Eakman, A. M., Ikiugu, M. N., Gribble, N., Asaba, E., Kottorp, A., Falkmer, O., Eklund, M., Ness, N. E., Balogh, S., Hynes, P., & Falkmer, T. (2023). Occupational therapy gender imbalance; revisiting a lingering issue. *Scandinavian Journal of Occupational Therapy*, *30*(7), 1113–1121. https://doi.org/10.1080/11038128.2023.2220912

National Center for Transgender Equality. (2016). *The report of the 2015 U.S. Transgender Survey*. Washington, DC: National Center for Transgender Equality. Retrieved from https://globalhealth.usc.edu/wp-content/uploads/2017/03/2015-us-transgender-survey-executive-summary.pdf

Pascale, A. B., & DeVita, J. M. (2024). Transgender college students' mental health: Comparing transgender students to their cisgender peers. *Journal of American College Health*, *72*(1), 135–141. https://doi.org/10.1080/07448481.2021.2024212

Price-Feeney, M., Green, A. E., & Dorison, S. (2020). Understanding the mental health of transgender and nonbinary youth. *Journal of Adolescent Health*, 66(6), 684–690. https://doi.org/10.1016/j.jadohealth.2019.11.314

Seibel, B. L., de Brito Silva, B., Fontanari, A. M. V., Catelan, R. F., Bercht, A. M., Stucky, J. L., … Costa, A. B. (2018). The impact of parental support on risk factors in the process of gender affirmation of transgender and gender diverse people. *Frontiers in Psychology*, 9, Article 399. https://doi.org/10.3389/fpsyg.2018.00399

Sievert, E. D., Schweizer, K., Barkmann, C., Fahrenkrug, S., & Becker-Hebly, I. (2021). Not social transition status, but peer relations and family functioning predict psychological functioning in a German clinical sample of children with Gender Dysphoria. *Clinical Child Psychology and Psychiatry*, 26(1), 79–95. https://doi.org/10.1177/1359104520964530

7 Mental Health and Biopsychosocial Aspects

Chapter Objectives

Upon completion of this chapter, the reader will be able to:

1. Understand the psychosocial impact of infertility and fertility treatments on women's mental health and occupational performance.
2. Explore occupational therapy approaches to supporting women undergoing fertility treatments, emphasizing emotional resilience and quality of life.
3. Discuss the role of occupational therapy in promoting maternal mental health during the breastfeeding period, addressing common challenges and interventions.
4. Identify effective occupational therapy strategies for managing menopausal symptoms, including physical, emotional, and social aspects.
5. Utilize appropriate assessments and interventions to support women experiencing menopause, enhancing their occupational engagement and quality of life.
6. Incorporate tailored interventions to address the unique needs of women at various stages of reproductive and maternal health, ensuring holistic and client-centered care.

Women's Sexual Health: A Biopsychosocial and OT Perspective

Women's sexual health encompasses a wide range of physical, emotional, and social factors that influence their overall well-being. Sexual health issues can significantly impact a woman's daily life, relationships, self-esteem, and mental health. From a biopsychosocial perspective, addressing sexual health involves understanding the interplay between biological factors (e.g., hormonal changes, physical health), psychological factors (e.g., mental health, body image), and social factors (e.g., relationship dynamics, cultural beliefs). The biopsychosocial approach recognizes that health and illness are influenced by a combination of these factors, and effective treatment requires addressing all three dimensions. OTPs can play a crucial role in addressing sexual health by providing holistic care that considers these biopsychosocial factors.

DOI: 10.4324/9781003531678-7

Education and Counseling

Providing education on sexual health topics, including anatomy, sexual response, and the impact of health conditions on sexual function. Counseling can help address psychological barriers to sexual health, such as anxiety, depression, or trauma.

Impact on Mental Health and Biopsychosocial Aspects: Improving knowledge and understanding of sexual health can empower women, reduce anxiety and misconceptions about sexual functioning, and promote a healthier body image. Counseling supports mental health by addressing emotional barriers, enhancing self-esteem, and fostering a positive sexual identity, thereby improving overall quality of life and intimate relationships.

Physical Interventions

Assisting with pelvic floor rehabilitation, pain management techniques, and ergonomic positioning during sexual activities to reduce discomfort and enhance pleasure.

Impact on Mental Health and Biopsychosocial Aspects: Addressing physical pain and discomfort during sexual activities can alleviate stress and anxiety related to sexual performance, improve physical comfort, and enhance intimate relationships. This can lead to increased sexual satisfaction and emotional well-being, promoting a healthier biopsychosocial balance.

Emotional Support

Offering a safe space for clients to discuss their sexual health concerns and providing strategies to improve body image and self-esteem.

Impact on Mental Health and Biopsychosocial Aspects: Emotional support helps women feel validated and understood, reducing feelings of isolation and shame. Improving body image and self-esteem can enhance overall mental health, increase participation in intimate relationships, and foster a positive sense of self.

Relationship and Communication Skills

Helping clients develop effective communication skills to discuss sexual needs and preferences with partners, enhancing intimacy and mutual understanding.

Impact on Mental Health and Biopsychosocial Aspects: Effective communication skills can improve relationship dynamics, reduce misunderstandings and conflicts, and strengthen emotional bonds. Enhanced intimacy and mutual understanding contribute to better mental health and overall well-being, creating a supportive social environment.

Adaptive Strategies

Recommending adaptive devices or positioning aids to support sexual activity for women with physical limitations.

Impact on Mental Health and Biopsychosocial Aspects: Adaptive strategies can enable women with physical limitations to engage in sexual activities comfortably, reducing frustration and enhancing sexual satisfaction. This promotes a positive sexual identity, supports emotional well-being, and facilitates meaningful participation in intimate relationships. Table 7.1 lists some sample scenarios in sexual counseling for women's health, OT interventions, and their impact on mental health and biopsychosocial aspects.

Table 7.1 Scenarios in sexual counseling for women's health, OT interventions, and their impact on mental health and biopsychosocial aspects

Scenario	OT Intervention	Specific Strategies and Examples	Impact on Mental Health and Biopsychosocial Aspects
Woman with hip replacement seeking safe sexual positions post-op	Safe and Comfortable Positioning	Teach safe sexual positions that avoid stress on the hip joint, such as side-lying or using pillows for support.	Reduces anxiety about injury, enhances physical comfort, improves sexual satisfaction, and fosters a positive self-image.
Postpartum woman struggling with sexual intimacy	Alternate Forms of Sexual Pleasure	Suggest non-penetrative sexual activities, using vibrators or other devices to enhance pleasure without discomfort.	Reduces pressure to resume penetrative sex, promotes sexual pleasure, and enhances emotional intimacy with partner, improving mental health.
Woman in a wheelchair looking for accessible sexual positions	Adaptive Techniques and Devices	Recommend positions that can be easily performed in a wheelchair, such as sitting on a sturdy surface or using support bars.	Enhances sexual satisfaction, reduces frustration, and promotes a positive sexual identity, supporting overall well-being.
Woman experiencing vaginal dryness during menopause	Managing Vaginal Dryness	Suggest using water-based lubricants or vaginal moisturizers to reduce discomfort.	Reduces pain during intercourse, improves sexual satisfaction, and enhances self-esteem and relationship satisfaction.
Woman experiencing painful sex (dyspareunia)	Pain Management Techniques	Teach relaxation techniques and use of dilators or gradual desensitization exercises to reduce pain.	Alleviates anxiety related to sexual activity, improves physical comfort, and enhances overall mental health and relationship quality.

Addressing sexual health from a biopsychosocial perspective is essential for improving the overall well-being of women. By understanding and addressing the multifaceted nature of sexual health, OTPs can provide holistic care that supports mental health, enhances self-esteem, and promotes satisfying intimate relationships. The interventions discussed not only help manage physical symptoms but also foster emotional and social well-being, leading to a more balanced and fulfilling life.

Coping with Stress of Infertility: OT Support

Infertility can be a significant source of stress, anxiety, and emotional pain for women, profoundly impacting their mental health and occupational performance. The emotional toll of infertility often includes feelings of grief, loss, inadequacy, and social isolation, which can lead to anxiety, depression, and strained relationships. Additionally, the rigorous and often invasive nature of infertility treatments can disrupt daily routines and occupational roles, affecting work performance, social participation, and engagement in leisure activities. OTPs are uniquely positioned to support women coping with infertility by addressing the biopsychosocial aspects of this experience, promoting emotional resilience, and enhancing overall well-being through tailored interventions.

The diagnosis of infertility can be an extremely confronting and challenging experience for clients. The emotional journey of infertility is often described as a "roller coaster" due to the fluctuating emotions associated with this condition. It is common for women to experience stress and sadness in what is often perceived as a life crisis. Approximately 1 in 6 couples worldwide face difficulty conceiving within the first 12 months of trying, though many eventually have children, some with and some without treatment. Infertility can evoke a range of emotions, including shock, anger, anxiety, fear, sadness, and guilt. OTPs play a critical role in helping women manage these complex emotional responses and the associated stress of infertility and its treatments.

Occupational Therapy Interventions

Occupational therapy interventions for women experiencing infertility focus on addressing the multifaceted challenges posed by this condition. OTPs employ a holistic approach to support emotional, psychological, and social well-being while enhancing occupational performance. By providing tailored interventions, OTPs help clients develop effective coping strategies, establish and maintain healthy routines, and foster resilience. These interventions are designed to mitigate the stress and anxiety associated with infertility, improve daily functioning, and promote a sense of control and empowerment. Through individualized care plans, OTPs aim to enhance clients' overall quality of life and support them in navigating the complex emotional landscape of infertility treatments.

Emotional Coping Strategies

Teaching emotional coping strategies tailored to the unique stressors of infertility can help women manage anxiety and emotional distress. These strategies might include:

- **Journaling**: Encouraging clients to express their thoughts and emotions through writing, which can help process feelings and reduce anxiety. This can be particularly helpful for reflecting on daily experiences and tracking emotional fluctuations.
- **Creative Arts**: Using art, music, or other creative outlets to express emotions and reduce stress. For example, creating a visual diary of their infertility journey can provide a therapeutic outlet for expressing complex emotions.
- **Supportive Listening**: Providing a non-judgmental space where clients can share their experiences and feelings openly, facilitating emotional release and validation.

Routine and Structure

Helping women establish and maintain daily routines that include self-care, leisure activities, and social engagement promotes overall well-being. Specific examples include:

- **Daily Planning**: Assisting clients in creating structured daily schedules that balance medical appointments, work, leisure, and self-care activities. Ensuring they have time for relaxation and enjoyment is crucial.
- **Role Management**: Helping clients identify and manage their roles and routines, such as balancing work and personal life while dealing with infertility treatments. This can involve creating routines that reduce stress and improve productivity.

- **Habits and Rituals**: Encouraging the development of positive habits and rituals that support mental health, such as mindfulness practices or bedtime routines that promote restful sleep.

Support Groups

Facilitating or connecting clients with support groups where they can share experiences and receive peer support is vital. Examples of this support include:

- **Peer-led Groups**: Organizing or recommending local or online peer-led support groups specifically for women experiencing infertility, where they can discuss coping strategies and share experiences.
- **Family Involvement**: Encouraging clients to involve family members in support groups to enhance understanding and provide a broader support network. This can also help family members learn how to better support their loved ones.

Education and Resources

Providing information on infertility treatments, coping strategies, and connecting clients with relevant resources and specialists empowers women. Examples include:

- **Resource Guides**: Developing comprehensive guides that include information on medical treatments, holistic approaches, and coping strategies. This can help clients make informed decisions about their care.
- **Specialist Referrals**: Referring clients to fertility specialists, mental health counselors, and other healthcare providers as needed to ensure they receive comprehensive care and support.

Occupational Engagement

Encouraging participation in meaningful activities and hobbies helps maintain a sense of purpose and joy during the infertility journey. Examples of occupational engagement include:

- **Leisure Activities**: Identifying and engaging in hobbies and interests that provide enjoyment and distraction, such as gardening, painting, or dancing. These activities can offer a sense of fulfillment and joy.
- **Community Involvement**: Encouraging participation in community events and volunteer opportunities to build social connections and enhance well-being. This can help clients feel more connected and supported.
- **Physical Activity**: Developing personalized exercise routines that promote physical health and reduce stress, such as yoga, swimming, or walking. Physical activity can also help improve mood and overall well-being.

Fertility Treatment and Occupational Therapy Support

Receiving fertility treatment presents unique stressors distinct from the diagnosis of infertility. Common fertility treatments such as in vitro fertilization (IVF), intrauterine insemination (IUI), and hormone therapies often involve physically and emotionally demanding medical procedures, financial burdens, and the uncertainty of outcomes, all of which can exacerbate stress, anxiety, and emotional pain. Side effects of these treatments can include hormonal fluctuations, mood swings, fatigue, and physical discomfort. These treatments can significantly disrupt daily routines, occupational roles, and social participation, adding layers of complexity to the client's life.

It is crucial for OTPs to recognize these unique challenges and provide targeted interventions to support women undergoing fertility treatments. The Fertility Quality of Life Questionnaire (FertiQoL) is a valuable tool that OTPs can use to assess the quality of life in individuals receiving fertility treatment. The FertiQoL includes a relational subscale that evaluates the impact of fertility issues on personal relationships, providing insights into the relational dynamics that might be affected by the stressors of treatment. This assessment helps OTPs understand the specific areas where clients may need support, allowing for the development of more precise and effective intervention strategies.

Using FertiQoL in Occupational Therapy

1. **Assessment of Relational Dynamics**

    - **Purpose**: Evaluate the impact of fertility treatment on personal relationships, including partner relationships, family dynamics, and social connections.
    - **Application**: Use the relational subscale of the FertiQoL to identify specific relational stressors and areas of concern, facilitating targeted interventions to improve relational well-being.

2. **Tailored Interventions**

    - **Emotional Support**: Provide counseling and supportive listening to address the emotional toll of fertility treatments, helping clients process their feelings and develop coping strategies.
    - **Routine Management**: Assist clients in creating structured daily routines that incorporate medical appointments, self-care activities, and relaxation techniques to manage stress effectively.
    - **Social Support and Peer Groups**: Facilitate connections with support groups where clients can share experiences and receive peer support, helping to reduce feelings of isolation and build a sense of community.
    - **Education and Resources**: Provide information on fertility treatments, potential side effects, and coping strategies, empowering clients to make informed decisions about their care.

By incorporating tools like the FertiQoL and focusing on the unique stressors of fertility treatment, OTPs can offer comprehensive support that addresses both the emotional and practical aspects of undergoing fertility treatments. This holistic approach ensures that clients receive the necessary support to navigate the challenges of fertility treatment, promoting resilience, enhancing quality of life, and fostering a sense of empowerment throughout their journey.

By addressing the multifaceted challenges of infertility through tailored interventions, OTPs can significantly enhance the mental health and well-being of women experiencing infertility. These strategies not only help in managing stress and emotional pain but also support women in maintaining their roles and routines, fostering resilience, and promoting a sense of control and empowerment. As we move forward, it is essential to consider how occupational therapy can further support women during their childbearing years, ensuring they feel empowered and supported throughout their journey.

Empowering Agency in Childbearing: OT Insights

Empowering women during the childbearing years involves supporting them in making informed choices, managing physical and emotional changes, and maintaining their roles and routines. Occupational therapy can play a significant role in ensuring women feel empowered and supported during this critical period. Research shows that women who feel empowered during childbirth report higher levels of satisfaction and lower levels of postpartum depression and anxiety. According to the World Health Organization (WHO), empowering women in their reproductive decisions can improve maternal and infant health outcomes. Moreover, studies have indicated that women who receive comprehensive prenatal education and support are more likely to have positive childbirth experiences, adhere to health-promoting behaviors, and experience lower levels of stress and anxiety during pregnancy and postpartum.

Prenatal Education

Providing education on pregnancy, labor, and delivery prepares women for the physical and emotional changes they may experience. Conducting or recommending childbirth classes that cover topics such as stages of labor, pain management techniques, and postpartum recovery can empower women with knowledge and confidence. Additionally, educating women on how to navigate the healthcare system, understand medical terminology, and advocate for their needs during pregnancy and childbirth can help reduce anxiety and improve communication with healthcare providers.

Decision-Making Support

Supporting women in making informed decisions about their pregnancy, childbirth, and postpartum care is crucial. This includes helping them understand their options and the potential outcomes of different choices. For instance, OTPs can assist women in creating birth plans that reflect their preferences and values, providing them with a sense of control and empowerment.

Physical Preparation

Developing exercise programs to enhance strength, flexibility, and endurance promotes a healthy pregnancy and facilitates recovery postpartum. Examples include teaching prenatal yoga poses that strengthen the body, improve flexibility, and promote relaxation. Designing safe strength training exercises to support muscle endurance and prepare the body for childbirth can also improve overall physical health and resilience.

Role Adaptation

Helping women adapt to new roles and routines associated with motherhood, including time management and balancing multiple responsibilities, ensures they can maintain their identity and well-being while embracing their new role. Teaching clients how to use planners and digital tools to manage their time effectively can help them balance work, childcare, and self-care. Assisting clients in negotiating role changes with family members and employers to balance caregiving and work responsibilities can reduce stress and improve family dynamics.

Emotional Support

Offering counseling to address fears, anxieties, and emotional adjustments related to pregnancy and motherhood provides a safe space for women to express their concerns and receive validation and support. Providing individual counseling sessions to discuss fears and anxieties about childbirth and motherhood can help women process their emotions and develop coping strategies. Facilitating group therapy sessions where expectant mothers can share experiences and support each other can provide a sense of community and shared understanding.

Occupational Balance

Helping women maintain a balance between self-care, childcare, work, and leisure activities supports overall well-being. Assisting clients in developing self-care routines that include rest, relaxation, and activities that bring joy can improve mental health and reduce burnout. Analyzing daily activities to identify opportunities for balance and integration of meaningful occupations can help women prioritize their time and energy effectively.

These strategies are summarized and further detailed in Table 7.2, highlighting specific interventions and their impact on women's psychosocial health.

By addressing the unique challenges of childbearing through tailored interventions, OTPs can significantly enhance the well-being and empowerment of women during

Table 7.2 Strategies for empowering women in childbearing: Interventions and their impact on women's psychosocial health

Area of Focus	Strategy	Example of Intervention	Impact on Women's Psychosocial Health
Prenatal Education	Childbirth Classes and Transition Preparation	Stages of labor, pain management, postpartum recovery, understanding new roles.	Enhances confidence, reduces anxiety, and prepares women mentally and physically for childbirth and motherhood.
Decision-Making Support	Birth Plan Development	Assisting in creating birth plans that reflect preferences and values.	Promotes a sense of control and empowerment, leading to reduced anxiety and increased satisfaction.
Physical Preparation	Exercise Programs	Prenatal yoga, strength training exercises.	Improves physical health, reduces pregnancy-related discomfort, and enhances mental well-being.
Role Adaptation	Time Management and Role Negotiation Tools	Planners, digital tools, role negotiation strategies.	Promotes effective role management, reduces stress, and enhances satisfaction with the motherhood experience.
Emotional Support	Counseling and Group Therapy	Individual counseling sessions, group therapy.	Provides a supportive environment to process emotions, enhancing mental health and emotional resilience.
Occupational Balance	Self-Care Routines and Activity Analysis	Developing self-care routines, analyzing daily activities.	Promotes balance, reduces burnout, and supports sustained well-being.

pregnancy and motherhood. These strategies not only support physical and emotional health but also foster greater occupational participation and performance by helping women maintain their daily routines and roles. By promoting a sense of control and confidence in managing the complexities of this life stage, occupational therapy can ensure that women continue to engage in meaningful activities, fulfill their responsibilities, and maintain a balanced lifestyle. Moving forward, it is essential to continue exploring how occupational therapy can further empower women in their childbearing years, enhancing their capacity to navigate this transformative period with confidence and resilience.

Managing Psychiatric Symptoms during Pregnancy: OT Interventions

Psychiatric conditions during pregnancy can have a profound impact on both the mother and the developing fetus. Women with pre-existing psychiatric conditions such as depression, anxiety, bipolar disorder, and schizophrenia may experience exacerbations of their symptoms during pregnancy. Additionally, new psychiatric conditions can arise during pregnancy, including antenatal depression and anxiety. According to the American College of Obstetricians and Gynecologists, approximately 14–23% of women will experience depressive symptoms while pregnant, and anxiety disorders are also highly prevalent. The presence of these conditions can negatively affect prenatal care adherence, maternal health behaviors, and overall pregnancy outcomes, making it essential for OTPs to address and manage these symptoms effectively.

The impact of psychiatric symptoms during pregnancy extends beyond mental health, significantly influencing occupational participation, engagement, and performance. Women may struggle with daily activities, maintaining employment, fulfilling social roles, and engaging in self-care and leisure activities (see Table 7.3). Addressing these challenges is crucial for promoting overall well-being and ensuring that women can maintain their roles and routines during this critical period.

Table 7.3 Occupational therapy interventions for managing psychiatric symptoms during pregnancy and their impact on mental health and occupational participation

Area of Focus	Strategy	Example of Intervention	Impact on Mental Health and Occupational Participation
Emotional and Psychological Support	Individual Counseling	Techniques using CBT, ACT, and MBSR approaches to address fears, anxieties, and emotional adjustments.	Reduces anxiety and depression, promotes healthier coping mechanisms, improves occupational engagement.
	Group Therapy	Support groups for pregnant women with similar challenges.	Provides peer support and a sense of community, reduces isolation, enhances social participation.
	Mindfulness and Relaxation Techniques	Incorporating mindfulness meditation, progressive muscle relaxation, and guided imagery into therapy sessions.	Reduces stress, promotes relaxation, enhances emotional well-being, improves participation in daily activities.

(Continued)

Table 7.3 (Contiuned)

Area of Focus	Strategy	Example of Intervention	Impact on Mental Health and Occupational Participation
Routine and Structure	Daily Planning	Developing daily schedules with balanced activities.	Reduces anxiety, improves mood stability, provides a sense of control, enhances occupational performance.
	Role Management	Navigating changing roles and responsibilities.	Ensures fulfillment of occupational roles while managing symptoms, supports role balance.
Occupational Engagement	Leisure Activities	Engaging in therapeutic hobbies such as knitting or gardening.	Improves mental health, provides a sense of purpose and fulfillment, enhances quality of life.
	Physical Activity	Prenatal yoga, swimming, or walking.	Enhances physical health, reduces anxiety, improves mood, promotes participation in physical activities.
Education and Resources	Resource Guides	Providing comprehensive guides on psychiatric conditions and coping strategies.	Empowers clients with knowledge, enhances self-management, supports informed decision-making.
	Specialist Referrals	Referring to mental health professionals for specialized care.	Ensures comprehensive and specialized treatment, addresses complex needs, enhances overall well-being.
Environmental Modifications	Home Assessments	Assessing and modifying home environment for stress reduction.	Creates a supportive and calming home environment, enhances comfort, promotes relaxation.
	Workplace Accommodations	Advocating for flexible work schedules and reduced workloads.	Supports continued employment, reduces work-related stress, promotes work-life balance.
Holistic Wellness Programs	Nutrition and Sleep	Educating on balanced diet and sleep hygiene.	Promotes overall health, reduces psychiatric symptoms, enhances daily functioning.
	Social Support Networks	Facilitating connections with community resources.	Provides additional emotional and social support, reduces feelings of isolation, enhances social engagement.

Emotional and Psychological Support

Providing emotional and psychological support is crucial for managing psychiatric symptoms during pregnancy. OTPs can offer:

- **Individual Counseling**: Facilitating one-on-one counseling sessions to discuss fears, anxieties, and emotional adjustments related to pregnancy. Techniques such as cognitive-behavioural therapy (CBT), acceptance and commitment therapy (ACT), and mindfulness-based stress reduction (MBSR) can help women develop healthier coping mechanisms.

- **Group Therapy**: Creating support groups for pregnant women experiencing similar challenges can provide a sense of community and shared understanding. Group sessions can focus on stress management techniques, mindfulness practices, and peer support.
- **Mindfulness and Relaxation Techniques**: Incorporating mindfulness meditation, progressive muscle relaxation, and guided imagery into therapy sessions to reduce stress and promote relaxation. These techniques can help women manage anxiety and improve their overall mental well-being.
- **Stress Management Strategies**: Teaching clients practical stress management strategies such as deep breathing exercises, progressive muscle relaxation, and guided imagery to help them cope with daily stressors. These techniques can be integrated into their daily routines to promote a sense of calm and control.

Routine and Structure

Establishing and maintaining a structured daily routine can help mitigate psychiatric symptoms by providing a sense of normalcy and control. OTPs can assist with:

- **Daily Planning**: Developing daily schedules that balance self-care, medical appointments, leisure activities, and social engagement. This structure can help reduce anxiety and improve mood stability.
- **Role Management**: Helping clients navigate their changing roles and responsibilities during pregnancy, ensuring they can fulfill their occupational roles while managing their symptoms effectively.

Occupational Engagement

Encouraging participation in meaningful activities can improve mental health and provide a sense of purpose. OTPs can promote occupational engagement by:

- **Leisure Activities**: Identifying and engaging in hobbies and interests that bring joy and relaxation. Activities such as gardening, knitting, or painting can serve as therapeutic outlets.
- **Physical Activity**: Developing exercise routines that are safe for pregnancy and beneficial for mental health. Prenatal yoga, swimming, or walking can improve mood, reduce anxiety, and enhance physical well-being.

Education and Resources

Providing education on psychiatric conditions and available resources empowers women to manage their symptoms effectively. OTPs can:

- **Resource Guides**: Create comprehensive guides that include information on psychiatric conditions, coping strategies, and support services. These guides can help clients understand their conditions and access appropriate resources.
- **Specialist Referrals**: Refer clients to mental health professionals, such as psychiatrists or psychologists, for specialized care and medication management as needed.

Environmental Modifications

Modifying the home and work environment to reduce stress and enhance comfort can be beneficial. OTPs can:

- **Home Assessments**: Conduct assessments to identify stressors in the home environment and recommend modifications, such as creating a quiet, relaxing space for mindfulness practices.
- **Workplace Accommodations**: Advocate for flexible work schedules, reduced workloads, or other accommodations to help clients manage their symptoms while maintaining employment.

Holistic Wellness Programs: Developing holistic wellness programs that incorporate physical, mental, and social health can be highly beneficial. OTPs can design programs that include:

- **Nutrition and Sleep**: Educating clients on the importance of a balanced diet and proper sleep hygiene for managing psychiatric symptoms. Collaborating with dietitians and sleep specialists to create individualized plans.
- **Social Support Networks**: Facilitating connections with community resources and support networks to provide additional emotional and social support.

By addressing the unique challenges of psychiatric symptoms during pregnancy through tailored interventions, OTPs can significantly enhance the well-being and empowerment of women. These strategies not only support physical and emotional health but also promote a sense of control and confidence in managing the complexities of this life stage. Addressing psychiatric symptoms effectively enables women to maintain their occupational roles and participation, ensuring they can navigate pregnancy with resilience and support.

OT Support for Breastfeeding and Maternal Mental Health

Breastfeeding has significant benefits for both mothers and infants, but it can also be a source of stress and anxiety for new mothers. According to the WHO, approximately 38% of infants are exclusively breastfed for the first six months of life globally. Despite its benefits, many mothers experience challenges such as pain, milk supply issues, and societal pressures, which can significantly impact their mental health and overall well-being. Studies indicate that up to 60% of mothers feel societal pressure to breastfeed, and approximately 50% face significant breastfeeding difficulties, including latching problems, insufficient milk supply, and physical discomfort. Additionally, about 30% of mothers report fear of judgment or criticism when they are unable to breastfeed or choose to supplement with formula. These challenges can disrupt daily routines, social participation, and occupational performance, leading to increased anxiety, depression, and feelings of inadequacy. OTPs are uniquely positioned to support mothers through these difficulties by providing comprehensive, holistic interventions that address the physical, emotional, and social aspects of breastfeeding.

Occupational Therapy Interventions

Occupational therapy interventions for breastfeeding and maternal mental health focus on providing comprehensive support to new mothers, addressing the physical, emotional, and social challenges associated with breastfeeding. OTPs employ a holistic approach to help mothers navigate the complexities of breastfeeding, ensuring that they receive the necessary education, emotional support, and practical strategies to enhance their overall well-being. By focusing on tailored interventions, OTPs can help mothers manage pain, overcome anxiety and depression, establish effective routines, and create supportive environments. These interventions aim to improve maternal mental health, promote positive breastfeeding experiences, and enhance the quality of life for both mother and baby.

Education and Counseling

OTPs can provide critical education on breastfeeding techniques, positions, and common challenges. For instance, they can demonstrate effective latching techniques to ensure the baby is feeding efficiently and the mother is comfortable. Counseling sessions can address anxiety and depression related to breastfeeding difficulties, offering a space for mothers to express concerns and develop coping strategies. Educating mothers about the benefits of breastfeeding and helping them manage expectations can reduce stress and empower them in their breastfeeding journey.

Example of OT Support for Latching

An OTP can help a mother understand how to recognize her baby's feeding cues and assist with positioning for a good latch. The OTP might demonstrate how to hold the baby in a cross-cradle position, supporting the baby's neck and shoulders to bring the baby gently to the breast, allowing the baby to latch deeply. They can also guide the mother to look for signs that the baby is latched correctly, such as a wide-open mouth, flanged lips, and rhythmic sucking and swallowing. Additionally, OTPs can teach mothers to watch for baby cues indicating hunger (e.g., rooting, sucking on hands) and fullness (e.g., turning away from the breast, decreased sucking). Table 7.4 highlights infant cues indicating hunger and fullness.

Positioning for Effective Latching

1. **Cross-Cradle Hold**: The mother supports the baby's neck and shoulders with the opposite arm to the breast being used, allowing better control of the baby's head for a deeper latch.
2. **Football Hold**: The baby is tucked under the mother's arm on the same side as the breast, allowing the baby to latch from the side, which can be useful for mothers recovering from a C-section.
3. **Side-Lying Position**: Both mother and baby lie on their sides facing each other, which can be comfortable for night feedings or mothers recovering from childbirth.

Table 7.4 Infant cues indicating hunger and fullness

Cues	Indicating Hunger	Indicating Fullness
Hands	Sucking on hands, fists clenched	Hands open and relaxed
Mouth	Rooting (turning head towards the breast), lip smacking	Decreased sucking, mouth relaxed
Face	Alert and active, looking around	Turning away from the breast, looking sleepy
Body Movements	Moving towards the breast, making sucking motions	Body relaxed, less movement

Mental Health and Biopsychosocial Aspects 237

Physical Interventions

In addition to positioning, OTPs can provide ergonomic support and teach techniques for managing physical discomfort associated with breastfeeding. For example, they can recommend ergonomic breastfeeding pillows and seating arrangements to reduce strain on the mother's back and arms. They can also provide guidance on techniques for managing breast pain and engorgement, such as gentle massage, warm compresses, and appropriate pumping schedules. Furthermore, developing personalized feeding schedules can help support milk production and prevent maternal fatigue.

Emotional Support

Creating a supportive environment where mothers can openly discuss their breastfeeding concerns is essential. OTPs can facilitate peer support groups, allowing mothers to share their experiences and tips, fostering a sense of community and mutual support. Addressing body image issues and self-esteem through counseling and supportive listening can help mothers feel more confident and less isolated. Encouraging positive self-talk and self-compassion can significantly enhance a mother's emotional well-being.

Routine and Structure

Helping mothers integrate breastfeeding into their daily routines without overwhelming their schedules is crucial. OTPs can assist in creating a balanced daily schedule that includes time for self-care and leisure activities, ensuring mothers can manage the demands of breastfeeding alongside other responsibilities. For instance, they can help mothers plan their day to include regular breaks for feeding, rest, and enjoyable activities. This structured approach can reduce anxiety, improve mood stability, and enhance overall occupational performance.

Environmental Modifications

Assessing the home environment and suggesting modifications to create a comfortable breastfeeding space can significantly impact a mother's breastfeeding experience. OTPs can recommend tools and equipment, such as breastfeeding pillows, supportive chairs, and breast pumps, to enhance comfort and efficiency. They can also ensure mothers have access to community resources, such as lactation consultants and breastfeeding support groups, to provide ongoing support and advice.

By providing comprehensive support that addresses physical, emotional, and social aspects, OTPs can significantly enhance maternal mental health and occupational performance, promoting a positive breastfeeding experience for both mother and baby.

Supporting Transition to Bottle Feeding and Psychosocial Support

OTPs also play a crucial role in supporting mothers who decide to transition from breastfeeding to bottle feeding. This decision can be fraught with emotional challenges, including feelings of guilt, societal judgment, and personal disappointment. OTPs can provide guidance and support during this transition by helping mothers establish effective bottle-feeding routines, ensuring that feeding remains a positive experience for both mother and baby.

238 Occupational Therapy and Women's Health

In addition to practical support, OTPs offer crucial psychosocial support to help mothers cope with the emotional aspects of stopping breastfeeding. This includes psychosocial counseling to address feelings of guilt and sadness, and reinforcing the message that "fed is best." By affirming that a well-fed baby and a mentally healthy mother are the ultimate goals, OTPs can help mothers feel more confident and supported in their decision. This holistic approach ensures that mothers receive the emotional and practical support needed to maintain their well-being and the health of their infants.

Rethinking Menopause: OT Approaches

Menopause is a natural phase in a woman's life, typically occurring between the ages of 45 and 55, characterized by the cessation of menstruation and a decline in reproductive hormones. According to the National Institute on Aging, approximately 1.3 million women in the United States enter menopause each year. Menopausal symptoms, such as hot flashes, sleep disturbances, mood swings, and cognitive changes, can significantly impact a woman's daily life and occupational performance. Figure 7.1 highlights common body changes during menopause. The transition through menopause can be a challenging period due to the combined physical, emotional, and social changes. Understanding the impact of these changes through a biopsychosocial lens is crucial for OTPs in supporting women through this transition.

A biopsychosocial approach considers the intricate interplay between biological, psychological, and social factors, providing a comprehensive framework for addressing the multifaceted challenges of menopause. This approach recognizes that menopausal symptoms are not just physiological but also deeply intertwined with mental health and social well-being. For many women, menopause can trigger feelings of anxiety, depression, and a diminished sense of identity and self-worth, further complicating the physical symptoms they experience. By adopting a biopsychosocial perspective, OTPs can offer holistic interventions that address the full spectrum of a woman's needs during menopause.

Mental health plays a critical role in the menopausal transition, as the hormonal fluctuations can exacerbate pre-existing conditions or lead to new onset anxiety and depression. Women may struggle with changes in mood, self-esteem, and body image, which can impact their social interactions and overall quality of life. The emotional strain of menopause can also disrupt daily routines and occupational roles, making it difficult for women to maintain their usual activities and responsibilities. Therefore, providing comprehensive mental health support and practical strategies to manage these changes is essential in helping women navigate this life stage effectively.

Occupational Therapy Interventions

Occupational therapy interventions for menopause focus on addressing the multifaceted challenges associated with this life stage. By providing education, emotional support, and practical strategies, OTPs help women manage symptoms, maintain their roles and routines, and enhance their overall quality of life. These interventions aim to mitigate the physical and emotional impacts of menopause, promoting resilience and a sense of control over the changes they are experiencing. OTPs use a holistic approach to support women in navigating this significant transition, ensuring they feel empowered and supported throughout their journey.

Mental Health and Biopsychosocial Aspects 239

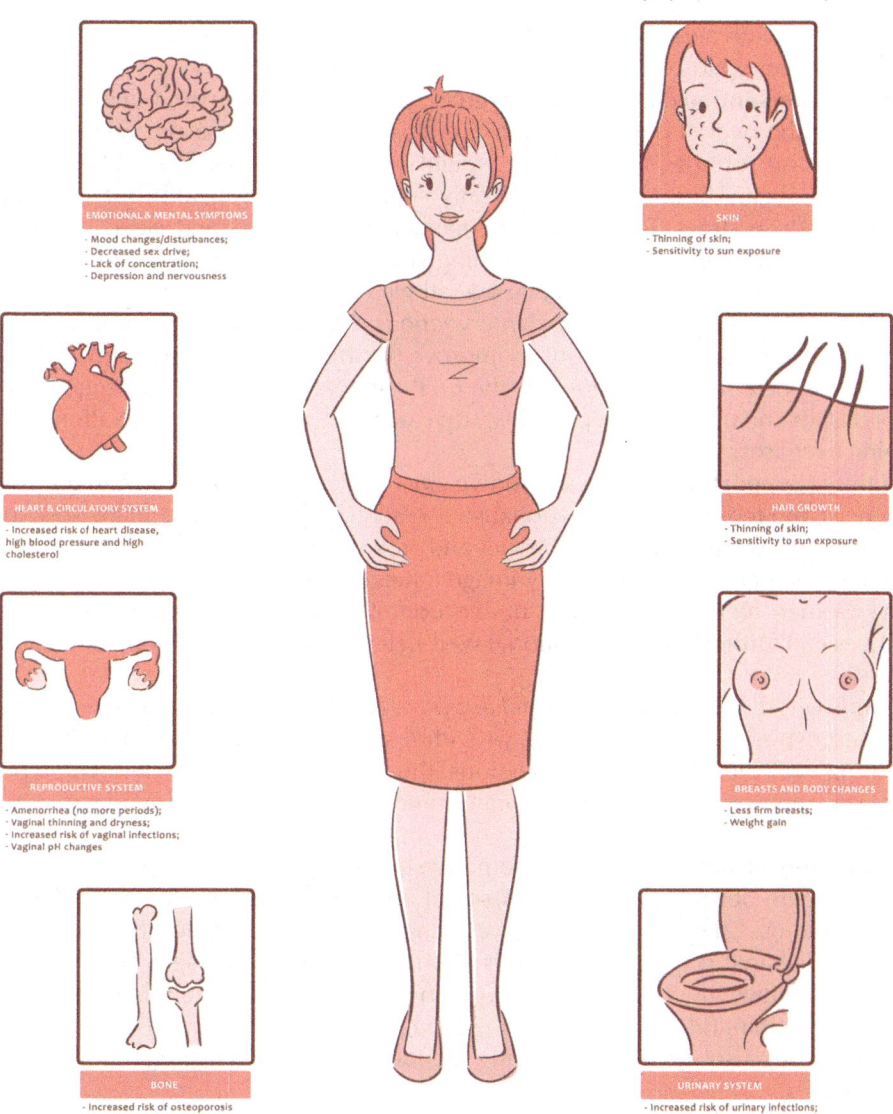

Figure 7.1 Body changes during menopause.

Education and Counseling: OTPs can provide essential education on menopause, its symptoms, and available treatments. For example, they can explain the physiological changes that occur during menopause and offer strategies for managing symptoms like hot flashes and mood swings. Counseling sessions can address anxiety, depression, and other emotional changes, helping women develop coping mechanisms and set realistic expectations. Educating women on self-advocacy and communication with healthcare providers can also enhance their ability to manage their health effectively.

Example of OT Support in Education and Counseling: An OTP might conduct a workshop on menopause, covering topics such as hormonal changes, symptom management, and healthy lifestyle choices. During one-on-one sessions, the OTP can provide personalized advice and support, helping women navigate the emotional and physical challenges of menopause.

Physical Interventions: Developing exercise programs to maintain bone density, muscle strength, and overall physical health is crucial during menopause. OTPs can design tailored exercise routines that include weight-bearing exercises like walking, strength training, and yoga. These activities not only support physical health but also improve mood and reduce stress. Techniques for managing hot flashes and sleep disturbances, such as relaxation exercises and establishing sleep hygiene practices, can also be integrated into therapy sessions to enhance overall well-being.

Example of OT Support in Physical Interventions: An OTP might design a weekly exercise plan that includes yoga sessions to improve flexibility and strength training exercises to maintain bone density. Additionally, the OTP can teach relaxation techniques to manage hot flashes and improve sleep quality, such as progressive muscle relaxation and deep breathing exercises.

Emotional Support: Creating a supportive environment where women can discuss their experiences and feelings about menopause is essential. OTPs can facilitate peer support groups, allowing women to share strategies and provide mutual encouragement. Individual counseling sessions can address body image issues, self-esteem, and emotional changes, helping women feel validated and understood. Teaching mindfulness and relaxation techniques can further support emotional well-being, reducing stress and enhancing coping skills.

Example of OT Support in Emotional Support: An OTP may facilitate a support group for women experiencing menopause, providing a space for them to share their stories and coping strategies. In individual sessions, the OTP can help women develop personalized relaxation routines that incorporate mindfulness practices to manage stress and anxiety.

Routine and Structure: Helping women establish and maintain daily routines that include self-care, leisure activities, and social engagement is vital for managing menopausal symptoms. OTPs can assist in developing structured schedules that balance work, family, and personal responsibilities. This approach can help manage changes in energy levels and cognitive function, ensuring women can continue to fulfill their roles and participate in meaningful activities. Time management strategies and role negotiation techniques can also be employed to support women in balancing their various responsibilities.

Example of OT Support in Routine and Structure: An OTP can help a client create a daily schedule that prioritizes self-care activities, such as regular exercise, adequate sleep, and leisure pursuits. The OTP might also work with the client to develop strategies for managing cognitive changes, such as using planners or digital reminders to stay organized and on track.

Environmental Modifications: Modifying the home and work environment to reduce stress and enhance comfort can significantly impact a woman's experience of menopause. OTPs can conduct home assessments to identify stressors and recommend modifications, such as creating a cool and relaxing space to manage hot flashes. Workplace accommodations, like flexible work schedules or reduced workloads, can also be advocated to help women maintain employment while managing symptoms. Ensuring access to community resources and support groups can provide additional emotional and social support.

Example of OT Support in Environmental Modifications: An OTP can conduct a home visit to suggest modifications such as installing blackout curtains to improve sleep quality and using fans or air conditioning to manage hot flashes. The OTP might also advocate for workplace adjustments, such as flexible hours or a cooler office environment, to help the client manage symptoms at work.

By addressing the unique challenges of menopause through tailored interventions, OTPs can significantly enhance the well-being and occupational performance of women during this life stage. These strategies not only support physical and emotional health but also promote a sense of control and confidence in managing the complexities of menopause. As a result, women can maintain their roles and routines, ensuring a balanced and fulfilling life.

Case Study in Mental Health and Psychosocial Aspects

Background and Medical History: The client is a 40-year-old woman who has been struggling with infertility for the past 3 years and is currently undergoing in vitro fertilization (IVF) treatment. She experiences significant emotional distress, including anxiety and depression, related to her infertility and the IVF process. The client is married, works full-time as a speech language pathologist and has reported increased difficulty in managing her professional responsibilities due to the stress and emotional burden of fertility treatments.

Prior Level of Function:

- **Occupational Performance**: The client was highly engaged in her role as a speech-language pathologist, effectively managing her workload and patient interactions.
- **Social Participation**: Actively involved in social activities and community events, regularly attending gatherings with friends and family.
- **ADLs and IADLs**: Independently managed all ADLs and IADLs.
- **Physical Health**: Lived a relatively sedentary lifestyle with limited physical activity.

Household Living Arrangements and Social History:

- **Living Arrangements**: Lives in a two-level home with her husband and their dog.
- **Social Support**: Strong marital relationship and supportive family network, although the stress of fertility treatments has strained some relationships.
- **Community Involvement**: Previously active in community service and local events, but participation has decreased due to the emotional and physical toll of fertility treatments.

Change in Functional Status and Challenges:

The client's emotional distress and the demanding nature of IVF treatments have significantly impacted her ability to engage in daily activities and fulfill her professional and social roles. Specific areas affected include:

- **Work**: Increased difficulty concentrating, preparing therapy plans, and managing patient sessions.
- **Social Activities**: Reduced participation in social gatherings and community events due to anxiety and emotional instability.

- **Health Management**: Challenges in managing medication adherence and maintaining a healthy routine due to the stress of IVF treatments.

Occupational Therapy Assessments:

- **Fertility Quality of Life (FertiQoL) Relational Subscale**: Low scores indicating poor quality of life related to the stressors of fertility treatment and its impact on personal relationships.
- **Canadian Occupational Performance Measure (COPM)**: Identified issues in self-care, productivity, and leisure activities.
- **Beck Depression Inventory (BDI)**: High scores reflecting significant depressive symptoms.
- **Generalized Anxiety Disorder-7 (GAD-7)**: High scores indicating moderate to severe anxiety symptoms.
- **Fatigue Severity Scale (FSS)**: High scores indicating severe fatigue impacting daily functioning.

Occupational Therapy Plan of Care and Goals

The client will receive skilled occupational therapy services once a week for 8 weeks to improve independence in ADLs, manage anxiety and depressive symptoms, and enhance quality of life.

Goals:

1. The client will increase COPM satisfaction scores related to self-care tasks by 30% within 8 weeks.
2. The client will report a 40% reduction in BDI scores through targeted emotional coping strategies within 8 weeks.
3. The client will implement stress management techniques to achieve a 30% reduction in GAD-7 scores within 8 weeks.
4. The client will improve relational quality of life, as indicated by a 25% increase in FertiQoL relational subscale scores within 8 weeks.
5. The client will demonstrate effective assertive communication skills in social interactions, as observed in three out of five role-playing sessions, within 8 weeks.
6. The client will engage in physical activity three times a week for 30 minutes each session, as reported in a physical activity log, within 8 weeks.

Occupational Therapy Interventions

The following interventions will be tailored to meet the client's specific needs and address the outlined goals:

Emotional and Psychological Support:

- Offer cognitive-behavioural therapy (CBT) sessions to address anxiety and depression, incorporating techniques to enhance emotional regulation.
- Facilitate peer support groups to provide a platform for sharing experiences and coping strategies.

- Teach relaxation techniques such as deep breathing and progressive muscle relaxation to manage emotional distress.

Self-Care Retraining:

- Provide training on cognitive techniques, such as positive self-talk and mindfulness, to encourage consistent engagement in self-care routines.
- Teach the use of adaptive equipment like ergonomic brushes and organizational tools to facilitate self-care tasks.

Health and Nutrition Management:

- Collaborate with a dietitian to develop a balanced meal plan that supports overall health and well-being.
- Educate the client on the importance of sleep hygiene and establish a bedtime routine to improve sleep quality.

Activity Modification and Energy Conservation:

- Educate the client on energy conservation techniques, such as scheduling high-energy tasks at peak times and incorporating frequent rest breaks.
- Advise on modifying activities at work to manage energy, such as arranging the workspace to minimize the need to lift heavy items.

Physical Activity Incorporation:

- Develop a tailored exercise routine that includes activities the client enjoys, such as walking, yoga, or light strength training, to be performed three times a week for 30 minutes each session.
- Monitor the client's progress through a physical activity log and adjust the routine as needed to maintain motivation and engagement.

Environmental Modifications:

- Suggest home modifications, such as creating a cool and relaxing space to manage fatigue.
- Advocate for workplace accommodations, such as flexible work schedules, to support the client in managing her symptoms at work.

Outcomes:

Post Treatment:

- **Self-Care Independence**: The client reported a significant increase in satisfaction with self-care tasks, achieving a 30% improvement in COPM scores.
- **Emotional Stability**: Notable reduction in depressive symptoms, evidenced by a 40% decrease in BDI scores. The client reported feeling more positive and engaged in her daily activities.
- **Routine Maintenance**: The client successfully maintained a consistent self-care routine, as recorded in her self-reported log.
- **Anxiety Management**: Achieved a 30% reduction in GAD-7 scores through the implementation of stress management techniques.

- **Relational Quality of Life**: Improved relational quality of life, indicated by a 25% increase in FertiQoL relational subscale scores.
- **Assertive Communication**: Demonstrated effective assertive communication skills in social interactions during role-playing sessions.
- **Physical Activity Engagement**: The client successfully incorporated physical activity into her routine, engaging in exercise three times a week for 30 minutes each session, as recorded in her physical activity log.

Follow-Up Visits:

- Continuously reinforce cognitive techniques and stress management strategies to ensure sustainability of improvements.
- Provide ongoing support and adjust the client's treatment plan based on her feedback and any changes in her symptoms.
- Monitor the client's adherence to health management routines and provide additional resources as needed.

The client demonstrated marked improvement in managing her infertility treatment-related stress and symptoms, enhancing her overall functionality and independence. She is now capable of performing daily tasks such as personal care and managing her professional responsibilities with greater efficiency and less anxiety. Through the collaborative and holistic approach of occupational therapy, the client has regained a better quality of life and improved her capacity to engage in meaningful activities.

Further Reading

Chauhan, A., & Potdar, J. (2022). Maternal mental health during pregnancy: A critical review. *Cureus*, 14(10), e30656. https://doi.org/10.7759/cureus.30656

Degirmenci Oz, S., Sezer, E., & Yildirim, D. (2024). The effect of occupational therapy on anxiety, depression, and psychological well-being in older adults: A single-blind randomized-controlled study. *European Geriatric Medicine*, 15(1), 217–223. https://doi.org/10.1007/s41999-023-00900-z

Gervais-Hupé, J., Filleul, A., Perreault, K., & Hudon, A. (2023). Implementation of a biopsychosocial approach into physiotherapists' practice: A review of systematic reviews to map barriers and facilitators and identify specific behavior change techniques. *Disability and Rehabilitation*, 45(14), 2263–2272. https://doi.org/10.1080/09638288.2022.2094479

Höhl, W., Moll, S., & Pfeiffer, A. (2017). Occupational therapy interventions in the treatment of people with severe mental illness. *Current Opinion in Psychiatry*, 30(4), 300–305. https://doi.org/10.1097/YCO.0000000000000339

Rocamora-Montenegro, M., Compañ-Gabucio, L. M., & Garcia de la Hera, M. (2021). Occupational therapy interventions for adults with severe mental illness: A scoping review. *BMJ Open*, 11(10), e047467. https://doi.org/10.1136/bmjopen-2020-047467

Romero-Ayuso, D. M., Toledano-González, A., Pinilla-Cerezo, M., Sánchez-Rodríguez, Ó., García-Arenas, J. J., Triviño-Juárez, J. M., & Ortíz-Rubio, A. (2024). Occupational balance and emotional regulation in people with and without serious mental illness. *Canadian Journal of Occupational Therapy. Revue Canadienne D'ergotherapie*, 91(1), 100–109. https://doi.org/10.1177/00084 174231178440

Sanders, T., & Lewis-Kipkulei, P. (2022). Occupational therapy interventions that address the psychosocial needs of clients with upper extremity injuries: A scoping review. *Journal of Allied Health*, 51(3), 220–228.

Sponseller, L., Silverman, F., & Roberts, P. (2021). Exploring the role of occupational therapy with mothers who breastfeed. *The American Journal of Occupational Therapy: Official Publication of the American Occupational Therapy Association*, 75(5), 7505205110. https://doi.org/10.5014/ajot.2021.041269

Vizheh, M., Rapport, F., Braithwaite, J., & Zurynski, Y. (2023). The impact of women's agency on accessing and using maternal healthcare services: A systematic review and meta-analysis. *International Journal of Environmental Research and Public Health, 20*(5), 3966. https://doi.org/10.3390/ijerph20053966

Woolley, H., Levy, E., Spector, S., Geneau, N., Castro, A., Rouleau, S., & Roy, L. (2020). "I'm not alone": Women's experiences of recovery oriented occupational therapy groups following depression. *Canadian Journal of Occupational Therapy. Revue Canadienne D'ergotherapie, 87*(1), 73–82. https://doi.org/10.1177/0008417419878916

Yuill, C., McCourt, C., Cheyne, H., & Leister, N. (2020). Women's experiences of decision-making and informed choice about pregnancy and birth care: A systematic review and meta-synthesis of qualitative research. *BMC Pregnancy and Childbirth, 20*(1), 343. https://doi.org/10.1186/s12884-020-03023-6

8 Cardiovascular Health

Chapter Objectives

Upon completion of this chapter, the reader will be able to:

1. Understand the prevalence, risk factors, and symptom presentations of various types of heart disease in women, and compare and contrast the differences in symptomatology and treatment responses between men and women.
2. Examine the role of occupational therapy in supporting women with heart disease through education on symptom recognition, lifestyle modifications, and stress management techniques, and develop skills in implementing energy conservation techniques, cardiac rehabilitation exercises, and ADL retraining specific to the needs of women with cardiovascular conditions.
3. Understand the psychosocial impact of heart disease on women, including higher rates of depression and anxiety, and implement psychosocial interventions such as support groups, peer mentoring, and therapeutic activities to improve self-esteem and social participation for women with heart disease.
4. Utilize wearable technology, telehealth platforms, and mobile health applications to enhance patient care and support women in monitoring their cardiovascular health, and educate clients on the use of remote monitoring software and smartwatches to track vital signs and detect warning signs of heart attack specific to women.
5. Identify high-risk populations for heart disease among women, including those with low socioeconomic status, family history, and comorbid conditions, and develop and implement targeted prevention strategies such as comprehensive health education, lifestyle modification programs, and early screening initiatives tailored to the needs of high-risk women.

Women and Heart Disease

Heart disease encompasses a range of conditions affecting the heart, including coronary artery disease, heart failure, arrhythmias, and valvular heart disease. It is the leading cause of death among women, accounting for approximately 1 in 4 female deaths in the United States. Despite its prevalence, heart disease in women is often underdiagnosed and

Cardiovascular Health

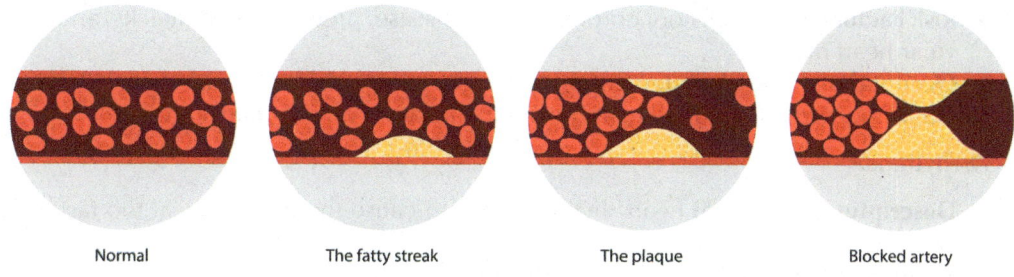

Normal   The fatty streak   The plaque   Blocked artery

Figure 8.1 Cholesterol is a waxy substance in the blood.

undertreated, partly due to differences in symptom presentation compared to men. Women are more likely to experience atypical symptoms such as fatigue, nausea, and shortness of breath rather than the classic chest pain, which can lead to delays in diagnosis and treatment.

Cholesterol is a waxy substance found in your blood that is essential for building healthy cells (see Figure 8.1). However, high levels of cholesterol can increase your risk of heart disease. Women are less likely to be treated with aspirin and statins to prevent future heart attacks, despite studies showing similar benefits in both genders. They are also less likely to undergo coronary bypass surgery due to factors such as less obstructive disease or smaller arteries with more small vessel disease. Additionally, women are less likely to be referred for cardiac rehabilitation, even though it can significantly improve health and aid in recovery from heart disease.

Understanding the specific types of heart disease that predominantly affect women is crucial for developing effective prevention and treatment strategies. By addressing these distinct forms of heart disease, OTPs can better support women in managing their cardiovascular health and improving their quality of life. Below, four primary types of heart disease prevalent in women are listed, highlighting symptoms, risk factors, and the role of occupational therapy interventions.

Types of Heart Disease in Women

1. **Coronary Artery Disease (CAD)**
   - **Description**: CAD is the most common type of heart disease, occurring when the coronary arteries become narrowed or blocked, reducing blood flow to the heart.
   - **Symptoms in Women**: Women often experience atypical symptoms such as jaw pain, shortness of breath, nausea, and fatigue.
   - **Risk Factors**: Hypertension, diabetes, smoking, high cholesterol, obesity, and physical inactivity.
   - **Occupational Therapy Interventions**: Education on symptom recognition, lifestyle modification programs, and stress management techniques.

2. **Heart Failure**
   - **Description**: A condition where the heart cannot pump enough blood to meet the body's needs.
   - **Symptoms in Women**: Shortness of breath, swelling in the legs, fatigue, and persistent coughing.

- **Risk Factors**: Hypertension, coronary artery disease, previous heart attacks, and valvular heart disease.
- **Occupational Therapy Interventions**: Energy conservation techniques, exercise programs to improve endurance, and patient education on self-management.

3. **Arrhythmias**
   - **Description**: Abnormal heart rhythms that can cause the heart to beat too fast, too slow, or irregularly.
   - **Symptoms in Women**: Palpitations, dizziness, fainting, and shortness of breath.
   - **Risk Factors**: Heart disease, high blood pressure, diabetes, and electrolyte imbalances.
   - **Occupational Therapy Interventions**: Stress management, biofeedback, and lifestyle education to manage triggers.

4. **Valvular Heart Disease**
   - **Description**: Disease that affects the valves of the heart, leading to improper blood flow.
   - **Symptoms in Women**: Fatigue, shortness of breath, and swollen ankles or feet.
   - **Risk Factors**: Age, history of rheumatic fever, and certain infections.
   - **Occupational Therapy Interventions**: Activity modification, education on signs and symptoms of valve disease, and adherence to medical treatments.

Impact on Daily Functioning

Women often face unique challenges related to their roles as caregivers, which can exacerbate the impact of heart disease. Balancing self-care with the care of others can lead to increased stress and fatigue, making it harder to adhere to treatment plans and participate in rehabilitation exercises. For example, the American Heart Association highlights that women frequently prioritize family responsibilities over their own health, which can delay recovery and increase the risk of recurrent cardiac events.

Additionally, the presentation of heart disease in women is often atypical, leading to delayed diagnosis and treatment. This delay can result in more severe physical limitations and a greater impact on occupational participation. Women are more likely to experience non-traditional symptoms such as shortness of breath, nausea, and back or jaw pain, which can be misattributed to other conditions.

Finally, the psychosocial impact of heart disease on women can be profound. Social isolation, changes in self-perception, and reduced engagement in social activities can lead to a decline in mental health and overall well-being. Women with heart disease often report feeling less supported by healthcare providers and family members, which can further contribute to emotional distress and reduced quality of life.

OT in Cardiac Rehabilitation for Women

Women often face different symptoms and psychosocial factors than men, requiring tailored interventions to ensure effective recovery and improved quality of life. Research indicates that women are less likely to be referred to cardiac rehabilitation programs compared to men and often face unique barriers, such as caregiving responsibilities and lower socioeconomic status, which can affect their participation and outcomes. Additionally, hormonal influences, functional capacity differences, and psychosocial factors play significant roles in how women experience and recover from heart disease.

Women are less likely to be referred to cardiac rehabilitation due to several factors, including gender biases in the healthcare system, the perception that heart disease is primarily a male issue, and women's own underestimation of their heart disease risk. Unique barriers such as caregiving responsibilities, which often take precedence over personal health, and lower socioeconomic status, which can limit access to healthcare and support services, further impact their participation in rehabilitation programs. Table 8.1 highlights key aspects such as symptom presentation, risk factors, and treatment outcomes, emphasizing the unique challenges women face in managing this condition.

Table 8.1 Key differences in heart disease between men and women and their implications for OT interventions

Aspect	Women	Men	Implications for OT Interventions
Symptom Presentation	Atypical symptoms such as fatigue, nausea, shortness of breath	More typical chest pain	Educate women on recognizing atypical symptoms and the importance of early medical intervention
Risk Factors	Higher prevalence of hypertension and diabetes	Higher prevalence of smoking and obesity	Tailor lifestyle modification programs to address specific risk factors more prevalent in women
Mortality Rate	Higher mortality rate after a heart attack; women are more likely to die within a year of their first heart attack	Lower mortality rate after a heart attack compared to women	Implement targeted interventions focusing on secondary prevention and close follow-up to manage risk factors and improve survival rates
Diagnosis	Often underdiagnosed; symptoms may be attributed to non-cardiac causes	More likely to be accurately diagnosed due to classic symptoms	Advocate for comprehensive diagnostic evaluations for women presenting with atypical symptoms
Treatment	Less likely to receive aggressive treatment and cardiac rehabilitation	More likely to receive aggressive treatment and follow-up care	Ensure that women receive referrals to cardiac rehabilitation and advocate for equal access to aggressive treatments
Psychosocial Impact	Higher rates of depression and anxiety post-heart attack; social and emotional factors play a significant role	Depression and anxiety are also concerns but may be less pronounced compared to women	Incorporate mental health support and psychosocial interventions tailored to women's needs, such as counseling and support groups
Outcomes	Generally poorer outcomes due to later diagnosis and less aggressive treatment	Better outcomes due to earlier diagnosis and treatment	Provide comprehensive follow-up care and support to improve long-term outcomes for women
MET Levels	Achieve lower MET levels on average; 2 METs lower than men for equivalent mortality risk	Achieve higher MET levels on average	Tailor cardiovascular fitness programs to account for lower MET levels in women, ensuring exercises are adjusted to their specific energy expenditure needs and functional capacity, such as low-impact aerobics

Unique Considerations in Cardiac Rehabilitation for Women

Cardiac rehabilitation for women requires a tailored approach that addresses hormonal influences, metabolic differences, and psychosocial factors. The protective effects of estrogen on the cardiovascular system diminish post-menopause, increasing heart disease risk due to declining estrogen levels. Hormonal changes also affect lipid profiles and blood pressure regulation, necessitating careful monitoring and tailored interventions.

1. **Hormonal Influences**
   - **Estrogen**: Estrogen has a protective effect on the cardiovascular system, but post-menopausal women face an increased risk of heart disease due to declining estrogen levels. Hormonal changes can also affect lipid profiles and blood pressure regulation.

2. **Metabolic Equivalents (METs)**
   While MET levels are generally the same for men and women in terms of energy expenditure, women may experience different physiological responses due to hormonal influences and body composition. Women often have a higher percentage of body fat and lower muscle mass, which can affect their cardiovascular fitness and rehabilitation outcomes. Women may achieve lower MET levels for the same activities compared to men indicating that women generally expend less energy or have lower cardiovascular fitness levels for the same activities compared to men. This difference is due to various factors such as body composition, muscle mass, and hormonal influences. Consequently, the same activity might feel just as challenging for women as it does for men, but women might need to approach it differently in a rehabilitation context to avoid overexertion and ensure effective recovery. This necessitates providing tailored interventions and gradual progression in exercise intensity. Table 8.2 highlights common MET levels for various activities and their differences for men and women.

Table 8.2 Common MET levels in cardiac rehabilitation and variations for women vs. men

MET Level	Activity	Men (METS)	Women (METS)	Implications for OT Interventions
1–2	Seated activities (e.g., reading, writing)	1.0–2.0	1.0–2.0	Ensure activities are not overly taxing, focus on seated exercises to build confidence and initial endurance.
2–3	Light housework (e.g., washing dishes)	2.5–3.0	2.0–2.5	Tailor tasks to avoid overexertion, provide energy conservation techniques for managing daily activities efficiently.
3–4	Walking slowly (2 mph)	3.0–3.5	2.5–3.0	Encourage gradual increase in walking speed and duration, monitor for signs of fatigue and adjust pace as needed.
4–5	Light gardening, pushing a lawnmower	4.0–5.0	3.5–4.0	Recommend modifications to gardening techniques to reduce strain, suggest frequent breaks and proper body mechanics.
5–6	Dancing, recreational swimming	5.0–6.0	4.5–5.0	Promote engagement in enjoyable activities to improve adherence, ensure activities are within safe exertion levels.
6+	Jogging, brisk walking (4 mph)	6.0+	5.0–6.0	Progress to higher intensity exercises carefully, emphasizing proper technique and safety to prevent overexertion.

3. Functional Capacity

- Studies show that women often have lower baseline functional capacity compared to men, which can influence their rehabilitation progress. This necessitates a more gradual and tailored approach in cardiac rehab programs for women.
- **Example**: An OTP could implement a graduated exercise program starting with low-intensity activities, progressively increasing as the woman's functional capacity improves. For instance, beginning with light stretching and short walks, then gradually introducing more intensive activities like resistance training or moderate aerobic exercises.

4. Psychosocial Factors

- Women are more likely to experience depression and anxiety post-heart attack or surgery, which can impact their recovery and participation in rehabilitation programs. Addressing these psychosocial factors is crucial for improving outcomes.
- **Example**: An OTP might incorporate mental health support into the rehabilitation plan by including regular check-ins, mindfulness training, and referrals to mental health professionals. They might also facilitate support groups where women can share their experiences and coping strategies.

By understanding these unique needs, OTPs can provide comprehensive, client-centered care that enhances recovery and promotes long-term cardiovascular health.

Individualized Assessment and Goal Setting

OTPs play a vital role in cardiac rehabilitation for women, addressing their unique physical, emotional, and social needs through individualized assessments and goal setting. Conducting a comprehensive assessment to identify specific barriers to recovery that women might face, such as balancing caregiving responsibilities or managing household tasks, is crucial. Setting personalized goals that are meaningful to the client, such as being able to return to caregiving roles or managing household tasks without fatigue, can enhance motivation and adherence to the rehabilitation program.

Energy Conservation Techniques

Energy conservation is essential for women in cardiac rehabilitation, especially since they often balance multiple roles. Teaching women how to manage their energy efficiently can help them maintain their roles at home and work without overwhelming fatigue. Practical strategies include planning and pacing activities, sitting during tasks when possible, and delegating heavy tasks to others.

   Example: Providing practical strategies such as planning and pacing activities, sitting during tasks when possible, and delegating heavy tasks to others.

   Practical Application: An OTP might help a client reorganize her home environment to reduce unnecessary movement and energy expenditure. For instance, placing commonly used items within easy reach in the kitchen or bathroom can help conserve energy for more essential activities.

Stress Management and Relaxation Techniques

Managing stress is crucial for women in cardiac rehabilitation due to the additional pressures they might face from societal expectations and family dynamics. Teaching relaxation techniques such as progressive muscle relaxation, guided imagery, or deep breathing exercises tailored to manage specific stressors related to their roles can be beneficial.

Example: Teaching relaxation techniques specifically targeted to manage stress related to caregiving roles, such as progressive muscle relaxation and guided imagery that focus on reducing anxiety and enhancing calmness.

Practical Application: An OTP can guide a client through progressive muscle relaxation exercises focusing on specific muscle groups that tend to hold tension, such as the shoulders and back. Additionally, the OTP might develop a personalized guided imagery script that the client can use during high-stress times, such as when juggling work and caregiving duties. The OTP can also provide resources for practicing these techniques at home, including audio recordings and written instructions.

Lifestyle Modification and Education

Education on heart-healthy lifestyles must be tailored to address the specific needs and challenges faced by women, particularly during hormonal changes such as menopause. Providing education on diet, exercise, and other lifestyle modifications that consider the hormonal changes and metabolic differences women experience is essential. A significant focus should be on strategies to reduce levels of cholesterol plaque in vessels, which is crucial for preventing heart disease (see Figure 8.2).

Example: Offering a tailored exercise program that includes weight-bearing exercises and resistance training to counteract bone density loss and manage weight gain associated with menopause.

Practical Application: An OTP might collaborate with a dietitian to develop a comprehensive meal plan that includes heart-healthy foods rich in phytoestrogens, such as flaxseeds and soy products, to help balance hormones and support cardiovascular health. The OTP can recommend specific exercises like brisk walking and resistance training to maintain cardiovascular fitness and manage weight effectively. The OTP can also educate the client on reading food labels and making healthier food choices when shopping. By analyzing the client's daily routine, OTPs can implement strategies to ensure good follow-through with the meal plan, such as scheduling specific times for meal preparation, creating grocery lists that prioritize heart-healthy ingredients, and providing tips for efficient and enjoyable cooking practices.

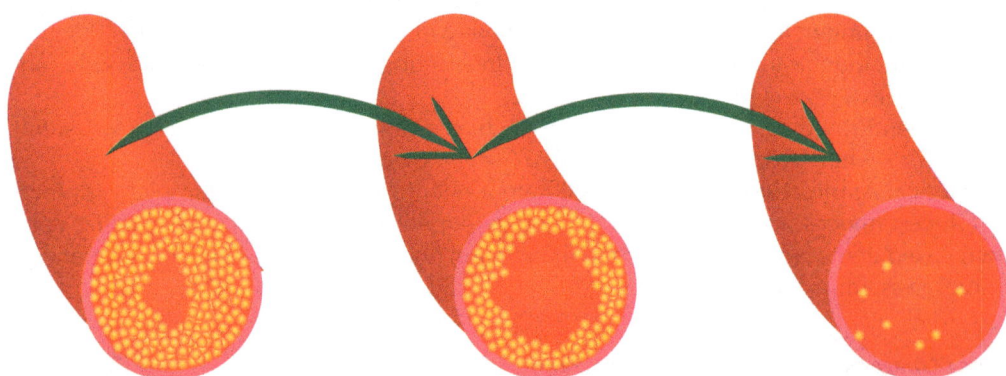

Figure 8.2 Reduced level of cholesterol plaque in blood vessels.

Social Support and Community Resources

Facilitating connections with support groups and community resources that specifically address the needs of women can enhance their recovery and provide emotional support. Connecting clients with women-specific cardiac support groups where they can share experiences and strategies for managing their condition is crucial.

Example: Connecting clients with women-specific cardiac support groups where they can share experiences and strategies for managing their condition.

Practical Application: An OTP might help a client find local or online support groups that provide peer support and shared experiences, which can reduce feelings of isolation and improve adherence to rehabilitation programs.

By addressing these unique challenges through tailored interventions, OTPs can significantly enhance the well-being and recovery outcomes for women in cardiac rehabilitation. These strategies not only support physical recovery but also promote emotional resilience and social engagement, ensuring a holistic approach to heart health.

Technology and Innovation in Heart Health

Technological advancements and innovative practices are revolutionizing heart health, offering new avenues for prevention, diagnosis, and treatment. These innovations are particularly impactful for women, who often experience different symptoms and risk factors for heart disease compared to men. For OTPs, understanding and integrating these technologies into their practice can enhance patient care, improve outcomes, and support women in maintaining their occupational roles and daily activities. Over the past 30 years, significant advancements in cardiovascular health have been made, yet women remain underdiagnosed, undertreated, and underrepresented in clinical trials. Utilizing digital health interventions (DHIs) and telemedicine can address these disparities by improving adherence to healthcare visits, monitoring, and promoting healthy behaviors. These technologies help mitigate geographical, structural, and financial barriers to care, which are crucial for women who often balance multiple roles and responsibilities.

Impact on Occupational Therapy Practice

Technological innovations in heart health can significantly enhance the way OTPs support women with heart disease. These advancements provide tools for more accurate assessments, personalized interventions, and ongoing monitoring, which are crucial for improving patient outcomes and ensuring that women can continue to engage in their meaningful occupations. Incorporating technology into OT practice allows for better management of cardiovascular health, tailored to the unique needs of women.

Key Technological Innovations

Wearable Technology

Wearable devices like fitness trackers and smartwatches can monitor heart rate, physical activity, and sleep patterns. These devices provide real-time data that helps in managing cardiovascular health, essential for women balancing multiple roles, such as work, caregiving, and household responsibilities. Research shows that women are often less likely to track their health stats manually due to busy schedules and multiple roles. Wearable technology automates this process, making it easier for women to stay informed about their health.

Practical Application: An OTP can use data from wearable devices to tailor exercise programs for women recovering from a heart attack, ensuring the intensity is appropriate and safe. For example, the OTP can adjust a woman's walking program based on her daily heart rate data, encouraging gradual increases in activity that align with her recovery goals and current capabilities.

Telehealth and Remote Monitoring

Telehealth platforms enable remote consultations and continuous monitoring of heart health, which is especially beneficial for women who might have responsibilities that limit their ability to attend in-person appointments. According to recent studies, women are more likely to have caregiving responsibilities that make attending regular appointments challenging. Telehealth provides a convenient solution, allowing women to receive care without disrupting their schedules.

Practical Application: OTPs can conduct virtual sessions to provide guidance, support, and education, ensuring continuous care and reducing the risk of hospital readmissions. For instance, an OTP can use telehealth to guide a woman through home-based exercises, monitor her progress, and make real-time adjustments to her rehabilitation plan.

Mobile Health Applications

Mobile apps offer educational resources, medication reminders, and tools for tracking symptoms and lifestyle changes, empowering women to take an active role in their heart health management. These tools are particularly useful for busy women who need to integrate health management into their daily routines. Studies have shown that women are more likely to adhere to health recommendations when they have easy access to information and reminders.

Practical Application: OTPs can recommend and teach clients how to use specific apps that support self-management, helping them integrate these tools into their daily routines. For example, an OTP might show a client how to use a nutrition app to track heart-healthy meals and ensure she is getting the necessary nutrients to support cardiovascular health.

Advanced Imaging and Diagnostic Tools

Technologies such as high-resolution imaging and genetic testing can lead to earlier and more accurate diagnoses of heart disease in women, who often present with atypical symptoms. Early diagnosis enables OTPs to develop and implement preventive and therapeutic interventions sooner, improving long-term outcomes.

Practical Application: For example, if advanced imaging detects early signs of heart disease, an OTP can work with a woman to develop a tailored exercise program and lifestyle changes to mitigate risks and prevent progression.

Assessments to Determine Technology Fit

To effectively integrate these technologies into practice, OTPs can use various assessments to determine a client's readiness and ability to use them. These assessments help evaluate a client's potential benefits from incorporating technology into their treatment plan.

1. **Technology Readiness Index (TRI)**
   - **Purpose**: Measures an individual's propensity to embrace and use new technologies.
   - **Application**: Helps determine a client's willingness and readiness to engage with health-related technologies such as wearables and mobile health apps.
   - **Example**: Administering the TRI to assess a client's openness to using a fitness tracker for monitoring physical activity and heart rate.

2. **Assessment of Motor and Process Skills (AMPS)**
   - **Purpose**: Evaluates a person's performance in daily activities to identify strengths and areas needing support.
   - **Application**: Assesses the client's ability to integrate technology into their daily routines, such as using a smartphone app to track medication adherence or physical activity.
   - **Example**: Using AMPS to evaluate how well a client can incorporate the use of a health app into their morning routine without disruption.

3. **Canadian Occupational Performance Measure (COPM)**
   - **Purpose**: Identifies problem areas in a client's life, evaluates performance and satisfaction, and measures changes over time.
   - **Application**: Identifies specific health management tasks that could be improved with technology and evaluates the client's satisfaction with these interventions.
   - **Example**: Using the COPM to set goals related to using a wearable device for managing heart disease and tracking progress.

4. **Self-Efficacy for Managing Chronic Disease Scale**
   - **Purpose**: Measures confidence in managing chronic disease.
   - **Application**: Evaluates a client's confidence in their ability to manage heart disease using technological interventions.
   - **Example**: Assessing a client's self-efficacy to determine if they feel capable of using a mobile health app for tracking dietary intake and physical activity.

Example of OT Intervention with Technology

Scenario: Assessing Readiness for Wearable Technology

1. **Assessment**: Administer the TRI to a female client recently diagnosed with heart disease to evaluate her openness and readiness to use wearable technology.
2. **Findings**: The TRI results indicate a high readiness and openness to using new technology.
3. **Intervention**: Introduce a fitness tracker that monitors heart rate, physical activity, and sleep patterns. Teach the client how to use the device and integrate it into her daily routine.
4. **Outcome**: Regular monitoring through the wearable device provides real-time data, allowing the OTP to tailor the client's exercise program and make necessary adjustments to ensure safety and effectiveness.

By leveraging technology and implementing targeted prevention strategies, OTPs can significantly contribute to the heart health of women. These approaches not only support physical health but also enhance occupational participation, ensuring that women can lead fulfilling and active lives. Women with busy lives and multiple responsibilities benefit greatly from these technologies, as they provide accessible and practical ways to monitor and improve their heart health, thus supporting their ability to engage in daily activities and maintain their various roles.

Heart Disease Prevention in High-Risk Populations

Heart disease is a leading cause of death among women, with certain populations being at a higher risk due to various genetic, socioeconomic, and lifestyle factors. High-risk populations include African American women, Hispanic women, women with low socioeconomic status, those with a family history of heart disease, and women with comorbid conditions such as diabetes and hypertension. According to the American Heart Association, African American women are nearly twice as likely to develop heart disease compared to white women, and Hispanic women are also at a significantly higher risk. Women from low socioeconomic backgrounds often face barriers such as limited access to healthcare, poor nutrition, and higher stress levels, which contribute to their increased risk of heart disease.

OTPs play a crucial role in heart disease prevention by addressing the specific needs and challenges of these high-risk populations. By providing targeted interventions and education, OTPs can help mitigate the impact of heart disease and promote healthier lifestyles. Table 8.3 highlights high-risk populations for heart disease.

Impact on Occupational Therapy Practice

High-risk populations often face unique challenges that can impact their ability to engage in meaningful occupations and maintain a healthy lifestyle. For example, women with low socioeconomic status may struggle to access healthy food, safe exercise environments,

Table 8.3 Overview and considerations of high-risk populations for heart disease in women

High-Risk Population	Description	Why They Are at Higher Risk
African American Women	Higher prevalence of hypertension, diabetes, and obesity	Genetic predisposition, socioeconomic factors, and limited access to preventive care
Hispanic Women	Higher rates of obesity and diabetes	Cultural dietary practices, socioeconomic barriers, and lower access to healthcare services
Women with Low Socioeconomic Status	Limited access to healthcare, healthy food, and safe places for physical activity	Financial constraints, lower health literacy, and increased stress levels due to economic instability
Women with Family History of Heart Disease	Genetic predisposition and shared lifestyle factors	Increased genetic risk, combined with potentially unhealthy lifestyle habits passed through generations
Women with Comorbid Conditions (e.g., Diabetes, Hypertension)	Increased risk due to compounded health issues	The presence of multiple health conditions increases the likelihood of heart disease and complicates management and treatment

and regular healthcare. African American and Hispanic women may experience cultural and linguistic barriers that affect their understanding and management of heart disease. OTPs can use their expertise to provide culturally sensitive interventions, advocate for better healthcare access, and support women in making sustainable lifestyle changes. These factors significantly influence their occupational participation and performance, making it essential for OTPs to tailor their interventions to address these barriers.

Prevention Strategies

Preventing heart disease in high-risk populations involves a multifaceted approach that addresses both individual and systemic factors. OTPs can implement a variety of prevention strategies to support women in these populations:

Comprehensive Health Education

Providing education on heart disease risk factors, healthy lifestyle choices, and the importance of regular medical check-ups is essential. Education should be culturally sensitive and tailored to the specific needs of high-risk populations.

- **Example**: Conducting community workshops on heart health that cover topics such as nutrition, physical activity, and smoking cessation. These workshops can be tailored to address cultural dietary practices and promote heart-healthy alternatives.
- **Practical Application**: An OTP might organize a heart health workshop for a community of Hispanic women, including information on traditional foods and healthier preparation methods, as well as culturally relevant physical activity recommendations.

Lifestyle Modification Programs

Developing and implementing programs that encourage physical activity, healthy eating, and stress management can significantly reduce the risk of heart disease. These programs should be accessible and consider the socioeconomic barriers faced by high-risk populations.

- **Example**: Creating a community-based exercise program that meets regularly to promote physical activity and provide social support.
- **Practical Application**: An OTP could collaborate with local community centers to establish a free or low-cost exercise program that includes regular group walks, yoga classes, and nutrition counseling.

Screening and Early Intervention

Regular screening for heart disease risk factors such as hypertension, high cholesterol, and diabetes can lead to early intervention and better health outcomes. OTPs can facilitate access to screening services and provide follow-up support.

- **Example**: Partnering with local health clinics to offer free blood pressure and cholesterol screenings during community events.
- **Practical Application**: An OTP can coordinate with a mobile health clinic to provide screenings at a community center, offering immediate feedback and referrals for further care if needed.

Enhancing Health Literacy

Improving health literacy among high-risk populations can empower women to make informed decisions about their health. This includes understanding medical information, navigating the healthcare system, and advocating for their health needs.

- **Example**: Developing easy-to-understand educational materials that explain heart disease risk factors and preventive measures in multiple languages.
- **Practical Application**: An OTP might create a series of bilingual pamphlets and videos that explain the importance of regular check-ups, medication adherence, and lifestyle changes in preventing heart disease.

Barriers and Solutions

When addressing heart disease prevention in high-risk populations, it is crucial to consider the various barriers these groups face. Socioeconomic, cultural, and psychosocial factors often hinder effective prevention and management of heart disease. OTPs can implement targeted solutions to overcome these barriers and enhance heart health outcomes for women.

1. **Socioeconomic Barriers**: High-risk populations often face financial constraints that limit access to healthy food, safe places for physical activity, and healthcare services.
   - **Solution**: Implementing community-based programs that provide affordable or free resources such as healthy food options, exercise facilities, and health services.
   - **Example**: Establishing a community garden that supplies fresh produce and offers nutrition education.
   - **Practical Application**: An OTP could work with local organizations to develop a community garden where women can learn about and grow their own heart-healthy foods, fostering a sense of empowerment and community involvement.
2. **Cultural and Language Barriers**: Cultural beliefs and language differences can hinder effective communication and access to healthcare.
   - **Solution**: Providing culturally sensitive care and employing bilingual health educators.
   - **Example**: Offering health education sessions in multiple languages and involving community leaders to bridge cultural gaps.
   - **Practical Application**: An OTP can collaborate with cultural liaisons to deliver heart health education in a way that respects cultural practices and uses the preferred language of the community.
3. **Psychosocial Barriers**: Stress, depression, and lack of social support can negatively impact heart health.
   - **Solution**: Integrating mental health support and fostering social connections through group activities.
   - **Example**: Creating support groups for women at risk of heart disease that focus on stress management and emotional well-being.
   - **Practical Application**: An OTP might facilitate a support group for women with high stress levels, providing a space to share experiences and learn coping strategies, thereby enhancing emotional support and reducing the risk of heart disease.

By addressing these barriers and implementing tailored prevention strategies, OTPs can play a vital role in reducing the risk of heart disease among high-risk populations. Through comprehensive education, lifestyle modifications, early screening, and culturally sensitive interventions, OTPs can empower women to take control of their heart health and improve their overall quality of life. By fostering a holistic approach to prevention, OTPs can ensure that women in high-risk groups receive the support and resources they need to maintain healthy and fulfilling lives.

Case Study in Cardiovascular Health

Background and Medical History: The client is a 52-year-old elementary school teacher diagnosed with coronary artery disease (CAD). The client has a history of hypertension and type 2 diabetes, both of which are managed with medication and lifestyle modifications. Recently, the client experienced a myocardial infarction (heart attack) and underwent angioplasty with stent placement to restore blood flow. Prior to the diagnosis, the client reported fatigue, shortness of breath, and occasional chest discomfort, which was attributed to stress and aging. Following the heart attack, the cardiologist recommended the client engage in activities at a moderate MET level of 3–5 to ensure safe physical exertion during recovery.

Prior Level of Function:

- Functioned independently in all areas of occupation.
- Engaged actively in teaching, managing a classroom, and participating in school events.
- Enjoyed gardening and walking the dog in the evenings.
- Managed household tasks and cooking for the family.

Household Living Arrangements and Social History:

- Lives with a partner in a suburban home.
- Has two grown children who visit occasionally.
- Active in the local community, attending church and participating in a book club.

Change in Functional Status and Challenges: The client's recent heart attack has significantly impacted the ability to engage in daily activities across various domains of life:

- **ADLs**: Experiences fatigue and shortness of breath, making it difficult to complete personal hygiene routines and dress independently.
- **Work**: Struggles with concentration and stamina, affecting the ability to manage a full day of teaching and administrative tasks.
- **Social Activities**: Reduced participation in community events and social gatherings due to fear of another cardiac event and physical limitations.
- **Health Management**: Needs to adhere to a complex medication regimen and incorporate dietary changes, facing challenges with meal planning and preparation.

OT Assessments:

- **Barthel Index**: The client scored 60 out of 100, indicating moderate assistance required for most ADLs due to physical limitations and fatigue.
- **Canadian Occupational Performance Measure (COPM)**: The client identified fatigue management, returning to work, and resuming gardening as top priorities. Satisfaction and performance scores were low in these areas.

- **Hospital Anxiety and Depression Scale (HADS)**: The client scored 12 on anxiety and 10 on depression, indicating moderate anxiety and mild depression impacting daily functioning.
- **Six-Minute Walk Test (6MWT)**: The client walked 300 meters, which is below average for their age and gender, indicating reduced cardiovascular endurance and functional capacity.
- **Cardiac Assessment**: The cardiologist recommended physical activity at a moderate MET level of 3–5 to ensure safe exertion levels during rehabilitation.

Occupational Therapy Plan of Care and Goals: The client will receive skilled occupational therapy services three times a week for 12 weeks to improve independence in ADLs, IADLs, and overall quality of life.

Goals:

1. Increase Barthel Index score to 80/100, demonstrating improved independence in personal care tasks within 12 weeks.
2. Implement energy conservation techniques to enable the client to complete a full day of teaching with minimal fatigue within 12 weeks.
3. Improve COPM performance and satisfaction scores by 30% in the areas of fatigue management, work, and gardening within 12 weeks.
4. Reduce HADS scores to below 8 for both anxiety and depression, indicating improved emotional well-being within 12 weeks.
5. Increase 6MWT distance to 400 meters, indicating improved cardiovascular endurance within 12 weeks for increased independence with community mobility.

Interventions: The following interventions will be tailored to meet the client's specific needs and address the outlined goals:

Energy Conservation Techniques:

- Educate the client on pacing activities, taking frequent breaks, and planning tasks to conserve energy throughout the day.
- Teach how to prioritize and delegate tasks both at home and work to manage fatigue effectively.

Cardiac Rehabilitation Exercises:

- Develop a graduated exercise program starting with low-intensity activities like walking and gradually increasing to moderate-intensity exercises (MET level 3–5).
- Incorporate resistance training and stretching exercises to improve cardiovascular fitness and muscle strength.

ADL Retraining:

- Provide guidance on adaptive techniques and use of assistive devices to enhance independence in personal hygiene and dressing.
- Educate the client on strategies to simplify household tasks and improve efficiency in meal preparation.

Stress Management and Relaxation Techniques:

- Implement cognitive-behavioural techniques to address anxiety related to the heart condition.

- Teach mindfulness and relaxation exercises such as deep breathing and progressive muscle relaxation to reduce stress and promote relaxation.

Health Management and Education:

- Provide education on heart-healthy nutrition and assist the client in meal planning to adhere to dietary recommendations.
- Educate the client on the warning signs of a heart attack in women, emphasizing differences compared to men, such as atypical symptoms like jaw pain, nausea, and fatigue.
- Teach the client to monitor her own vitals during functional activities using remote monitoring software or a smart watch.
- Monitor medication adherence and collaborate with the healthcare team to ensure optimal management of the client's conditions.

Work Reintegration:

- Develop a phased return-to-work plan, gradually increasing teaching hours and responsibilities.
- Adapt the work environment to reduce physical strain, such as using ergonomic furniture and organizing the classroom efficiently.

Psychosocial Interventions:

- Facilitate support groups or peer mentoring to provide emotional support and share coping strategies with others who have experienced similar health challenges.
- Engage in therapeutic activities to improve self-esteem and social participation.

Outcomes:

Post Treatment:

- **Energy Conservation and Fatigue Management**: Demonstrated significant improvement in managing fatigue, as indicated by a 30% increase in COPM scores and a Barthel Index score improvement from 60 to 85.
- **Cardiac Fitness**: Successfully completed a graduated exercise program, achieving higher endurance and strength levels, as evidenced by an increase in 6MWT distance from 300 meters to 420 meters, enabling resumption of walking the dog and light gardening activities.
- **Emotional Well-being**: Achieved reduced anxiety and depression scores on the HADS, reflecting improved emotional resilience and coping skills.
- **Work and Social Participation**: Successfully reintegrated into the teaching role with adapted strategies, managing a full workday without significant fatigue. Increased participation in community events and social gatherings, demonstrating improved confidence and engagement.

Follow-Up Visits:

- Continued reinforcement of energy conservation techniques and stress management strategies to sustain progress.
- Ongoing support in managing the heart condition, adjusting therapy goals as needed.

- Regular monitoring of cardiovascular fitness and emotional well-being indicators, adapting interventions to promote long-term health and functional independence.

At the conclusion of therapy, the client demonstrated marked improvements across various domains, showcasing enhanced resilience and adaptive skills in managing cardiovascular health. Significant progress was noted in fatigue management, cardiac fitness, and emotional well-being, enabling the client to engage more fully in professional and personal life. The client's commitment to therapy and collaboration with the occupational therapy team resulted in sustainable improvements, highlighting the capacity for growth and resilience in the face of health challenges.

Further Reading

Borg, S., Öberg, B., Nilsson, L., Alfredsson, J., Söderlund, A., & Bäck, M. (2023). Effectiveness of a behavioral medicine intervention in physical therapy on secondary psychological outcomes and health-related quality of life in exercise-based cardiac rehabilitation: A randomized, controlled trial. *BMC Sports Science, Medicine & Rehabilitation*, 15(1), 42. https://doi.org/10.1186/s13102-023-00647-x

Bracewell, N. J., Plasschaert, J., Conti, C. R., Keeley, E. C., & Conti, J. B. (2022). Cardiac rehabilitation: Effective yet underutilized in patients with cardiovascular disease. *Clinical Cardiology*, 45(11), 1128–1134. https://doi.org/10.1002/clc.23911

Ekblom, Ö., Cider, Å., Hambraeus, K., Bäck, M., Leosdottir, M., Lönn, A., & Börjesson, M. (2022). Participation in exercise-based cardiac rehabilitation is related to reduced total mortality in both men and women: Results from the SWEDEHEART registry. *European Journal of Preventive Cardiology*, 29(3), 485–492. https://doi.org/10.1093/eurjpc/zwab083

Garcia, M., Miller, V. M., Gulati, M., Hayes, S. N., Manson, J. E., Wenger, N. K., Bairey Merz, C. N., Mankad, R., Pollak, A. W., Mieres, J., Kling, J., & Mulvagh, S. L. (2016). Focused cardiovascular care for women: The need and role in clinical practice. *Mayo Clinic Proceedings*, 91(2), 226–240. https://doi.org/10.1016/j.mayocp.2015.11.001

Ghisi, G. L. M., Kin, S. M. R., Price, J., Beckie, T. M., Mamataz, T., Naheed, A., & Grace, S. L. (2022). Women-focused cardiovascular rehabilitation: An International Council of Cardiovascular Prevention and Rehabilitation clinical practice guideline. *The Canadian Journal of Cardiology*, 38(12), 1786–1798. https://doi.org/10.1016/j.cjca.2022.06.021

He, J., Zhu, Z., Bundy, J. D., Dorans, K. S., Chen, J., & Hamm, L. L. (2021). Trends in cardiovascular risk factors in US adults by race and ethnicity and socioeconomic status, 1999–2018. *JAMA*, 326(13), 1286–1298. https://doi.org/10.1001/jama.2021.15187

Ivey, S. L., Hanley, H. R., Taylor, C., Stock, E., Vora, N., Woo, J., Johnson, S., Bairey Merz, C. N., & Right Care Women's Cardiovascular Writing Group (2022). Early identification and treatment of women's cardiovascular risk factors prevents cardiovascular disease, saves lives, and protects future generations: Policy recommendations and take action plan utilizing policy levers. *Clinical Cardiology*, 45(11), 1100–1106. https://doi.org/10.1002/clc.23921

Khadanga, S., Gaalema, D. E., Savage, P., & Ades, P. A. (2021). Underutilization of cardiac rehabilitation in women: Barriers and solutions. *Journal of Cardiopulmonary Rehabilitation and Prevention*, 41(4), 207–213. https://doi.org/10.1097/HCR.0000000000000629

Norris, J. (2018). Cognitive function in cardiac patients: Exploring the occupational therapy role in lifestyle medicine. *American Journal of Lifestyle Medicine*, 14(1), 61–70. https://doi.org/10.1177/1559827618757189

Tang, L. H., Doherty, P., Skou, S. T., & Harrison, A. (2023). Optimal outcomes from cardiac rehabilitation are associated with longer-term follow-up and risk factor status at 12 months: An observational registry-based study. *International Journal of Cardiology*, 386, 134–140. https://doi.org/10.1016/j.ijcard.2023.05.028

Tessler, J., & Bordoni, B. (2023). Cardiac rehabilitation. In *StatPearls*. StatPearls Publishing.

9 Sleep, Weight, and Lifestyle Factors in Women's Health

Chapter Objectives

Upon completion of this chapter, the reader will be able to:

1. Understand the physiological, psychological, and social impacts of sleep, weight, and lifestyle factors on women's health.
2. Identify common sleep disorders affecting women and their implications on daily functioning and occupational performance.
3. Discuss the role of occupational therapy in assessing and addressing sleep disturbances in women.
4. Define obesity and understand its multifaceted impact on women's health, including associated chronic conditions.
5. Identify common assessments and interventions used by OTPs to address obesity and weight management in women.
6. Apply occupational therapy frameworks and approaches to effectively support women with eating-related disorders.
7. Develop personalized intervention plans that incorporate physical activity and healthy lifestyle choices to enhance overall well-being.

Sleep and Women's Health

Sleep is a fundamental aspect of health, essential for physical, mental, and emotional well-being. A typical sleep episode consists of multiple cycles, each lasting about 90 minutes. These cycles include two main types of sleep: Non-Rapid Eye Movement (NREM) sleep and Rapid Eye Movement (REM) sleep.

1. NREM Sleep

- **Stage 1 (Light Sleep):** This initial stage of light sleep lasts about 5–10 minutes, where the body transitions from wakefulness to sleep.
- **Stage 2 (Light Sleep):** This stage comprises about 50% of the sleep cycle, lasting around 20 minutes per cycle. Heart rate slows, and body temperature drops.

- **Stage 3 (Deep Sleep)**: Also known as slow-wave sleep, this stage is crucial for restorative processes such as tissue repair and growth. It typically makes up about 20% of total sleep time.

2. **REM Sleep**
   - REM sleep occurs about 90 minutes after falling asleep and recurs approximately every 90 minutes, making up about 20–25% of total sleep time. This stage is marked by vivid dreams, rapid eye movements, and increased brain activity.

The structure of sleep, known as sleep architecture, can be illustrated by a hypnogram, which shows the progression of sleep stages throughout the night. Understanding these fundamentals helps in comprehending how disturbances can affect overall health.

Sleep Requirements for Women

The amount of sleep required varies by age, and both the quantity and quality of sleep are crucial for health. Here are the recommended hours of sleep for different age groups:

- School-age Children (6–13 years): 9–11 hours per night.
- Teenagers (14–17 years): 8–10 hours per night.
- Young Adults (18–25 years): 7–9 hours per night.
- Adults (26–64 years): 7–9 hours per night, although some individuals may require as few as 6 hours or as many as 10 hours per night.
- Older Adults (65+ years): 7–8 hours per night.

While the quantity of sleep is important, the quality of sleep is equally, if not more, significant. High-quality sleep involves uninterrupted sleep cycles, particularly ensuring sufficient deep NREM and REM sleep stages, which are vital for physical restoration and cognitive functioning.

Melatonin and Cortisol in Circadian Rhythm

The circadian rhythm, an internal process that regulates the sleep-wake cycle, is influenced by the fluctuations of hormones such as melatonin and cortisol. Melatonin, a hormone that promotes sleep, typically reaches its highest levels between 6 PM and 6 AM, aiding in the onset and maintenance of sleep. In contrast, cortisol, known as the "stress hormone," peaks around 7 AM, helping to wake the body and prepare for the day. Understanding these hormonal patterns is crucial for addressing sleep disturbances and improving overall sleep quality (see Figure 9.1).

Effects of Sleep Duration

Shorter sleep duration, such as sleeping for only five hours per night, often results in significantly less time spent in REM sleep and deep NREM sleep. These stages are critical for cognitive function, emotional regulation, and physical recovery. Consequently, individuals with limited sleep duration may experience increased sleep fragmentation and reduced overall sleep quality. In contrast, sleeping for the recommended 7 to 8 hours per night allows for more complete sleep cycles, ensuring adequate time in both REM and NREM

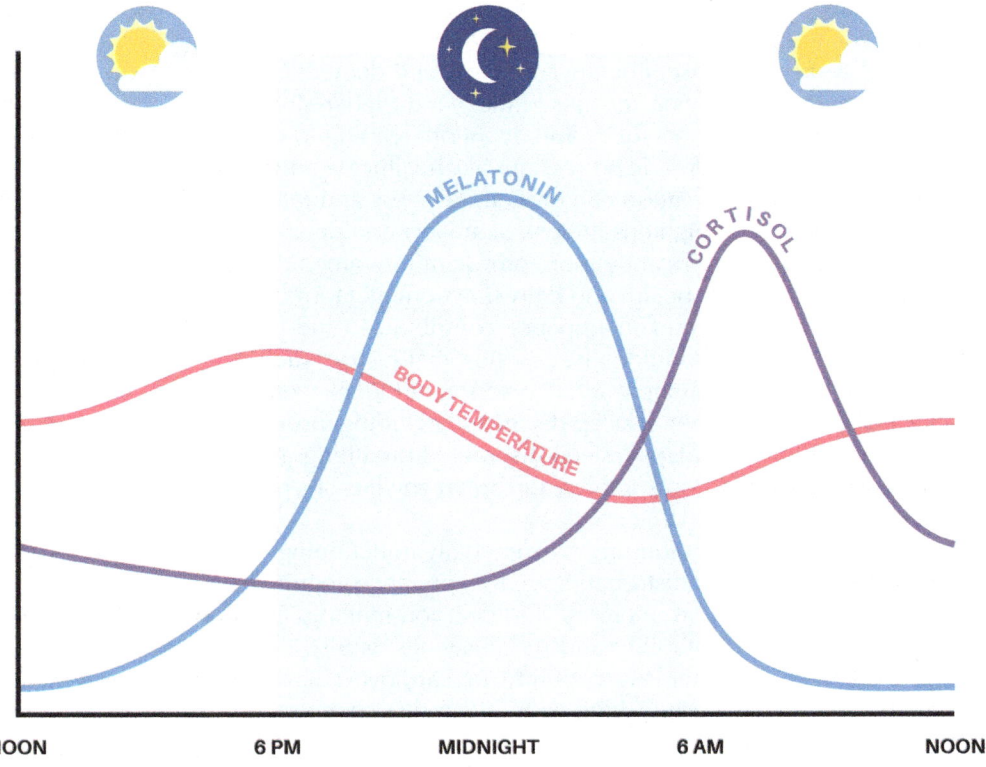

Figure 9.1 Melatonin and cortisol fluctuations along circadian rhythm.

sleep stages. This duration supports optimal physical, mental, and emotional health by providing sufficient restorative deep sleep and cognitive benefits from REM sleep.

Impact of Sleep Disturbances on Women's Health and Daily Functioning

Sleep disturbances disproportionately impact women due to various physiological, hormonal, and psychosocial factors. Hormonal changes during menstruation, pregnancy, and menopause can lead to significant sleep disturbances. For example, fluctuations in estrogen and progesterone levels affect sleep patterns, making women more susceptible to conditions like insomnia and sleep apnea. Pregnancy often brings about a decline in sleep quality due to physical discomfort, hormonal changes, and increased frequency of urination. During menopause, hot flashes and night sweats can significantly disrupt sleep.

Physiological differences also play a role in how sleep affects women differently from men. For instance, sleep deprivation impacts women's metabolism more severely, increasing the risk of metabolic disorders. Additionally, women's immune systems may be more sensitive to sleep deprivation, leading to a higher susceptibility to infections. Psychosocial factors, such as caregiving responsibilities and stress, further contribute to sleep disturbances in women. These factors can lead to higher rates of depression, anxiety, and cardiovascular diseases among women who experience chronic sleep disturbances.

Working while sleep-deprived significantly impairs job performance and overall health, particularly for women. Lack of sleep causes overworked neurons, resulting in slower cognitive processing, impaired physical reactions, and emotional exhaustion. These immediate effects disrupt productivity, while chronic sleep deprivation increases risks of obesity, heart disease, cognitive decline, and dementia. Women, who often face hormonal changes, caregiving responsibilities, and higher stress levels, are particularly vulnerable. Sleep loss hinders focus and attention, leading to errors and slower reaction times, which can be hazardous in professions like healthcare and transportation. Emotional instability from sleep deprivation can exacerbate stress and interfere with sleep, creating a detrimental cycle that heightens the risk of anxiety and depression.

Sleep disorders are significantly more prevalent in women compared to men, impacting various aspects of their health and daily functioning. Hormonal fluctuations related to menstruation, pregnancy, and menopause contribute to the higher incidence of sleep disturbances in women. Additionally, psychosocial factors such as caregiving responsibilities and higher rates of anxiety and depression further exacerbate sleep issues. Women are affected by several common sleep disorders, including insomnia, sleep apnea, restless legs syndrome (RLS), narcolepsy, sleep-disordered breathing, movement disorders, REM sleep behavior disorder, parasomnias, circadian rhythm sleep disorder, and shift work sleep disorder (see Table 9.1).

Sleep disorders can profoundly impact daily functioning and overall well-being. Women with chronic sleep disturbances may experience cognitive impairment, including difficulty with concentration, memory, and decision-making. Emotional instability, characterized by increased irritability and mood swings, is also common. Physically, these women may face a greater susceptibility to cardiovascular diseases, obesity, and a weakened immune response. Additionally, sleep disturbances can lead to reduced productivity, affecting efficiency at work or school and making it challenging to manage daily responsibilities.

Table 9.1 Common sleep disorders in women

Disorder	Causes	Description
Insomnia	Hormonal changes, stress, anxiety	Difficulty falling asleep, staying asleep, or waking up too early
Sleep Apnea	Obesity, menopause, anatomical factors	Repeated interruptions in breathing during sleep
Restless Legs Syndrome (RLS)	Iron deficiency, pregnancy, genetics	Uncontrollable urge to move legs, often accompanied by uncomfortable sensations
Narcolepsy	Genetics, autoimmune factors	Sudden attacks of sleep and excessive daytime drowsiness
Sleep-Disordered Breathing	Obesity, anatomical issues	Abnormal breathing patterns during sleep, including snoring and apnea
Movement Disorders	Parkinson's disease, restless legs	Involuntary movements that disrupt sleep
REM Sleep Behavior Disorder	Neurological conditions	Acting out dreams during REM sleep
Parasomnia	Stress, PTSD, medication side effects	Abnormal behaviors during sleep, such as sleepwalking and night terrors
Circadian Rhythm Sleep Disorder	Shift work, jet lag, lifestyle factors	Misalignment between sleep-wake patterns and the natural light-dark cycle
Shift Work Sleep Disorder	Irregular work hours	Sleep problems due to working non-traditional hours, leading to insomnia or excessive sleepiness

The rise of digital connectivity has blurred the boundaries between work and home life, making it difficult to mentally detach from work-related stress. This detachment is essential for reducing the negative effects of work stress and ensuring quality sleep. However, many jobs, especially those with high demands or irregular hours, challenge this balance. Professions requiring constant availability or shift work often result in sleep disorders. Given these challenges, it is crucial for women to prioritize consistent, quality sleep to maintain health and productivity. Addressing sleep health is vital for enhancing women's well-being and occupational performance, given their unique physiological and psychosocial stressors.

Assessments and Interventions

Addressing sleep disorders in women requires a comprehensive approach that includes appropriate assessments and targeted interventions. OTPs play a crucial role in evaluating sleep disturbances and developing personalized treatment plans. Given the prevalence of sleep disorders in women and their impact on various aspects of health, it is essential for OTPs to routinely inquire about clients' sleep habits and issues during evaluations. Sleep disturbances can contribute to a wide range of problems seen in occupational therapy, such as pain, headaches, and impaired daily functioning. During the interview portion of the evaluation, OTPs can use both informal and formal questions to gather detailed information about a client's sleep. Informal questions might include:

- "Can you describe your typical sleep routine?"
- "How many hours of sleep do you usually get each night?"
- "Do you have difficulty falling asleep or staying asleep?"
- "How do you feel when you wake up in the morning?"
- "Do you take naps during the day? If so, how often?"

Table 9.2 outlines some key assessments used to identify sleep issues and potential interventions that can be implemented to improve sleep quality and overall well-being.

By using these assessments, OTPs can develop personalized intervention plans to improve sleep hygiene, address specific sleep disorders, and ultimately enhance the overall health and well-being of women.

Table 9.2 Assessments and interventions for sleep disorders in women

Assessment	Description	Interventions
Pittsburgh Sleep Quality Index (PSQI)	Self-rated questionnaire assessing sleep quality and disturbances over one month	Sleep hygiene education, cognitive-behavioural therapy
Epworth Sleepiness Scale (ESS)	Measures daytime sleepiness to identify potential sleep disorders	Recommendations for sleep environment modifications
Insomnia Severity Index (ISI)	Evaluates severity of insomnia symptoms and their impact on daily life	Stress management techniques, relaxation exercises
Sleep Diary	Daily log of sleep patterns, duration, and quality	Personalized sleep routine development
Actigraphy	Non-invasive monitoring of rest/activity cycles using a wrist-worn device	Activity scheduling to regulate sleep patterns

Common Interventions

Several interventions are commonly used to improve sleep quality and address sleep disorders. These interventions focus on modifying behaviors, environments, and cognitive patterns to promote better sleep as an occupation.

1. **Sleep Hygiene Education**: Sleep hygiene education involves teaching individuals about healthy sleep habits and routines. This includes maintaining a consistent sleep schedule, creating a comfortable sleep environment, limiting exposure to screens before bedtime, and avoiding caffeine and heavy meals close to bedtime. By adopting these practices, women can establish a more conducive environment for sleep, improving both the duration and quality of their rest.
2. **Sleep Restriction Therapy**: Sleep restriction therapy aims to consolidate sleep by limiting the amount of time spent in bed to the actual amount of sleep obtained. Initially, this may involve reducing the time in bed to match the average sleep duration, gradually increasing it as sleep efficiency improves. This intervention helps regulate the sleep-wake cycle and reduces sleep fragmentation, leading to more restorative sleep.
3. **Cognitive Behavioural Therapy for Insomnia (CBT-I)**: CBT-I is a structured program that helps individuals identify and replace thoughts and behaviors that cause or worsen sleep problems with habits that promote sound sleep. CBT-I addresses the underlying cognitive and behavioural aspects of insomnia, such as negative sleep thoughts and poor sleep habits. Research has shown CBT-I to be highly effective in treating chronic insomnia, often more so than medication. Further training is required to utilize CBT-I techniques.
4. **Relaxation Techniques**: Techniques such as progressive muscle relaxation, deep breathing exercises, and mindfulness meditation can help reduce anxiety and stress, which are common contributors to sleep disturbances. These techniques promote a state of relaxation that is conducive to falling and staying asleep.
5. **Environmental Modifications**: Modifying the sleep environment can significantly impact sleep quality. This includes optimizing the bedroom for sleep by controlling light, noise, and temperature. Using blackout curtains, white noise machines, and maintaining a cool room temperature are examples of effective environmental modifications.
6. **Physical Activity**: Regular physical activity can improve sleep quality and reduce the time it takes to fall asleep. Encouraging women to engage in moderate aerobic exercise, such as walking or swimming, can help regulate sleep patterns and enhance overall well-being.
7. **Performance Patterns**: Habits and Routines: Establishing sleep-friendly habits and routines is crucial for maintaining healthy sleep patterns. According to the Occupational Therapy Practice Framework (OTPF), performance patterns include habits, routines, roles, and rituals. These patterns play a significant role in how individuals manage their daily activities, including sleep.
    - **Habits**: Developing consistent habits, such as going to bed and waking up at the same time every day, can strengthen the body's internal clock and improve sleep quality.
    - **Routines**: Creating a bedtime routine that includes relaxing activities, such as reading or taking a warm bath, can signal to the body that it is time to wind down and prepare for sleep.

- **Roles**: Recognizing and balancing roles within daily life, such as caregiving responsibilities, work, and personal time, can help reduce stress and promote better sleep.
- **Rituals**: Engaging in calming pre-sleep rituals, such as meditation or gentle stretching, can help create a peaceful transition from wakefulness to sleep.

These performance patterns can be incorporated into intervention plans to help women establish and maintain sleep-friendly habits and routines. By enhancing sleep quality through these interventions, women can experience better physical health, emotional stability, and cognitive function, which in turn positively impacts their daily lives and overall well-being.

These interventions not only address the specific sleep disorder but also contribute to the holistic improvement of sleep as an occupation. By enhancing sleep quality, women can experience better physical health, emotional stability, and cognitive function, which in turn positively impacts their daily lives and overall well-being.

OT Approaches to Eating-Related Disorders, Obesity, and Weight Management

Eating-related disorders and obesity are significant public health issues that affect millions of women worldwide. According to the National Eating Disorders Association, approximately 20 million women in the United States will experience an eating disorder at some point in their lives. These conditions can lead to severe health complications, including cardiovascular disease, diabetes, and psychological distress. OT plays a critical role in addressing these issues by helping women develop healthier eating habits, manage weight, and improve their overall well-being.

Eating-Related Disorders in Women

Eating-related disorders, such as anorexia nervosa, bulimia nervosa, and binge-eating disorder, are prevalent among women and can have devastating physical and psychological effects. These disorders often co-occur with other mental health conditions, such as depression and anxiety, further complicating treatment and recovery. Additionally, conditions like avoidant/restrictive food intake disorder (ARFID) and other specified feeding or eating disorder (OSFED) also significantly impact women's health.

Eating disorders are significantly more common in women than in men. Studies suggest that approximately 90% of those diagnosed with eating disorders are women. The lifetime prevalence rates for eating disorders in women are estimated at 0.9% for anorexia nervosa, 1.5% for bulimia nervosa, and 3.5% for binge-eating disorder. In contrast, the rates for men are 0.3%, 0.5%, and 2.0%, respectively. These disorders often begin in adolescence and young adulthood, although they can occur at any age.

Age Groups Impacted by Eating Disorders

Eating disorders can affect women of all ages, but they most commonly begin in adolescence and young adulthood.

- **Adolescents (12–18 years)**: This group is at a high risk for developing eating disorders due to body image issues, peer pressure, and the onset of puberty.
- **Young Adults (18–25 years)**: The transition to adulthood, academic pressures, and social expectations can trigger or exacerbate eating disorders.

Table 9.3 Common eating-related disorders in women

Disorder	Causes	Description
Anorexia Nervosa	Genetic, environmental, psychological	Characterized by an intense fear of gaining weight and a distorted body image, leading to restricted food intake
Bulimia Nervosa	Genetic, environmental, psychological	Involves cycles of binge eating followed by compensatory behaviors such as vomiting or excessive exercise
Binge-Eating Disorder	Genetic, environmental, psychological	Recurrent episodes of eating large quantities of food without subsequent purging behaviors
Avoidant/Restrictive Food Intake Disorder (ARFID)	Sensory issues, negative experiences with food	Avoidance or restriction of food intake, leading to nutritional deficiencies
Other Specified Feeding or Eating Disorder (OSFED)	Varies	Symptoms do not meet the full criteria for other eating disorders but still cause significant distress
Pica	Nutritional deficiencies, mental health conditions	Persistent eating of non-food substances (e.g., dirt, clay, paper)
Rumination Disorder	Lack of stimulation, stress, neglect	Repeated regurgitation of food, which may be re-chewed, re-swallowed, or spit out

- **Adults (26–40 years)**: Career pressures, pregnancy, and postpartum body changes can influence eating behaviors and body image.
- **Middle-aged and Older Women (40+ years)**: Menopause and aging can also lead to or worsen eating disorders, although they are less common in this age group compared to younger women (Table 9.3).

Causes of Eating Disorders in Women

The etiology of eating disorders in women is multifactorial, involving a complex interplay of genetic, biological, psychological, and sociocultural factors:

- **Genetic Factors**: Family history of eating disorders or other mental health conditions increases the risk.
- **Biological Factors**: Hormonal changes, particularly during puberty, pregnancy, and menopause, can influence eating behaviors.
- **Psychological Factors**: Low self-esteem, perfectionism, and a history of trauma or abuse are significant contributors.
- **Sociocultural Factors**: Societal pressure to conform to ideal body shapes, exposure to media emphasizing thinness, and cultural norms play a substantial role.

The OTPs Role within Eating Disorder Treatment

OTPs are integral to the multidisciplinary treatment team for individuals with eating disorders. OTPs focus on enhancing the individual's overall function and quality of life by addressing the physical, psychological, and social aspects of eating disorders.

Occupational Therapy Frameworks Used with Women with Eating Disorders

Several occupational therapy frameworks have been effective in treating women with eating disorders:

1. **Model of Human Occupation (MOHO)**: MOHO emphasizes understanding the individual's volition, habituation, performance capacity, and environmental influences on their behaviors. This model helps OTPs create personalized interventions that address the motivations and habits associated with eating disorders.
2. **Person-Environment-Occupation (PEO) Model**: This model focuses on the dynamic interaction between the person, their environment, and their occupations. It is useful in identifying and modifying environmental factors that contribute to disordered eating behaviors.
3. **Cognitive Behavioural Framework**: This approach addresses the cognitive distortions and behaviors associated with eating disorders. OTPs use techniques such as cognitive restructuring and behavioural experiments to help individuals develop healthier thoughts and behaviors.

Effective Approaches in Occupational Therapy for Eating Disorders

Occupational therapy offers a range of effective approaches to address the multifaceted needs of individuals with eating disorders. These approaches focus on educating clients, developing essential skills, and creating supportive environments to foster recovery and enhance quality of life. By utilizing evidence-based strategies and personalized interventions, OTPs can help clients develop healthier relationships with food, improve body image, and build resilience against the triggers and challenges associated with eating disorders.

1. **Psychoeducation**: Educating clients about the physical and psychological effects of eating disorders, nutrition, and healthy eating habits.
2. **Skills Training**: Teaching coping strategies, stress management techniques, and social skills to improve emotional regulation and interpersonal relationships.
3. **Meal Planning and Support**: Assisting with meal planning, grocery shopping, and cooking to promote healthy eating habits and reduce anxiety around food.
4. **Body Image Interventions**: Activities and discussions aimed at improving body image and self-esteem.
5. **Mindfulness and Relaxation Techniques**: Techniques such as mindfulness meditation, progressive muscle relaxation, and deep breathing exercises to reduce anxiety and improve emotional regulation.
6. **Routine and Structure**: Helping clients establish healthy routines and daily structures to support recovery and prevent relapse.

By utilizing these frameworks and approaches, OTPs can play a crucial role in the treatment and recovery of women with eating disorders, addressing both the psychological and practical aspects of these complex conditions. Through a comprehensive and individualized approach, occupational therapy can significantly enhance the quality of life and functional outcomes for women struggling with eating disorders.

Table 9.4 Factors contributing to obesity in women

Factor	Description
Genetic Predisposition	Family history of obesity increases risk
Behavioural Factors	Poor dietary habits, lack of physical activity
Environmental Influences	Access to unhealthy foods, socioeconomic status
Psychological Factors	Stress, depression, emotional eating

Obesity and Weight Management

Obesity is a complex and multifaceted condition characterized by an excessive accumulation of body fat. While it is often defined by a body mass index (BMI) of 30 or higher, other measures are also important in assessing obesity. For instance, visceral fat—fat stored around internal organs—can be a more accurate indicator of health risks than BMI alone. Additionally, waist circumference is a critical measure, with a waist measurement of 35 inches or more in women indicating a higher risk of obesity-related health conditions. The development of obesity is influenced by a combination of genetic, behavioural, and environmental factors. These can include poor diet, lack of physical activity, genetic predisposition, and socioeconomic status (see Table 9.4).

Obesity is a major public health concern because it significantly increases the risk of various chronic health conditions, such as type 2 diabetes, hypertension, cardiovascular diseases, certain cancers, and musculoskeletal disorders like osteoarthritis. In women, obesity is particularly concerning as it is linked to several gender-specific health issues. For instance, obesity can complicate pregnancy, leading to gestational diabetes, pre-eclampsia, and increased risk of cesarean delivery. Postmenopausal women with obesity are also at a higher risk for breast cancer and endometrial cancer. Additionally, the excess weight places extra stress on joints, leading to conditions such as osteoarthritis, which can severely impact mobility and quality of life.

Given the broad range of health issues associated with obesity, effective weight management strategies are essential. These strategies can include dietary modifications, increased physical activity, behavioural interventions, and sometimes medical or surgical treatments. Occupational therapy plays a crucial role in weight management by promoting healthy lifestyle changes and supporting individuals in developing sustainable habits.

Impact on Daily Functioning and Occupational Performance

Eating-related disorders and obesity can profoundly impact daily functioning and occupational performance. Women with these conditions may often experience:

- **Physical Health Issues**: Women with eating disorders or obesity face a heightened risk of chronic diseases, reduced physical stamina, and mobility issues. For example, obesity is associated with a 50–100% increased risk of premature death compared to individuals with a healthy weight. Chronic conditions such as cardiovascular diseases, type 2 diabetes, and certain cancers are more prevalent among obese individuals. Additionally, the physical strain from excess weight can lead to musculoskeletal problems like osteoarthritis, further limiting mobility and physical activity.

- **Emotional and Psychological Distress**: Low self-esteem, anxiety, depression, and social isolation are common among women with eating-related disorders and obesity. Approximately 50–70% of individuals with eating disorders also have a lifetime prevalence of anxiety disorders. The stigma associated with obesity can lead to significant emotional distress, diminished quality of life, and increased risk of mental health issues. Women may struggle with body image issues and feel a pervasive sense of shame and guilt related to their eating habits and body size.
- **Occupational Challenges**: Difficulties in managing daily routines, maintaining employment, and engaging in social activities are significant for women with eating disorders and obesity. Obesity-related health issues can result in increased absenteeism and decreased productivity at work. Women with severe obesity may face discrimination in the workplace, further affecting their occupational performance and opportunities. The economic cost of obesity in the United States is estimated to be $147 billion annually, including medical expenses and lost productivity. Additionally, individuals with binge-eating disorder often report impaired social and occupational functioning, leading to a reduced quality of life.

Assessments and Interventions

OTPs utilize various assessments and interventions to help women manage eating-related disorders and obesity (see Table 9.5). These interventions focus on promoting healthy eating habits, increasing physical activity, and addressing the psychological aspects of these conditions.

Common Interventions

OTPs provide a range of interventions to support women with eating-related disorders and obesity. While OTPs collaborate closely with dietitians, their role focuses on facilitating

Table 9.5 Assessments and interventions for eating-related disorders and obesity

Assessment	Description	Interventions	Used for
Eating Disorder Inventory (EDI)	Measures psychological and behavioural traits common in eating disorders	Cognitive-behavioural therapy, nutritional counseling, mindful eating practices	Eating Disorders
24-Hour Food Recall	Records all foods and beverages consumed in the past 24 hours	Personalized meal planning, ADL/IADL retraining (e.g., grocery shopping, meal preparation)	Eating Disorders, Obesity
Body Mass Index (BMI)	Calculates body fat based on height and weight	Diet modification/nutrition management, physical activity programs, therapeutic exercises	Obesity
Physical Activity Log	Tracks daily physical activities	Exercise prescription, activity scheduling, therapeutic exercises	Obesity
Beck Depression Inventory (BDI)	Assesses symptoms of depression, which can co-occur with eating disorders	Psychotherapy, stress management techniques, sensory modulation activities	Eating Disorders

healthy eating habits and routines through practical, everyday activities. Here are some specific interventions and delineations:

1. **Nutritional Counseling**: While OTPs do not provide in-depth nutritional counseling like dietitians, they play a crucial role in educating clients about healthy eating habits. This includes teaching clients how to plan and prepare balanced meals, read food labels, and make healthier food choices. OTPs can also grade interventions based on individual needs, such as increasing daily or weekly food intake for those with restrictive eating disorders or reducing caloric intake for weight management. OTPs work alongside dietitians to ensure that the nutritional plans align with the client's health goals. They may implement the dietitian's recommendations into the client's daily routines and activities, helping clients adhere to their nutritional plans effectively.
2. **Cognitive-Behavioural Therapy (CBT)**: CBT is an effective approach for addressing the psychological aspects of eating-related disorders and obesity. It helps individuals identify and change negative thought patterns and behaviors related to food, body image, and self-esteem. OTPs use CBT techniques to reduce symptoms of depression and anxiety, promoting healthier eating habits and weight management.
3. **Mindful Eating Practices**: Mindful eating encourages individuals to focus on the sensory experience of eating, such as the taste, smell, and texture of food. This practice can help reduce binge eating and promote healthier food choices. OTPs teach mindful eating techniques to help women develop a more positive relationship with food.
4. **Physical Activity Programs**: Regular physical activity is essential for managing weight and improving overall health. OTPs design individualized exercise programs that consider the client's physical capabilities, preferences, and lifestyle. These programs can include aerobic exercises, strength training, and flexibility exercises to promote physical fitness and well-being.
5. **Behavioural Modification**: Behavioural modification involves identifying and changing unhealthy eating and activity habits. Techniques such as goal setting, self-monitoring, and positive reinforcement motivate individuals to adopt healthier behaviors. OTPs support clients in developing and maintaining these changes over time.
6. **ADL/IADL Retraining**: ADL and IADL retraining help clients develop skills for independent living. Specific activities might include:
   - **Meal Preparation**: Teaching clients how to prepare healthy meals.
   - **Grocery Shopping**: Educating clients on how to choose nutritious foods and manage a shopping list.
   - **Time Management**: Helping clients incorporate regular physical activity and meal planning into their daily routines.
7. **Therapeutic Exercises**: Therapeutic exercises tailored to the individual's needs can help improve physical health and manage weight. These may include aerobic exercises, strength training, and flexibility exercises to improve cardiovascular fitness, build muscle mass, and enhance range of motion.
8. **Sensory Modulation Activities**: Sensory modulation helps clients regulate their emotional responses and manage stress, which can influence eating behaviors. Activities may include deep pressure stimulation (e.g., using weighted blankets), calming sensory input (e.g., listening to soothing music), and tactile activities (e.g., clay modeling).

9. **Stress Management Techniques**: Stress can significantly impact eating behaviors and weight. Techniques such as relaxation exercises, deep breathing, and mindfulness meditation can help reduce stress and its negative effects on eating habits. OTPs integrate these techniques into treatment plans to support overall mental health and well-being.
10. **Performance Patterns**: Establishing healthy habits and routines is crucial for managing eating-related disorders and obesity. According to the Occupational Therapy Practice Framework (OTPF), performance patterns include habits, routines, roles, and rituals. Interventions include:

    - **Habits**: Developing consistent habits, such as regular meal times and portion control, can support healthy eating behaviors.
    - **Routines**: Creating structured daily routines that incorporate balanced meals and physical activity can help maintain a healthy lifestyle.
    - **Roles**: Recognizing and balancing roles within daily life, such as caregiving responsibilities and personal time, can reduce stress and support healthy behaviors.
    - **Rituals**: Engaging in positive rituals, such as family meals or cooking healthy recipes, can foster a supportive environment for healthy eating.

These interventions not only address specific eating-related issues and obesity but also contribute to the holistic improvement of overall health and well-being. By enhancing eating habits and physical activity, women can experience better physical health, emotional stability, and cognitive function, which in turn positively impacts their daily lives and overall well-being.

Promoting Physical Activity and Healthy Lifestyle Choices

Physical activity and healthy lifestyle choices are crucial components of overall well-being and play a significant role in preventing and managing various health conditions, including cardiovascular diseases, diabetes, and mental health disorders. For women, engaging in regular physical activity and maintaining healthy lifestyle choices can enhance quality of life, improve physical and mental health, and reduce the risk of chronic diseases. OTPs are uniquely positioned to support women in integrating physical activity and healthy habits into their daily routines.

Importance of Physical Activity

Physical activity is essential for maintaining physical fitness, mental health, and overall quality of life. The World Health Organization recommends that adults engage in at least 150 minutes of moderate-intensity aerobic activity or 75 minutes of vigorous-intensity aerobic activity per week, along with muscle-strengthening activities on two or more days per week. Only 22.9% of American adults meet the recommended physical activity guidelines for both aerobic and muscle-strengthening activities. Women are less likely than men to meet physical activity guidelines, with only 18% of women engaging in regular physical exercise.

Barriers to Physical Activity for Women

Women may face unique barriers to engaging in physical activity, including:

- **Time Constraints**: Balancing work, family, and personal responsibilities can make it challenging to find time for exercise.
- **Safety Concerns**: Concerns about personal safety can limit opportunities for outdoor physical activities.
- **Socioeconomic Factors**: Limited access to safe and affordable exercise facilities and resources.
- **Health Issues**: Chronic health conditions, pain, and physical limitations can impede the ability to engage in regular physical activity.

Impact on Daily Functioning and Occupational Performance

Physical inactivity can significantly impact daily functioning and occupational performance. Women who do not engage in regular physical activity may experience reduced physical health, including an increased risk of chronic diseases, reduced stamina, and mobility issues. Additionally, they may face higher rates of mental health issues such as depression, anxiety, and stress. These physical and mental health challenges can lead to occupational challenges, including decreased energy levels, reduced productivity, and difficulties in managing daily routines and responsibilities. Overall, the lack of regular physical activity can have profound effects on women's overall well-being and ability to perform everyday tasks effectively.

Assessments and Interventions

OTPs utilize various assessments to evaluate physical activity levels and barriers to healthy lifestyle choices, followed by targeted interventions to promote these behaviors. The assessments help identify the specific needs and challenges faced by women, allowing OTPs to develop personalized intervention plans. See Table 9.6 for an overview of these tools and their corresponding interventions.

By using these assessments, OTPs can develop personalized intervention plans to address the unique needs and challenges faced by women.

Table 9.6 Assessments and interventions for promoting physical activity and healthy lifestyle choices

Assessment	Description	Interventions
Physical Activity Readiness Questionnaire (PAR-Q)	Assesses readiness for physical activity and identifies potential risks	Tailored exercise programs, gradual activity progression
Activity Log	Tracks daily physical activities	Personalized exercise routines, activity scheduling
Health-Promoting Lifestyle Profile (HPLP-II)	Measures health-promoting behaviors in areas such as nutrition, physical activity, and stress management	Lifestyle coaching, goal setting
Barriers to Physical Activity Questionnaire	Identifies perceived barriers to physical activity	Problem-solving strategies, environmental modifications

Interventions

To promote physical activity and healthy lifestyle choices among women, OTPs can implement a variety of interventions. These interventions focus on enhancing motivation, reducing barriers, and integrating physical activity into daily routines. The goal is to help women develop sustainable, health-promoting habits that fit their individual lifestyles and preferences. Below are some common interventions used by OTPs to support physical activity and healthy living.

1. **Exercise Prescription and Physical Activity Programs**: OTPs can design individualized exercise programs that consider the client's physical capabilities, preferences, and lifestyle. These programs can include:
   - **Aerobic Exercises**: Such as walking, cycling, or swimming to improve cardiovascular fitness.
   - **Strength Training**: Using weights or resistance bands to build muscle mass and enhance metabolic health.
   - **Flexibility and Balance Exercises**: Such as yoga or tai chi to improve range of motion, balance, and reduce the risk of falls.

2. **Lifestyle Coaching**: Lifestyle coaching involves working with clients to set realistic goals, develop action plans, and monitor progress. This intervention helps clients overcome barriers to physical activity and establish sustainable healthy habits. OTPs can provide motivation, support, and accountability to help clients achieve their health goals.

3. **Environmental Modifications**: Modifying the environment to make physical activity more accessible and enjoyable can significantly impact engagement. Examples include:
   - **Creating Safe Exercise Spaces**: Ensuring that the home or community environment is safe for physical activity.
   - **Providing Access to Equipment**: Recommending and facilitating access to affordable exercise equipment, such as resistance bands or yoga mats.
   - **Community Resources**: Connecting clients with local resources, such as parks, recreational centers, and fitness classes.
   - **Behavioural Strategies**: Behavioural strategies can help clients adopt and maintain physical activity and healthy lifestyle choices. Techniques include:
   - **Goal Setting**: Setting specific, measurable, achievable, relevant, and time-bound (SMART) goals to guide physical activity.
   - **Self-Monitoring**: Encouraging clients to track their physical activity and progress using journals or mobile apps.
   - **Positive Reinforcement**: Using rewards and positive feedback to motivate and reinforce healthy behaviors.

4. **ADL/IADL Integration**: Incorporating physical activity into ADLs and IADLs can make it easier for clients to stay active. Examples include:
   - **Active Transportation**: Encouraging walking or cycling for short trips instead of driving.
   - **Household Activities**: Promoting physically active chores, such as gardening, cleaning, or carrying groceries.
   - **Leisure Activities**: Identifying and engaging in physically active hobbies, such as dancing, hiking, or playing sports.

5. **Health Education and Counseling**: Providing education on the benefits of physical activity and healthy lifestyle choices is essential. OTPs can educate clients on topics such as:

   - **Nutritional Guidelines**: Understanding the role of nutrition in overall health and physical activity.
   - **Stress Management**: Techniques for managing stress and its impact on health and physical activity.
   - **Sleep Hygiene**: The importance of sleep in supporting physical activity and overall well-being.

6. **Social Support and Community Engagement**: Encouraging clients to seek social support and engage in community activities can enhance motivation and adherence to physical activity routines. OTPs can facilitate:

   - **Group Exercise Classes**: Joining or forming exercise groups to promote social interaction and accountability.
   - **Family Involvement**: Involving family members in physical activity and healthy lifestyle changes.
   - **Community Programs**: Participating in local health promotion programs, events, and workshops.

By incorporating these interventions, OTPs can help women overcome barriers to physical activity, establish healthy habits, and improve their overall well-being. Promoting physical activity and healthy lifestyle choices not only enhances physical health but also contributes to emotional stability, cognitive function, and quality of life.

Unhealthy Lifestyle Choices and Their Impact

In addition to promoting physical activity, OTPs also address unhealthy lifestyle choices that negatively impact health. Unhealthy lifestyle choices are a significant concern among women and are linked to numerous adverse health outcomes. For example, sedentary behavior and poor dietary habits can lead to obesity, which affects 40% of American women and increases the risk of type 2 diabetes, heart disease, and certain cancers. Smoking is responsible for nearly 1 in 5 deaths among women in the United States and significantly increases the risk of respiratory diseases and cardiovascular problems. Excessive alcohol consumption is associated with higher rates of liver disease, mental health issues, and accidents, with about 13% of women reporting binge drinking. Additionally, lack of sleep, which affects approximately 30% of women, is linked to higher risks of chronic health conditions such as hypertension, depression, and cognitive impairment.

Common unhealthy lifestyle choices include:

- **Sedentary Behavior**: Extended periods of inactivity can lead to weight gain, cardiovascular issues, and decreased muscle strength.
- **Poor Dietary Habits**: Consuming high-calorie, low-nutrient foods can contribute to obesity, diabetes, and other chronic diseases.
- **Smoking**: Tobacco use is a leading cause of various health problems, including respiratory issues and heart disease.
- **Excessive Alcohol Consumption**: Can lead to liver disease, mental health issues, and increased risk of accidents.

- **Lack of Sleep**: Insufficient sleep is linked to a higher risk of chronic health conditions, mental health issues, and impaired cognitive function.

Promoting Healthy Lifestyle Choices

OTPs help women replace unhealthy habits with healthier alternatives, promoting overall health and well-being. Healthy lifestyle choices are essential for preventing chronic diseases, enhancing mental health, and improving quality of life. By adopting healthier habits, women can reduce their risk of numerous health issues and achieve better physical and emotional health.

Some healthy lifestyle choices include:

- **Regular Physical Activity**: Incorporating exercise into daily routines. Engaging in at least 150 minutes of moderate-intensity aerobic activity per week can significantly reduce the risk of chronic diseases and improve mental health.
- **Balanced Diet**: Eating a variety of nutrient-rich foods and maintaining portion control. Consuming a diet rich in fruits, vegetables, whole grains, and lean proteins supports overall health and helps manage weight.
- **Adequate Sleep**: Ensuring 7–9 hours of quality sleep per night. Good sleep hygiene practices, such as maintaining a regular sleep schedule and creating a restful environment, are crucial for physical and mental health.
- **Stress Management**: Practicing relaxation techniques and maintaining a balanced life. Techniques such as mindfulness, yoga, and deep breathing exercises can help reduce stress and improve emotional resilience.
- **Avoiding Tobacco and Limiting Alcohol**: Reducing or eliminating smoking and moderating alcohol intake. Quitting smoking and limiting alcohol consumption can significantly decrease the risk of various health problems.

By integrating these interventions and promoting healthy lifestyle choices, OTPs can significantly enhance women's overall well-being, helping them lead healthier and more fulfilling lives. Promoting physical activity and healthy lifestyle choices not only enhances physical health but also contributes to emotional stability, cognitive function, and quality of life.

Substance Use in Women's Health

Substance use, including alcohol, tobacco, prescription medications, and illicit drugs, poses significant health risks for women. Substance use disorders (SUDs) affect millions of women worldwide, with significant variations in prevalence based on age, socioeconomic status, and cultural background. According to the National Institute on Drug Abuse (NIDA), women are more likely than men to experience chronic pain and be prescribed prescription pain relievers, increasing the risk of misuse and addiction. Additionally, women are more susceptible to the adverse effects of alcohol and other substances due to biological differences in body composition and metabolism. Approximately 19.5 million women (or 15.4%) aged 18 and older reported past-month use of illicit drugs in the United States in 2020. Women are also more likely than men to develop co-occurring mental health disorders, such as depression and anxiety, which can exacerbate substance use. Pregnant women who use substances face higher risks of complications, including preterm birth, low birth weight, and neonatal abstinence syndrome (NAS).

Factors Contributing to Substance Use in Women

Several factors contribute to substance use in women, including:

- **Biological Factors**: Women may experience more intense cravings and are more likely to relapse following treatment due to hormonal fluctuations and other physiological differences.
- **Psychosocial Factors**: Trauma, domestic violence, and social pressures can increase the likelihood of substance use. Women often use substances as a coping mechanism for stress, anxiety, and depression.
- **Socioeconomic Factors**: Limited access to healthcare, education, and economic opportunities can contribute to substance use. Women in lower socioeconomic groups are at higher risk for substance use disorders.
- **Cultural Factors**: Cultural norms and stigma surrounding substance use can impact a woman's willingness to seek help and adhere to treatment.

Impact on Daily Functioning and Occupational Performance

Substance use can profoundly impact a woman's daily functioning and occupational performance. Women with substance use disorders may experience physical health issues such as an increased risk of chronic diseases, weakened immune system, and reproductive health problems. Mental health issues, including higher rates of depression, anxiety, and other mental health disorders, are also common. Occupational challenges, such as difficulties maintaining employment, managing household responsibilities, and fulfilling social roles, can arise. Additionally, substance use can strain relationships with family and friends, lead to social isolation, and result in potential involvement with the criminal justice system.

Assessments and Interventions

OTPs utilize various assessments and interventions to support women in overcoming substance use disorders. These interventions focus on promoting recovery, enhancing daily functioning, and supporting healthy lifestyle choices (see Table 9.7).

Table 9.7 Assessments and interventions for substance use in women

Assessment	Description	Interventions
Substance Use Disorder Diagnostic Scale (SUDDS)	Evaluates the severity and impact of substance use disorders	Individualized treatment planning, motivational interviewing techniques
CAGE Questionnaire	A brief screening tool for identifying potential alcohol problems	Brief interventions, referral to specialized treatment
Alcohol Use Disorders Identification Test (AUDIT)	Assesses alcohol consumption, drinking behaviors, and alcohol-related problems	Education on safe drinking limits, cognitive-behavioural strategies
Beck Depression Inventory (BDI)	Assesses symptoms of depression, which often co-occur with substance use disorders	Psychosocial counseling, stress management techniques
Canadian Occupational Performance Measure (COPM)	Evaluates clients' self-perception of performance in daily activities and satisfaction with performance	Goal setting, ADL/IADL retraining, occupational engagement

Sleep, Weight, and Lifestyle Factors 281

By using these assessments, OTPs can develop personalized intervention plans to address the unique needs and challenges faced by women with substance use disorders.

Interventions

To support women in overcoming substance use disorders and promoting overall health, OTPs can implement a variety of interventions. These interventions focus on enhancing motivation, reducing barriers, and integrating recovery into daily routines. Below are some common interventions used by OTPs to support recovery and healthy living:

1. **Motivational Interviewing**: Motivational interviewing is a client-centered counseling approach that helps individuals explore and resolve ambivalence about changing substance use behaviors. This technique enhances motivation and commitment to recovery by empowering clients to set and achieve their own goals.
2. **Cognitive-Behavioural Therapy (CBT)**: CBT is an effective approach for addressing the psychological aspects of substance use disorders. It helps individuals identify and change negative thought patterns and behaviors related to substance use. CBT can reduce symptoms of depression and anxiety, promoting healthier coping mechanisms and relapse prevention.
3. **ADL/IADL Retraining**: ADL and IADL retraining can help clients develop skills for independent living. Specific activities might include:
    - **Household Management**: Teaching clients how to manage daily tasks such as cooking, cleaning, and budgeting.
    - **Vocational Rehabilitation**: Assisting clients in developing job skills and seeking employment.
    - **Time Management**: Helping clients organize their time to balance recovery activities, work, and personal responsibilities.
4. **Stress Management Techniques**: Stress can significantly impact substance use behaviors. Techniques such as relaxation exercises, deep breathing, and mindfulness meditation can help reduce stress and its negative effects on substance use. OTPs can integrate these techniques into treatment plans to support overall mental health and well-being.
5. **Environmental Modifications**: Modifying the environment to reduce triggers and support recovery can significantly impact engagement and success. Examples include:
    - **Creating Safe and Supportive Environments**: Ensuring that the home or community environment is conducive to recovery and free from triggers.
    - **Providing Access to Resources**: Recommending and facilitating access to support groups, counseling services, and community resources.
    - **Community Resources**: Connecting clients with local resources, such as support groups, rehabilitation centers, and healthcare providers.
6. **Health Education and Counseling**: Providing education on the risks of substance use and the benefits of recovery is essential. OTPs can educate clients on topics such as:
    - **Nutritional Guidelines**: Understanding the role of nutrition in supporting recovery and overall health.
    - **Sleep Hygiene**: The importance of sleep in supporting recovery and overall well-being.
    - **Safe Medication Use**: Educating clients on the safe use of prescription medications and the risks of misuse.

282   Occupational Therapy and Women's Health

7. **Performance Patterns: Habits, Roles, and Routines**: Establishing healthy habits, roles, and routines is crucial for supporting recovery and promoting overall well-being. OTPs can help clients identify and modify unhealthy patterns and replace them with healthier ones. Specific strategies include:

- **Habit Formation**: Encouraging the development of positive habits, such as regular exercise, healthy eating, and consistent sleep routines.
- **Role Identification and Management**: Assisting clients in identifying and balancing their roles, such as worker, parent, or student, to reduce stress and promote a balanced lifestyle.
- **Routine Development**: Creating structured daily routines that incorporate healthy activities and coping mechanisms, which can help prevent relapse and support long-term recovery.
- **Healthy Coping Skills**: Teaching clients effective coping skills to manage stress, anxiety, and triggers without resorting to substance use.

8. **Social Support and Community Engagement**: Encouraging clients to seek social support and engage in community activities can enhance motivation and adherence to recovery plans. OTPs can facilitate:

- **Support Groups**: Joining or forming support groups to promote social interaction and accountability.
- **Family Involvement**: Involving family members in the recovery process to provide support and encouragement.
- **Community Programs**: Participating in local recovery programs, events, and workshops.

By incorporating these interventions, OTPs can help women overcome substance use disorders, establish healthy habits, and improve their overall well-being. Promoting recovery and healthy lifestyle choices not only enhances physical health but also contributes to emotional stability, cognitive function, and quality of life.

Case Studies in Sleep, Weight, and Lifestyle Factors

CASE A: Anorexia Nervosa

Background and Medical History: The client is a 19-year-old college student diagnosed with anorexia nervosa. The client has a history of frequent hospital admissions due to severe weight loss and complications arising from malnutrition. The client's medical history includes childhood trauma from being in an abusive relationship in high school, which has contributed to ongoing struggles with low self-esteem and body image issues. The client recently took a year off from college to focus on recovery but continues to face challenges with food intake and overall health.

Prior Level of Function:

- Functioned independently in all areas of occupation.
- Engaged actively in college studies, participating in campus activities, and socializing with friends.
- Enjoyed running and yoga as part of a daily exercise routine.
- Managed personal care and household tasks independently.

Household Living Arrangements and Social History:

- Lives with parents and a younger sibling in a suburban home.
- Has a supportive relationship with family members but often feels overshadowed by the sibling, exacerbating low self-esteem.
- Active in the local community, previously volunteered at a community center.

Change in Functional Status and Challenges: The client's anorexia nervosa has significantly impacted the ability to engage in daily activities across various domains of life:

- **ADLs**: Struggles with maintaining personal hygiene routines and dressing independently due to extreme fatigue, anxiety, and cognitive distortions such as rumination and obsessive thoughts about body image and food.
- **Education**: Took a year off from college due to physical and mental health challenges, including obsession regarding food and body weight; aims to return but feels apprehensive about managing academic pressures.
- **Social Activities**: Reduced participation in social events and community activities due to fear of eating in public, body image issues, and obsessive thoughts about food and weight.
- **Health Management**: Faces significant challenges with increasing food intake, adhering to a structured meal plan, and managing stress and anxiety due to constant preoccupation with body weight and food intake.

OT Assessments:

- **Barthel Index**: The client scored 50 out of 100, indicating significant assistance required for most ADLs due to anxiety, fatigue, and cognitive distortions such as rumination.
- **Canadian Occupational Performance Measure (COPM)**: The client identified meal planning, returning to college, and resuming social activities as top priorities. Satisfaction and performance scores were low in these areas.
- **Hospital Anxiety and Depression Scale (HADS)**: The client scored 16 on anxiety and 14 on depression, indicating severe anxiety and moderate depression impacting daily functioning.
- **Eating Disorder Inventory (EDI)**: High scores in areas of body dissatisfaction, drive for thinness, and perfectionism.
- **Nutritional Assessment**: Conducted in collaboration with a dietitian to evaluate dietary intake and nutritional status.

Occupational Therapy Plan of Care and Goals: The client will receive skilled occupational therapy services three times a week for 12 weeks to improve independence in ADLs, IADLs, and overall quality of life.

Goals:

1. Identify and incorporate at least three food items from different food groups that the client is willing to eat within 4 weeks.
2. Gradually increase food intake to achieve 50% of a balanced meal at least once a week within 8 weeks.
3. Increase Barthel Index score to 70/100, demonstrating improved independence in personal care tasks within 12 weeks.

4. Improve COPM performance and satisfaction scores by 30% in the areas of meal planning, education, and social participation within 12 weeks.
5. Reduce HADS scores to below 10 for both anxiety and depression, indicating improved emotional well-being within 12 weeks.
6. Develop a phased return-to-college plan, gradually increasing study hours and academic responsibilities within 12 weeks.

Interventions: The following interventions will be tailored to meet the client's specific needs and address the outlined goals:

Graded Meal Planning and Intake:

- Collaborate with a dietitian to develop a comprehensive meal plan, starting with small, frequent meals and gradually increasing portion sizes.
- Provide education on balanced nutrition and the importance of regular meals for recovery.
- Identify and incorporate food items from different food groups that the client is willing to eat.
- Use food diaries and nutritional tracking apps to monitor intake and progress.

ADL Retraining:

- Provide guidance on adaptive techniques and use of assistive devices to enhance independence in personal hygiene and dressing.
- Educate the client on strategies to simplify household tasks and improve efficiency in meal preparation.

Psychosocial Education and Skills Training:

- Educate the client about the physical and psychological effects of anorexia nervosa.
- Teach coping strategies and stress management techniques to improve emotional regulation.
- Facilitate body image interventions, including activities and discussions aimed at improving self-esteem.

Social and Community Engagement:

- Encourage participation in social activities and community events to reduce isolation.
- Facilitate support groups or peer mentoring to provide emotional support and share coping strategies.

Health Management and Education:

- Monitor medication adherence and collaborate with the healthcare team to ensure optimal management of the client's conditions.
- Provide education on recognizing and managing symptoms of anxiety and depression.

Phased Return-to-College Plan:

- Develop a gradual plan for returning to college, starting with part-time study and increasing to full-time as the client's health improves.
- **Collaborate** with college staff to ensure accommodations are in place to support the client's academic success.

Outcomes:

Post Treatment:

- **Meal Planning and Nutritional Intake**: Demonstrated significant improvement in meal planning and food intake, as indicated by a 30% increase in COPM scores and a Barthel Index score improvement from 50 to 70.
- **Emotional Well-being**: Achieved reduced anxiety and depression scores on the HADS, reflecting improved emotional resilience and coping skills.
- **Education and Social Participation**: Successfully reintegrated into academic activities with adapted strategies, managing a part-time study schedule without significant fatigue. Increased participation in community events and social gatherings, demonstrating improved confidence and engagement.

Follow-Up Visits:

- Continued reinforcement of nutritional education and stress management strategies to sustain progress.
- Ongoing support in managing the eating disorder, adjusting therapy goals as needed.
- Regular monitoring of nutritional intake, emotional well-being, and academic performance indicators, adapting interventions to promote long-term health and functional independence.

At the conclusion of therapy, the client demonstrated marked improvements across various domains, showcasing enhanced resilience and adaptive skills in managing anorexia nervosa. Significant progress was noted in meal planning, emotional well-being, and academic engagement, enabling the client to resume education and participate more fully in social activities. The client's commitment to therapy and collaboration with the occupational therapy team resulted in sustainable improvements, highlighting the capacity for growth and resilience in the face of health challenges.

CASE B: Sleep Issues and Substance Abuse Recovery

Background and Medical History: The client is a 23-year-old female in recovery for substance abuse, specifically heroin. She has a history of frequent hospital admissions due to complications related to substance abuse and severe sleep disturbances. The client has struggled with sleep issues, experiencing insomnia and irregular sleep patterns, exacerbated by her substance use. She has a supportive relationship with her grandmother, but it has been strained due to her substance abuse. Currently, the client is unemployed and temporarily sleeping on a friend's couch after being asked to leave her grandmother's home.

Prior Level of Function:

- Functioned independently in all areas of occupation.
- Lived with her grandmother and contributed to household tasks.
- Was employed part-time and engaged in social activities with friends.
- Managed personal care and household tasks independently.

Household Living Arrangements and Social History:

- Temporarily staying on a friend's couch in an urban setting.
- Previously lived with her grandmother in a suburban home.
- Has a supportive but strained relationship with her grandmother due to substance abuse.
- No significant employment or educational engagement due to health challenges.

Change in Functional Status and Challenges:

The client's substance abuse and sleep disturbances have significantly impacted her ability to engage in daily activities across various domains of life:

- **ADLs**: Struggles with maintaining personal hygiene routines and dressing independently due to extreme fatigue and anxiety.
- **Employment**: Unemployed and lacks the energy and motivation to seek work due to sleep disturbances and substance abuse recovery.
- **Social Activities**: Reduced participation in social events and community activities due to fear of judgment and low self-esteem.
- **Health Management**: Faces significant challenges with managing sleep patterns, adhering to recovery plans, and managing stress and anxiety.

OT Assessments:

- **Barthel Index**: The client scored 50 out of 100, indicating significant assistance required for most ADLs due to anxiety, fatigue, and cognitive distortions related to substance abuse.
- **Pittsburgh Sleep Quality Index (PSQI)**: Assesses sleep quality and disturbances, indicating severe sleep issues impacting daily functioning.
- **Substance Abuse Subtle Screening Inventory (SASSI)**: Identifies the probability of substance dependence and guides treatment planning.
- **Patient Health Questionnaire-9 (PHQ-9)**: Assesses the severity of depression symptoms impacting the client's daily functioning.
- **Quality of Life Scale (QoLS)**: Measures the client's perceived quality of life in various domains.

Occupational Therapy Plan of Care and Goals: The client will receive skilled occupational therapy services three times a week for 12 weeks to improve independence in ADLs, IADLs, and overall quality of life.

Goals:

1. Identify and incorporate at least three healthy sleep hygiene practices within 4 weeks.
2. Increase sleep duration to at least 6 hours per night within 8 weeks.
3. Increase Barthel Index score to 70/100, demonstrating improved independence in personal care tasks within 12 weeks.
4. Improve sleep quality scores on the PSQI by 30% within 12 weeks.
5. Reduce PHQ-9 scores to below 10, indicating improved emotional well-being within 12 weeks.
6. Develop a phased plan to seek employment, gradually increasing job search activities and responsibilities within 12 weeks.

7. Implement relapse prevention strategies and develop healthy coping skills to replace substance use habits, reducing the risk of relapse within 12 weeks.

Interventions: The following interventions will be tailored to meet the client's specific needs and address the outlined goals:

Graded Sleep Hygiene Practices:

- Educate the client on sleep hygiene practices, such as establishing a regular sleep schedule, creating a restful environment, and limiting caffeine intake.
- Implement a sleep diary to track sleep patterns and identify areas for improvement.
- Use relaxation techniques such as deep breathing and progressive muscle relaxation to improve sleep quality.

ADL Retraining:

- Provide guidance on adaptive techniques and use of assistive devices to enhance independence in personal hygiene and dressing.
- Educate the client on strategies to simplify household tasks and improve efficiency in daily routines.

Motivational Interviewing and Skills Training:

- Use motivational interviewing to enhance the client's motivation and commitment to behavior change, focusing on sleep hygiene and substance abuse recovery.
- Teach coping strategies and stress management techniques to improve emotional regulation and reduce reliance on substances.
- Facilitate body image and self-esteem interventions, including activities and discussions aimed at improving self-perception.

Social and Community Engagement:

- Encourage participation in social activities and community events to reduce isolation.
- Facilitate support groups or peer mentoring to provide emotional support and share coping strategies.

Health Management and Education:

- Monitor medication adherence and collaborate with the healthcare team to ensure optimal management of the client's conditions.
- Provide education on recognizing and managing symptoms of anxiety and depression.
- Collaborate with substance abuse counselors to support recovery efforts.

Employment Readiness Plan:

- Develop a gradual plan for seeking employment, starting with part-time job search activities and increasing to full-time as the client's health improves.
- Collaborate with job placement services to identify suitable employment opportunities.

Relapse Prevention:

- Implement relapse prevention strategies, including identifying triggers and developing a plan to manage them.
- Teach healthy coping skills to replace substance use habits, such as engaging in physical activities, creative pursuits, and relaxation techniques.

Outcomes:

Post Treatment:

- **Sleep Quality and Duration**: Demonstrated significant improvement in sleep quality and duration, as indicated by a 30% improvement in PSQI scores and achieving at least 6 hours of quality sleep per night.
- **Emotional Well-being**: Achieved reduced anxiety and depression scores on the PHQ-9, reflecting improved emotional resilience and coping skills.
- **ADL Independence**: Improved Barthel Index score from 50 to 70, demonstrating greater independence in personal care tasks.
- **Employment and Social Participation**: Successfully initiated job search activities with adapted strategies, managing a part-time job search schedule without significant fatigue. Increased participation in community events and social gatherings, demonstrating improved confidence and engagement.
- **Relapse Prevention**: Successfully implemented relapse prevention strategies, reducing the risk of relapse and demonstrating the use of healthy coping skills.

Follow-Up Visits:

- Continued reinforcement of sleep hygiene education and stress management strategies to sustain progress.
- Ongoing support in managing substance abuse recovery, adjusting therapy goals as needed.
- Regular monitoring of sleep quality, emotional well-being, and employment search activities, adapting interventions to promote long-term health and functional independence.

At the conclusion of therapy, the client demonstrated marked improvements across various domains, showcasing enhanced resilience and adaptive skills in managing sleep issues and substance abuse recovery. Significant progress was noted in sleep hygiene practices, emotional well-being, and employment readiness, enabling the client to pursue job opportunities and participate more fully in social activities. The client's commitment to therapy and collaboration with the occupational therapy team resulted in sustainable improvements, highlighting the capacity for growth and resilience in the face of health challenges.

Further Reading

Akbarfahimi, M., Nabavi, S. M., Kor, B., Rezaie, L., & Paschall, E. (2020). The effectiveness of occupational therapy-based sleep interventions on quality of life and fatigue in patients with multiple sclerosis: A pilot randomized clinical trial study. *Neuropsychiatric Disease and Treatment, 16*, 1369–1379. https://doi.org/10.2147/NDT.S249277

American Occupational Therapy Association. (2020). Occupational therapy practice framework: Domain and process (4th ed.). *American Journal of Occupational Therapy, 74*(Supplement_2), 7412410010p1–7412410010p87. https://doi.org/10.5014/ajot.2020.74S2001

Gronski, M. (2022). Occupational therapy interventions to support sleep in children from birth to age 5 years. *The American Journal of Occupational Therapy: Official Publication of the American Occupational Therapy Association, 76*(5), 7605390010. https://doi.org/10.5014/ajot.2022.049552

Henderson, S. (1999). Frames of reference utilized in the rehabilitation of individuals with eating disorders. *Canadian Journal of Occupational Therapy, 66*(1). https://doi.org/10.1177/000841749906600105

Jessen-Winge, C., Ilvig, P. M., Jonsson, H., Fritz, H., Lee, K., & Christensen, J. R. (2021). Obesity treatment: A role for occupational therapists? *Scandinavian Journal of Occupational Therapy*, *28*(6), 471–478. https://doi.org/10.1080/11038128.2020.1712472

Ludwig, R., Eakman, A., Bath-Scheel, C., & Siengsukon, C. (2022). How occupational therapists assess and address the occupational domain of sleep: A survey study. *The American Journal of Occupational Therapy: Official Publication of the American Occupational Therapy Association*, *76*(6), 7606345010. https://doi.org/10.5014/ajot.2022.049379

Mack, R. A., Stanton, C. E., & Carney, M. R. (2023). The importance of including occupational therapists as part of the multidisciplinary team in the management of eating disorders: A narrative review incorporating lived experience. *Journal of Eating Disorders*, *11*(1), 37. https://doi.org/10.1186/s40337-023-00763-6

Muntefering, C., Fields, B., & Christensen, J. R. (2023). Going beyond management and maintenance: Occupational therapy's role in primary prevention for adults at risk of obesity. *The American Journal of Occupational Therapy: Official Publication of the American Occupational Therapy Association*, *77*(5), 7705347020. https://doi.org/10.5014/ajot.2023.050154

Patel, A. K., Reddy, V., Shumway, K. R., & Araujo, J. F. (2024). Physiology, sleep stages. In *StatPearls*. StatPearls Publishing. Retrieved from https://www.ncbi.nlm.nih.gov/books/NBK526132/

Polo, K. M., Hunter, E. G., & Morikawa, S. (2023). Interventions to improve sleep for people living with or beyond cancer (2018–2022). *The American Journal of Occupational Therapy: Official Publication of the American Occupational Therapy Association*, *77*(Suppl 1), 7710393360. https://doi.org/10.5014/ajot.2023.77S10036

Schwartz, J., & Proffitt, R. (2024). Cautioning the role of occupational therapy in addressing obesity. *The American Journal of Occupational Therapy: Official Publication of the American Occupational Therapy Association*, *78*(2), 7802050010. https://doi.org/10.5014/ajot.2024.050653

10 Oncology in Women's Health

Chapter Objectives

Upon completion of this chapter, the reader will be able to:

1. Describe the impact of oncological conditions, specifically breast, lung, and gynecological cancers, on the occupational performance and daily lives of women.
2. Identify common physical, emotional, and psychosocial challenges faced by women undergoing cancer treatment.
3. Analyze the role of occupational therapy in managing symptoms related to cancer and its treatments, such as fatigue, lymphedema, and cognitive impairments.
4. Discuss the application of evidence-based occupational therapy interventions tailored to the needs of women with cancer.
5. Evaluate case studies to understand the practical application of occupational therapy strategies in enhancing the quality of life for women with cancer.
6. Develop skills to create personalized care plans that incorporate patient-centered goals and culturally sensitive interventions for women dealing with cancer.
7. Advocate for the integration of occupational therapy services in oncology care teams to ensure comprehensive support for women throughout their cancer journey.

OT in Management of Breast Cancer

Breast cancer is the most frequently diagnosed cancer among women, representing a significant health concern globally. Each year, over 2 million new cases are reported worldwide, making it a major focus of public health initiatives. In the United States, approximately 1 in 8 women will develop invasive breast cancer during their lifetime. Mortality rates have been declining due to advances in early detection and treatment, with the 5-year relative survival rate for localized breast cancer at approximately 99%. Despite these improvements, disparities persist, with higher incidence and mortality rates observed among African American women compared to Caucasian women, highlighting the need for equitable healthcare access and targeted interventions.

The American Cancer Society (ACS) currently recommends that women begin monthly breast self-examinations at the age of 20 years, ideally performed approximately one week following menses. Between the ages of 20 and 39 years, every woman should have a clinical breast exam (CBE) every three years. This exam, performed by a healthcare professional, is designed to feel for lumps and document changes in the size or shape of the breasts. At age 40 years, CBEs should be performed yearly. Additionally, at age 40, women should begin having a yearly mammogram. A mammogram, a radiograph of the breast, can often detect a tumor not yet palpable and is used to diagnose early signs of breast cancer. The use of screening mammography has been shown to reduce death from the disease by approximately 20–35% in women ages 50 to 69 years and approximately 20% in women ages 40 to 49 years. The earlier a breast cancer is detected, the less the need for aggressive therapeutic treatment, the fewer the overall side effects of those treatments, and the greater the chance for survival.

Breast cancer profoundly impacts a woman's quality of life, encompassing physical, emotional, and psychological domains. Physically, women may experience pain, fatigue, and lymphedema as a result of the disease and its treatments. Emotionally, the diagnosis often leads to anxiety, depression, and a pervasive fear of recurrence. Body image concerns and changes in sexual health can affect self-esteem and intimate relationships. Additionally, the ability to engage in daily activities, work, and social roles is frequently compromised, leading to a sense of loss of independence and identity. Long-term survivors may continue to face challenges such as chronic pain, cognitive changes, and persistent fatigue, further affecting their overall well-being.

Body Image Concerns in Women with Breast Cancer

Body image concerns are relatively common in patients with various types of cancer and other medical conditions. Disturbances in body image have been observed in patients with breast cancer, cervical cancer, and head and neck cancers. Additionally, side effects of cancer treatment, such as alopecia, have been associated with increased body image concerns.

Certain characteristics of diseases and associated treatments can also contribute to body image concerns. For example, disease activity, chronicity, treatment type, treatment complications, and presenting symptoms in various medical conditions can affect individuals' body image. Notably, treatment and improvement in disease activity do not always lead to improvements in body image. In some cases, treatment can worsen body image; for instance, increased body dissatisfaction has been reported after mastectomy in breast cancer patients. Conversely, some medical treatments can effectively reduce body image concerns.

Demographic, sociocultural, and psychosocial factors are significant risk factors for body image concerns. Women, Caucasian individuals, and men who identify as gay or bisexual are generally more at risk for body image concerns. Sociocultural factors, such as greater media consumption and exposure, have also been linked to increased body image concerns. Internalization of societal norms regarding thinness and perceived sociocultural pressure for thinness are strongly related to increased body image concerns.

In the context of breast cancer, body image disturbances can significantly impact a patient's emotional well-being and quality of life. Understanding and addressing these concerns is crucial for providing comprehensive care and support to breast cancer patients, helping them navigate the physical and psychological challenges associated with their condition and treatment.

292 *Occupational Therapy and Women's Health*

Anatomy of the Breast

The breast is primarily composed of lobes, lobules, and ducts, all embedded within fatty and connective tissue. Each breast contains 15–20 lobes, subdivided into smaller lobules responsible for milk production. The milk travels through ducts to the nipple, which is surrounded by the pigmented areola. Additionally, the breast contains a network of blood vessels and lymphatic channels, including lymph nodes located in the armpit, chest, and collarbone regions. Breast cancer typically originates in the ducts (ductal carcinoma) or lobules (lobular carcinoma) and can metastasize to nearby lymph nodes and other parts of the body via the lymphatic and vascular systems (Figure 10.1).

Pathology of Breast Cancer

The fundamental difference between normal cells and cancerous cells lies in their growth and replication processes. Normal cells follow a carefully regulated cell cycle, ensuring that cell growth equals cell death, thereby maintaining tissue homeostasis. These cells have built-in mechanisms to control their division and repair any damage that occurs. When cells become damaged beyond repair, they undergo programmed cell death (apoptosis), preventing the accumulation of faulty cells.

In contrast, cancerous cells lose these regulatory mechanisms. They undergo uncontrolled growth and division, ignoring signals that normally inhibit cell proliferation or trigger apoptosis. As a result, cancerous cells accumulate, forming a tumor mass. This tumor can invade and destroy normal tissues, competing for space and nutrients, and eventually spreading to other parts of the body.

Breast cancer is a type of cancer that often develops slowly, sometimes spreading microscopically years before it becomes detectable. Studies suggest that many breast cancers may be present for years before they are palpable or visible on mammograms. Diagnosing breast cancer typically involves performing a biopsy on palpable or

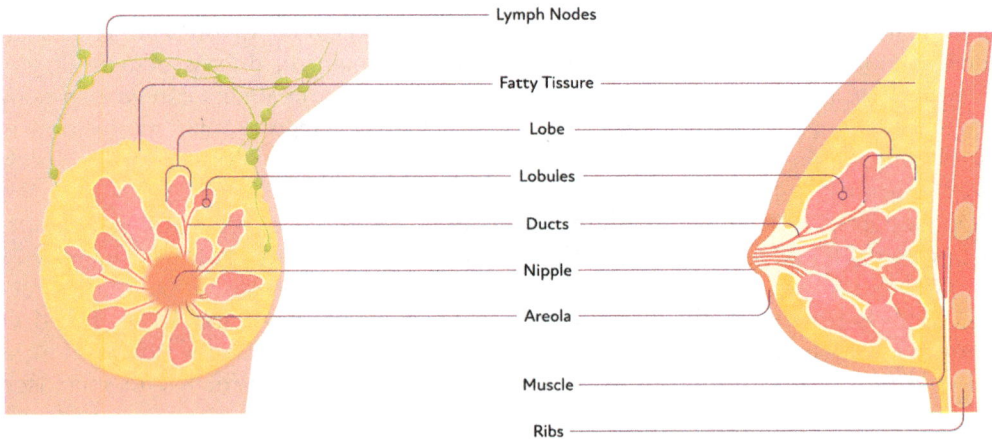

Figure 10.1 Anatomy of the breast.

suspicious mammographic lesions. Indications for a biopsy include a persistent breast mass, thickened breast tissue, bloody nipple discharge, nipple retraction, or other notable changes. Even non-palpable but suspicious mammographic abnormalities can necessitate a biopsy.

Once breast cancer is diagnosed, staging is a critical next step. Staging involves classifying the cancer based on its extent, which is essential for determining the most appropriate treatment and predicting the patient's prognosis. Breast cancer staging is most commonly performed using the TNM (Tumor, Nodes, Metastasis) classification system developed by the American Joint Commission on Cancer. This system considers the size of the tumor, the involvement of regional lymph nodes, and the presence of distant metastasis (see Table 10.1).

This classification is crucial as it guides the choice of treatment and helps predict the patient's prognosis (Figure 10.2).

Table 10.1 TNM staging of breast cancer

Stage	Description
Stage 0	Also known as DCIS (ductal carcinoma in situ). This is a non-invasive cancer confined to the milk ducts of the breast. "In situ" means "in place," indicating that these abnormal cancer cells have not spread beyond this original site. Non-invasive breast cancer is very treatable when caught at this stage.
Stage 1	Invasive breast cancer where cancer cells are invading the surrounding breast tissue.
1A	The tumor measures up to 2 centimeters and has not spread outside of the breast.
1B	Small groups of cancer cells (no larger than 2 millimeters) are found in the lymph nodes, or there is both a tumor (not greater than 2 cm) in the breast and cancer cells (no larger than 2 mm) in the lymph nodes.
Stage 2	
2A	No breast tumor but cancer cells (larger than 2 mm) found in the lymph nodes. Tumor smaller than 2 cm and has spread to lymph nodes. Tumor between 2 and 5 cm but has not spread to lymph nodes.
2B	Tumor between 2 and 5 cm with spread to lymph nodes. Tumor larger than 5 cm but no lymph node involvement.
Stage 3	
3A	No tumor or tumor of any size and spread to 4–9 lymph nodes. Tumor larger than 5 cm with small groups of breast cancer cells (no greater than 2 mm) found in lymph nodes. Tumor larger than 5 cm with spread to 1–3 lymph nodes.
3B	Tumor may be any size and has spread to the skin or chest wall resulting in swelling or an ulcer. May have spread to up to 9 lymph nodes. Inflammatory breast cancer may be staged as 3B and will manifest symptoms such as redness, warmth, and swelling.
3C	No tumor or tumor of any size with spread to chest wall or skin. Has spread to 10 or more axillary lymph nodes. Has spread to lymph nodes below or above the collarbone. Has spread to lymph nodes near the breastbone.
Stage 4	Advanced or metastatic breast cancer that has spread beyond the breast and lymph nodes. Common areas of metastasis are lungs, brain, liver, skin, bones, or distant lymph nodes.

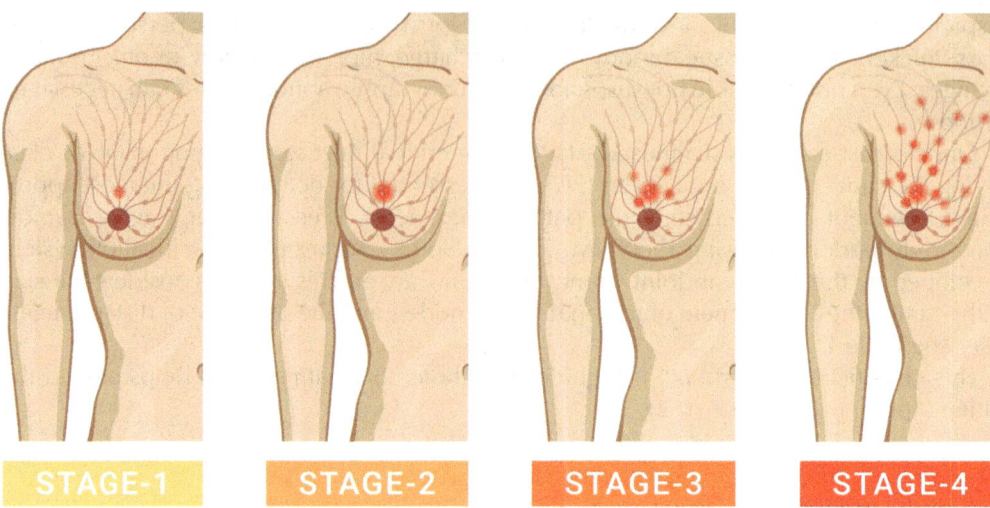

Figure 10.2 Stages of breast cancer.

Medical Management of Breast Cancer

The management of breast cancer involves a multifaceted approach, including diagnostics and various treatment modalities. Each treatment can have side effects that impact participation in occupations or occupational functioning.

- **Diagnosis**: Standard diagnostic tools include mammograms, ultrasounds, and biopsies. Magnetic resonance imaging (MRI) may be employed for high-risk patients to enhance detection.
- **Surgery**: Surgical options range from lumpectomy (removal of the tumor and some surrounding tissue) to mastectomy (complete removal of one or both breasts). Sentinel lymph node biopsy or axillary lymph node dissection may also be performed to assess the spread of cancer. Surgery can lead to pain, limited range of motion, and lymphedema. These side effects can impact ADLs, such as dressing, bathing, and household chores, due to restricted arm and shoulder movement.
- **Radiation Therapy**: Often administered post-surgery to eliminate residual cancer cells and reduce recurrence risk. Fatigue is a common side effect of radiation therapy. This fatigue can significantly reduce overall energy levels, making it challenging to maintain work, social, and leisure activities.
- **Chemotherapy**: Utilizes cytotoxic drugs to kill cancer cells, often used preoperatively (neoadjuvant) to shrink tumors or postoperatively (adjuvant) to decrease recurrence. Fatigue, decreased functional capacity, and anemia are common side effects. These can lead to difficulties in performing both physical and cognitive tasks, impacting occupational performance and the ability to sustain employment or engage in social activities.
- **Hormonal Therapy**: Effective for hormone receptor-positive breast cancers, it blocks hormones that fuel cancer growth. Side effects may include hot flashes, joint pain, and mood changes. These symptoms can interfere with sleep, reduce mobility, and affect emotional well-being, thereby impacting occupational engagement and quality of life.

- **Targeted Therapy**: Focuses on specific molecular targets associated with cancer, such as HER2-positive breast cancers. May cause heart problems and skin issues. Cardiac side effects can limit physical endurance, affecting the ability to perform vigorous activities or exercises.
- **Immunotherapy**: Aims to enhance the immune system's ability to recognize and attack cancer cells. Can cause immune-related adverse effects like inflammation of organs (e.g., colitis, pneumonitis). These side effects can lead to chronic fatigue and require frequent medical visits, disrupting daily routines and occupational roles.

Post-operative care is critical and includes wound management, pain control, occupational therapy, physical therapy, and monitoring for complications such as infection or lymphedema. Regular follow-up is essential to detect any recurrence early and manage side effects that could impair occupational functioning.

The side effects of breast cancer treatments can lead to physical limitations, fatigue, cognitive impairments, and emotional distress. These issues can interfere with:

- **Work**: Reduced capacity to meet job demands, necessitating adjustments or time off.
- **ADLs**: Challenges in performing self-care tasks due to pain, fatigue, or limited mobility.
- **Social Participation**: Decreased ability to engage in social activities due to fatigue or emotional distress.
- **Leisure Activities**: Reduced involvement in hobbies and recreational activities that require physical or mental energy.

Addressing these side effects through a comprehensive rehabilitation approach, including occupational therapy, can help mitigate their impact and enhance overall functioning and quality of life.

Symptoms and Barriers to Occupational Performance for Women with Breast Cancer

Common symptoms of breast cancer include:

- A lump or mass in the breast or underarm area.
- Changes in the size, shape, or appearance of the breast.
- Dimpling or puckering of the skin.
- Nipple retraction or inversion.
- Redness, scaliness, or thickening of the nipple or breast skin.
- Unusual nipple discharge.
- Persistent localized pain in the breast.

Symptoms indicative of metastatic breast cancer include bone pain, fatigue, shortness of breath, and weight loss, reflecting the spread of cancer to other parts of the body. Women with breast cancer face numerous barriers to occupational performance, including:

Physical Barriers:

- **Fatigue and Weakness**: Treatment-related fatigue and muscle weakness can significantly impact daily activities and occupational roles. One of the most pervasive symptoms, cancer-related fatigue (CRF) can affect concentration, motivation, and the ability to perform daily activities.

- **Pain and Lymphedema**: Post-surgical pain and the risk of lymphedema (swelling due to lymph fluid buildup) can limit arm movement and functional abilities.
- **Limited Range of Motion**: Surgical interventions often result in reduced shoulder and arm mobility, affecting tasks such as dressing, grooming, and household chores.
- **Neuropathy**: Chemotherapy-induced peripheral neuropathy can cause numbness and tingling in the hands and feet, impairing fine motor skills and balance.

Emotional and Psychological Barriers:

- **Anxiety and Depression**: The psychological burden of a breast cancer diagnosis and treatment can lead to significant emotional distress, impacting motivation and engagement in daily activities.
- **Body Image and Self-Esteem Issues**: Changes in appearance due to surgery and treatment can affect self-confidence and social interactions.

Social and Role-Based Barriers:

- **Disruption of Roles**: The demands of treatment and recovery can interfere with roles as caregivers, professionals, and community members, leading to a sense of role loss and isolation.
- **Work-Related Challenges**: Absenteeism, decreased productivity, and the need for workplace accommodations can affect employment status and financial stability.

Cognitive Barriers:

- **"Chemo Brain"**: Cognitive changes associated with chemotherapy, such as memory lapses and difficulty concentrating, can impact work performance and daily functioning.

Addressing these barriers through comprehensive, evidence-based occupational therapy interventions is crucial to enhancing the quality of life and functional outcomes for women with breast cancer. Strategies may include energy conservation techniques, pain management, lymphedema prevention exercises, adaptive equipment, psychological support, and vocational rehabilitation.

Interventions

OTPs are integral to the multidisciplinary care team for women with breast cancer, addressing both physical and psychosocial challenges. Their interventions are aimed at enhancing functional abilities, managing symptoms, and improving quality of life through personalized, evidence-based approaches. Given the complexity and individual variability of breast cancer, OTPs tailor their interventions to meet the specific needs of each patient, focusing on both pre-surgery preparation and post-surgery recovery (see Table 10.2). Occupational therapy intervention for women with breast cancer surgery focuses on addressing pain, limited shoulder motion, edema, and fatigue. It begins with pre-surgical evaluations and education on exercises and lymphedema management. Post-surgery, occupational therapy aids in improving ROM and function. Management of integumentary changes includes desensitization techniques and soft tissue mobilization. Continuous stretching and flexibility exercises are essential to prevent long-term ROM restrictions and complications during radiation therapy.

Table 10.2 OT interventions for women with breast cancer

Intervention	Pre-Surgery	Post-Surgery
Education on Surgical Procedures and Expectations	Providing detailed information about the upcoming surgery, what to expect during recovery, and how to prepare the home environment for post-surgical needs. Discussing potential side effects and complications, as well as strategies to manage them.	N/A
Energy Conservation Techniques	Developing individualized energy management plans that include pacing activities, setting priorities, and scheduling regular rest periods to help patients conserve energy and minimize fatigue.	Addressing cancer-related fatigue through education on sleep hygiene, stress management techniques, and activity modification. Helping patients develop strategies to balance activity and rest effectively.
Exercise and Physical Conditioning	Designing prehabilitation programs that focus on strengthening and conditioning the body in preparation for surgery. This includes cardiovascular exercises, strength training, and flexibility exercises.	Implementing individualized exercise programs to improve shoulder and arm mobility. Includes gentle stretching and strengthening exercises tailored to the patient's specific needs and recovery progress.
Psychosocial Support	Providing counseling and resources to address anxiety and emotional stress related to the upcoming surgery. Techniques such as mindfulness, relaxation exercises, and cognitive-behavioural strategies to manage pre-surgical anxiety.	Continuing to provide emotional support, facilitating support groups, and connecting patients with mental health resources. Encouraging participation in meaningful activities and social interactions to promote well-being.
Pain Management	Addressing pre-surgical pain related to the tumor through appropriate pain management strategies. Educating patients on pain management techniques that may be useful post-surgery.	Utilizing skilled myofascial release and gentle massage techniques to alleviate post-surgical pain and reduce scar tissue formation. Teaching relaxation techniques and guided imagery to help manage chronic pain.
Management of Chemotherapy-Induced Peripheral Neuropathy	N/A	Providing interventions to manage sensory changes and improve fine motor skills. Includes desensitization techniques, adaptive equipment for tasks such as buttoning and writing, and balance training to prevent falls.
Body Image and Self-Esteem	Addressing pre-surgical body image concerns through counseling and support. Preparing patients for potential changes in appearance and discussing coping strategies.	Offering counseling on cosmetic options, such as breast prosthetics and wigs, to help patients cope with changes in appearance. Supporting patients in exploring new ways to engage in social and intimate relationships.

Lymphedema Management

Lymphedema is a common concern for women undergoing breast cancer treatment. OTPs provide specialized interventions to prevent and manage lymphedema, including:

1. **Manual Lymphatic Drainage**: Performing manual lymphatic drainage to reduce swelling and promote lymphatic flow. This technique involves gentle, rhythmic massaging movements to stimulate the lymphatic system.
2. **Compression Therapy**: Educating patients on the use of compression garments to manage lymphedema. OTPs provide guidance on proper fitting and usage of these garments to ensure effectiveness and comfort.
3. **Exercise and Movement**: Designing exercise programs that include gentle, low-impact movements to promote lymphatic drainage and maintain range of motion. Specific exercises are tailored to each patient's condition and needs.
4. **Education and Self-Management**: Teaching patients how to monitor for signs of lymphedema, proper skin care, and techniques to reduce the risk of infection. Empowering patients with self-management strategies helps them take an active role in their care.

By providing specialized, evidence-based interventions, OTPs can significantly enhance the quality of life and functional outcomes for women with breast cancer. This comprehensive approach ensures that patients receive the support they need at each stage of their treatment and recovery, addressing the unique challenges posed by breast cancer and its treatments. Further detail on lymphedema management within occupational therapy will be discussed later in this chapter.

OT in Management of Lung Cancer

Lung cancer is one of the leading causes of cancer-related deaths among women worldwide. Each year, over 1.6 million new cases are diagnosed globally, and it poses significant public health challenges. In the United States, lung cancer is the second most common cancer in women, with a high mortality rate largely due to late-stage diagnosis. Early detection and effective treatment are crucial for improving survival rates.

The American Cancer Society (ACS) recommends annual lung cancer screening for adults aged 55 to 74 years with a history of heavy smoking. This screening is typically performed using low-dose computed tomography (LDCT), which can detect early-stage lung cancer that may not be visible on standard chest X-rays. Early detection can significantly reduce mortality rates by enabling timely intervention and treatment.

Lung cancer significantly impacts a woman's quality of life, affecting physical, emotional, and psychological well-being. Physically, women may experience symptoms such as chronic cough, chest pain, and shortness of breath. These symptoms, along with treatment side effects like fatigue and weakness, can severely limit daily activities and occupational roles. Emotionally, the diagnosis often leads to anxiety, depression, and stress, further complicating recovery and overall well-being.

Anatomy and Pathology of Lung Cancer

The lungs are a pair of spongy, air-filled organs located in the chest, responsible for gas exchange—oxygenating the blood and removing carbon dioxide. Lung cancer typically originates in the epithelial cells lining the bronchi and parts of the lung. There are two main types of lung cancer: Non-small cell lung cancer (NSCLC), which is the most common, and small cell lung cancer (SCLC), known for its rapid growth and early metastasis.

Lung cancer develops when cells in the lungs undergo genetic mutations that disrupt the normal cell cycle. These mutations lead to uncontrolled cell proliferation, forming a mass or tumor that can invade nearby tissues and spread to other parts of the body. Diagnosis often involves imaging studies such as chest X-rays, CT scans, and biopsies to confirm the presence of cancer and determine its type.

Staging of Lung Cancer Using the TNM System

Staging is essential for determining the extent of lung cancer and guiding treatment decisions. While the TNM classification system, developed by the American Joint Committee on Cancer, is widely used, other staging methods also exist. Understanding the stage of lung cancer helps in predicting prognosis and planning the appropriate therapeutic interventions. OT involvement may vary based on the stage, focusing on enhancing quality of life, functional independence, and managing symptoms (see Table 10.3).

Medical Management of Lung Cancer

Significant considerations for women with lung cancer include unique psychosocial and biological factors. Women may experience different patterns of symptoms and responses to treatment compared to men. Hormonal influences can affect the progression of the disease, and women might also face specific psychosocial challenges, such as

Table 10.3 Staging of lung cancer using the TNM System

Stage	Description	Role of OT
Stage 0	Carcinoma in situ (non-invasive cancer confined to the lung's epithelial layer).	Focus on education and preventive measures, including lifestyle modifications and early interventions to support lung health and overall well-being.
Stage I	Localized cancer, with the tumor confined to the lung.	Assist in managing mild symptoms, providing strategies to maintain independence in daily activities, and supporting mental health through the initial treatment phase.
Stage II	Cancer has spread to nearby lymph nodes.	Address functional limitations caused by treatment side effects, such as fatigue and pain, through energy conservation techniques, adaptive equipment, and psychosocial support.
Stage III	Cancer has spread to the chest wall, diaphragm, or mediastinum.	Provide comprehensive rehabilitation to manage more pronounced symptoms, enhance mobility, and improve participation in meaningful activities. This includes coordination with other healthcare providers for holistic care.
Stage IV	Advanced cancer with metastasis to distant organs such as the brain, bones, liver, or adrenal glands.	Focus on palliative care, optimizing comfort, and supporting patients and their families in managing advanced disease symptoms. This involves adaptations for daily living, pain management, and emotional support.

maintaining their roles within the family and managing the impact of the disease on their self-image and emotional well-being. Diagnosis and medical treatment include:

- **Diagnostic Tools**: Standard tools include chest X-rays, CT scans, and biopsies. PET scans and MRI may also be used to assess the extent of the disease.
- **Surgery**: Options include lobectomy (removal of a lobe), pneumonectomy (removal of an entire lung), and wedge resection (removal of a small part of the lung).
- **Radiation Therapy**: Often used post-surgery to destroy any remaining cancer cells and reduce recurrence risk.
- **Chemotherapy**: Uses cytotoxic drugs to kill cancer cells, often administered in cycles to shrink tumors and manage symptoms.
- **Targeted Therapy**: Focuses on specific genetic mutations associated with lung cancer, such as EGFR and ALK mutations.
- **Immunotherapy**: Enhances the immune system's ability to recognize and attack cancer cells.

Symptoms and Barriers to Occupational Performance for Women with Lung Cancer

Women with lung cancer face several barriers to occupational performance due to the symptoms of the disease and the side effects of its treatment. These barriers can be physical, emotional, psychological, social, role-based, and cognitive. Common symptoms of lung cancer include:

- Persistent cough.
- Chest pain.
- Shortness of breath.
- Wheezing.
- Coughing up blood.
- Fatigue and weight loss.

Barriers to Occupational Performance

Physical Barriers:

- **Fatigue and Weakness**: Treatment-related fatigue and muscle weakness can significantly impact daily activities and occupational roles.
- **Pain**: Persistent chest pain and discomfort can limit functional abilities.
- **Shortness of Breath**: Breathing difficulties can affect mobility and physical endurance.

Emotional and Psychological Barriers:

- **Anxiety and Depression**: The psychological burden of a lung cancer diagnosis can lead to significant emotional distress.
- **Stress**: The impact of treatment and disease progression can cause high levels of stress.

Social and Role-Based Barriers:

- **Disruption of Roles**: Treatment and recovery can interfere with roles as caregivers, professionals, and community members.

- **Work-Related Challenges**: Absenteeism and the need for workplace accommodations can affect employment status and financial stability.

Cognitive Barriers:

- **Cognitive Changes**: Cognitive impairments associated with lung cancer treatments can affect work performance and daily functioning.

Addressing these barriers requires a holistic approach, where OTPs play a crucial role by providing tailored interventions to enhance quality of life, promote independence, and facilitate engagement in meaningful activities. OTPs implement targeted strategies and therapeutic techniques to manage symptoms, support mental health, and adapt daily routines. In the following sections, we will explore specific interventions that OTPs can employ to support women with lung cancer in overcoming these barriers and improving their overall occupational performance.

Interventions by OTPs

OTPs are essential in managing the complex needs of women with lung cancer. Interventions are tailored to enhance functional abilities, manage symptoms, and improve quality of life. These interventions often differ pre-surgery and post-surgery, addressing the specific challenges encountered at each stage (see Table 10.4).

Transitioning from pre-surgical to post-surgical care, OTPs adapt their interventions to meet the evolving needs of women with lung cancer. By focusing on personalized care plans, OTPs ensure that patients receive comprehensive support throughout their cancer journey, facilitating improved outcomes and enhanced quality of life. Through these efforts, occupational therapy not only aids in physical recovery but also fosters emotional well-being, promoting a more comprehensive and patient-centered model of care.

OT in Management of Gynecological Cancers

Gynecological cancers, encompassing cervical, ovarian, uterine, and vulvar cancers, represent a significant health concern for women globally. These cancers originate in the female reproductive organs and each type presents unique challenges and impacts on a woman's quality of life. According to the World Health Organization (WHO), over 1 million women are diagnosed with gynecological cancers each year worldwide, with substantial morbidity and mortality rates. In the United States, the American Cancer Society (ACS) estimates that approximately 110,000 women will be diagnosed with a form of gynecological cancer annually, and over 30,000 will succumb to these diseases.

Cervical cancer, often linked to human papillomavirus (HPV) infection, remains a leading cause of cancer-related deaths in women, particularly in developing countries where screening programs are less prevalent. Ovarian cancer, known for its subtle symptoms and late-stage diagnosis, has one of the highest mortality rates among gynecological cancers. Uterine (endometrial) cancer is the most common gynecological cancer in developed countries and is often detected early due to abnormal bleeding, leading to better prognosis and survival rates. Vulvar cancer, although less common, can significantly impact a woman's sexual health and body image due to the nature of its treatment.

Table 10.4 OT Interventions for women with lung cancer pre- and post-surgery

Intervention	Pre-Surgery	Post-Surgery
Education on Surgical Procedures and Expectations	Providing detailed information about the upcoming surgery, what to expect during recovery, and how to prepare the home environment for post-surgical needs. Discussing potential side effects and complications, as well as strategies to manage them.	Reinforcing information on recovery expectations and managing any new concerns or complications that arise post-surgery.
Energy Conservation Techniques	Developing individualized energy management plans that include pacing activities, setting priorities, and scheduling regular rest periods to help patients conserve energy and minimize fatigue.	Continuing to address cancer-related fatigue through education on sleep hygiene, stress management techniques, and activity modification. Helping patients develop strategies to balance activity and rest effectively.
Exercise and Physical Conditioning	Designing prehabilitation programs that focus on strengthening and conditioning the body in preparation for surgery. This includes cardiovascular exercises, strength training, and flexibility exercises.	Implementing individualized exercise programs to improve shoulder and arm mobility and overall physical endurance. Includes gentle stretching and strengthening exercises tailored to the patient's specific needs and recovery progress.
Psychosocial Support	Providing counseling and resources to address anxiety and emotional stress related to the upcoming surgery. Techniques such as mindfulness, relaxation exercises, and cognitive-behavioural strategies to manage pre-surgical anxiety.	Continuing to provide emotional support, facilitating support groups, and connecting patients with mental health resources. Encouraging participation in meaningful activities and social interactions to promote well-being.
Pain Management	Addressing pre-surgical pain related to the tumor through appropriate pain management strategies. Educating patients on pain management techniques that may be useful post-surgery.	Utilizing skilled techniques to manage post-surgical pain and reduce discomfort. This may include relaxation techniques, guided imagery, and physical modalities such as myofascial release and gentle massage.
Management of Chemotherapy-Induced Peripheral Neuropathy	N/A	Providing interventions to manage sensory changes and improve fine motor skills. This may include desensitization techniques, adaptive equipment for daily tasks such as buttoning and writing, and balance training to prevent falls.
Body Image and Self-Esteem	Addressing pre-surgical body image concerns through counseling and support. Preparing patients for potential changes in appearance and discussing coping strategies.	Offering counseling and support to address changes in appearance and self-image. Helping patients explore new ways to engage in social and intimate relationships.

These cancers not only affect the physical health of women but also their emotional, psychological, and social well-being. The impact on quality of life can be profound, with symptoms and treatments often causing significant disruptions to daily activities and roles.

The ACS recommends regular screening for certain gynecological cancers to facilitate early detection and treatment. Pap smears are recommended every three years for women aged 21 to 29, and every five years for women aged 30 to 65, combined with HPV testing. For women at high risk of ovarian and uterine cancers, regular pelvic exams and transvaginal ultrasounds may be advised. Early detection through these screenings can significantly improve treatment outcomes and survival rates.

Anatomy and Pathology of Gynecological Cancers

Gynecological cancers originate in the female reproductive organs. These include:

Cervical Cancer:

- **Origin**: Begins in the cervix, the lower part of the uterus that connects to the vagina.
- **Cause**: Often linked to human papillomavirus (HPV) infection.
- **Pathology**: Develops when HPV infection causes genetic mutations in cervical cells, leading to abnormal cell growth and the potential to invade nearby tissues and spread to other parts of the body.

Ovarian Cancer:

- **Origin**: Starts in the ovaries, which are responsible for producing eggs and hormones.
- **Cause**: The exact cause is unknown, but risk factors include genetic mutations (such as BRCA1 and BRCA2), family history, and age.
- **Pathology**: Characterized by subtle symptoms, such as bloating and pelvic pain, making it often diagnosed at a later stage. Cancer cells can spread within the pelvis and abdomen.

Uterine (Endometrial) Cancer:

- **Origin**: Begins in the lining of the uterus (endometrium).
- **Cause**: Linked to hormonal imbalances, particularly excess estrogen, and other risk factors like obesity and diabetes.
- **Pathology**: Often detected early due to abnormal uterine bleeding, leading to prompt diagnosis and treatment. Cancer cells grow in the endometrial lining and can invade the muscular layer of the uterus and beyond.

Vulvar Cancer:

- **Origin**: Begins in the external genitalia (vulva).
- **Cause**: Risk factors include HPV infection, smoking, and a history of precancerous conditions or other genital cancers.
- **Pathology**: Typically presents as a lump, sore, or ulcer on the vulva. Cancer cells can invade nearby structures and spread to lymph nodes and other areas.

Gynecological cancers develop when cells in these areas undergo genetic mutations, leading to uncontrolled growth and the potential to invade nearby tissues and spread to other parts of the body. Diagnosis often involves a combination of imaging studies, biopsies, and blood tests to confirm the presence and type of cancer.

Table 10.5 Staging of gynecological cancers

Cancer Type	Stage 0	Stage 1	Stage 2	Stage 3	Stage 4
Cervical Cancer	Carcinoma in situ.	Confined to the cervix.	Spread beyond the cervix but not to pelvic wall.	Spread to the pelvic wall or lower third of the vagina.	Spread to nearby organs or distant parts of the body.
Ovarian Cancer	N/A	Confined to the ovaries.	Spread to pelvic organs.	Spread to abdominal cavity.	Distant metastasis.
Uterine Cancer	N/A	Confined to the uterus.	Spread to the cervix.	Spread to nearby tissues (pelvic area).	Spread to bladder, bowel, or distant parts of the body.
Vaginal Cancer	Carcinoma in situ.	Confined to the vaginal wall.	Spread to the tissues around the vagina.	Spread to the pelvic wall.	Spread to distant organs.
Vulvar Cancer	Carcinoma in situ (rare).	Confined to the vulva.	Spread to nearby structures.	Spread to lymph nodes.	Spread to upper urethra, bladder, or distant organs.

Notes
- **Stage 0:** Generally refers to carcinoma in situ, where abnormal cells are present but have not yet invaded deeper tissues. This stage is less common in ovarian and uterine cancers but can occur in cervical, vaginal, and vulvar cancers.
- **Stage 1:** Cancer is localized to the organ of origin.
- **Stage 2:** Cancer has spread to nearby tissues or organs within the pelvis.
- **Stage 3:** Cancer has spread more extensively within the pelvis or to regional lymph nodes.
- **Stage 4:** Cancer has spread to distant organs or parts of the body outside the pelvis.

Staging of Gynecological Cancers

Staging is crucial for determining the extent of gynecological cancers and guiding treatment decisions. Table 10.5 outlines the most common gynecological cancers and their typical staging.

Medical Management of Gynecological Cancers

The management of gynecological cancers involves a multifaceted approach, including:

- **Diagnosis**: Standard tools include Pap smears, HPV testing, pelvic exams, ultrasounds, CT scans, MRIs, and biopsies. Side effects from diagnostic procedures can include discomfort, bleeding, and anxiety.
- **Surgery**: Options vary by cancer type but may include hysterectomy (removal of the uterus), oophorectomy (removal of the ovaries), or radical surgeries for more advanced stages. Side effects may include pain, risk of infection, and hormonal changes.
- **Radiation Therapy**: Often used post-surgery to eliminate residual cancer cells and reduce recurrence risk. Side effects can include fatigue, skin irritation, and changes to the bowel and bladder function.
- **Chemotherapy**: Uses cytotoxic drugs to kill cancer cells, often administered in cycles. Side effects include nausea, vomiting, hair loss, fatigue, anemia, and increased risk of infection.

- **Hormonal Therapy**: Effective for hormone receptor-positive cancers, blocking hormones that fuel cancer growth. Side effects may include hot flashes, weight gain, and mood changes.
- **Targeted Therapy**: Focuses on specific genetic mutations associated with cancer. Side effects can include rash, diarrhea, and liver problems.
- **Immunotherapy**: Enhances the immune system's ability to recognize and attack cancer cells. Side effects can include fatigue, skin reactions, and flu-like symptoms.

Symptoms and Barriers to Occupational Performance for Women with Gynecological Cancers

Women with gynecological cancers experience various symptoms and face numerous barriers to occupational performance, significantly impacting their ability to participate and engage in daily activities and roles. Common symptoms of gynecological cancers include:

- Abnormal bleeding or discharge.
- Pelvic pain or pressure.
- Abdominal swelling.
- Changes in bowel or bladder habits.
- Itching or burning of the vulva.
- Pain during intercourse.

Women with gynecological cancers face numerous barriers to occupational performance, including:

Physical Barriers:

- **Fatigue and Weakness**: Treatment-related fatigue and muscle weakness can significantly impact daily activities and occupational roles, making it challenging to maintain energy levels for work, household tasks, and recreational activities.
- **Pain**: Persistent pain can limit functional abilities, affecting mobility, endurance, and the ability to perform ADLs such as dressing, bathing, and cooking.
- **Bowel and Bladder Issues**: Changes in bowel and bladder function can lead to frequent bathroom trips, discomfort, and reduced mobility, impacting participation in social events, work, and community activities.

Emotional and Psychological Barriers:

- **Anxiety and Depression**: The psychological burden of a cancer diagnosis can lead to significant emotional distress, affecting motivation, concentration, and the ability to engage in meaningful activities.
- **Body Image and Self-Esteem Issues**: Changes in appearance and function due to surgery and treatment can affect self-confidence, leading to withdrawal from social interactions and intimate relationships, and impacting overall mental health.

Social and Role-Based Barriers:

- **Disruption of Roles**: Treatment and recovery can interfere with roles as caregivers, professionals, and community members, leading to feelings of inadequacy and loss of identity. Women may struggle to fulfill their responsibilities and maintain relationships.

- **Work-Related Challenges**: Absenteeism and the need for workplace accommodations can affect employment status and financial stability. The inability to perform job duties effectively can lead to job loss or the need to reduce work hours, creating economic and social strain.

Impact on Occupational Participation and Engagement

The symptoms and side effects of medical treatments for gynecological cancers can profoundly affect a woman's ability to participate in and engage with her usual occupations. Fatigue and pain can reduce the capacity for physical activities, while emotional distress and changes in body image can diminish social interactions and participation in community life. Bowel and bladder issues can create discomfort and embarrassment, leading to avoidance of public places or social events. Disruptions in roles and work-related challenges can lead to a loss of purpose and financial insecurity, further exacerbating emotional and psychological barriers. Addressing these barriers through supportive care and tailored interventions can help women manage symptoms, maintain their roles, and improve their quality of life.

Interventions by OTPs

OTPs are essential in managing the complex needs of women with gynecological cancers. Interventions are tailored to enhance functional abilities, manage symptoms, and improve quality of life (see Table 10.6).

Table 10.6 Pre-surgery and post-surgery interventions

Intervention	Pre-Surgery	Post-Surgery
Education on Surgical Procedures and Expectations	Providing detailed information about the upcoming surgery, what to expect during recovery, and how to prepare the home environment for post-surgical needs. Discussing potential side effects and complications, as well as strategies to manage them.	Reinforcing information on recovery expectations and managing any new concerns or complications that arise post-surgery.
Energy Conservation Techniques	Developing individualized energy management plans that include pacing activities, setting priorities, and scheduling regular rest periods to help patients conserve energy and minimize fatigue.	Continuing to address cancer-related fatigue through education on sleep hygiene, stress management techniques, and activity modification. Helping patients develop strategies to balance activity and rest effectively.
Exercise and Physical Conditioning	Designing prehabilitation programs that focus on strengthening and conditioning the body in preparation for surgery. This includes cardiovascular exercises, strength training, and flexibility exercises.	Implementing individualized exercise programs to improve mobility and overall physical endurance. Includes gentle stretching and strengthening exercises tailored to the patient's specific needs and recovery progress.

(Continued)

Table 10.6 (Continued)

Intervention	Pre-Surgery	Post-Surgery
Psychosocial Support	Providing counseling and resources to address anxiety and emotional stress related to the upcoming surgery. Techniques such as mindfulness, relaxation exercises, and cognitive-behavioural strategies to manage pre-surgical anxiety.	Continuing to provide emotional support, facilitating support groups, and connecting patients with mental health resources. Encouraging participation in meaningful activities and social interactions to promote well-being.
Pain Management	Addressing pre-surgical pain related to the tumor through appropriate pain management strategies. Educating patients on pain management techniques that may be useful post-surgery.	Utilizing skilled techniques to manage post-surgical pain and reduce discomfort. This may include relaxation techniques, guided imagery, and physical modalities such as myofascial release and gentle massage.
Sexual Health Interventions	Providing education and counseling to address potential impacts on sexual health and intimacy. Discussing ways to maintain sexual health and intimacy during and after treatment.	Offering counseling and support for sexual health concerns. Providing strategies and adaptive devices to improve comfort and intimacy, such as lubricants, vaginal dilators, and pelvic floor exercises. Encouraging open communication with partners about changes and expectations.
Management of Chemotherapy-Induced Peripheral Neuropathy	N/A	Providing interventions to manage sensory changes and improve fine motor skills. This may include desensitization techniques and adaptive equipment for daily tasks such as buttoning and writing, and balance training to prevent falls.
Adaptive Equipment for Bowel and Bladder Management	N/A	Recommending and training in the use of adaptive equipment to manage bowel and bladder issues, such as portable commodes, raised toilet seats, and incontinence products. Providing strategies to maintain hygiene and dignity.
Body Image and Self-Esteem	Addressing pre-surgical body image concerns through counseling and support. Preparing patients for potential changes in appearance and discussing coping strategies.	Offering counseling and support to address changes in appearance and self-image. Helping patients explore new ways to engage in social and intimate relationships.

OTPs have a crucial role in addressing the multifaceted challenges faced by women with gynecological cancers. By offering personalized interventions from pre-surgical preparation to post-surgical recovery, OTPs enhance physical rehabilitation, emotional resilience, and social reintegration. Working alongside urogynecologists, urologists, and other specialists, they manage fatigue, pain, sexual health, and adaptive equipment use, ensuring women navigate their cancer journey with greater independence and confidence. This holistic, multidisciplinary approach empowers women to reclaim their roles, improve their quality of life, and foster a sense of normalcy and well-being during and after cancer treatment.

OT for Women with Lymphedema

Lymphedema is a chronic condition characterized by the accumulation of lymphatic fluid in the interstitial tissue, leading to swelling, most commonly in the arms or legs. This condition frequently arises as a complication following cancer treatments, particularly those involving the removal of lymph nodes or radiation therapy. Women are more likely to develop lymphedema than men, largely due to breast cancer treatments, which are a primary cause. Gynecological cancer treatments can also lead to lymphedema in the lower extremities. Although less common, lymphedema can also occur in women with lung cancer, typically arising from surgery or radiation that affects the lymphatic drainage in the chest or upper body.

Lymphedema can be categorized into primary and secondary types. Primary lymphedema is due to congenital malformations of the lymphatic system, while secondary lymphedema is acquired, often resulting from surgery, radiation therapy, infection, or trauma. In the context of cancer, secondary lymphedema is more common, resulting from lymph node dissection or radiation that disrupts normal lymphatic drainage.

Lymphedema can have profound physical, emotional, and psychological effects on women. Physically, it can cause discomfort, pain, restricted range of motion, and increased susceptibility to infections like cellulitis. Emotionally and psychologically, it can lead to distress, anxiety, depression, and body image issues due to the visible swelling and changes in appearance.

Impact on Women's Health

Women are particularly vulnerable to the effects of lymphedema due to the high incidence of breast and gynecological cancers, which often require extensive lymph node removal and radiation therapy. The visible and physical changes caused by lymphedema can severely impact a woman's quality of life, affecting her ability to perform daily activities and participate in social and occupational roles. The chronic nature of lymphedema means that women must often manage the condition long-term, necessitating ongoing support and intervention.

Stages of Lymphedema

Lymphedema is typically classified into four stages based on severity, each impacting a person's ability to perform ADLs and IADLs to varying degrees.

Stage 0 (Latent Stage):

- **Description**: No visible swelling despite impaired lymphatic function. This stage can last months or years before progressing.
- **Impact on ADLs/IADLs**: Minimal impact. Individuals may not experience noticeable symptoms, allowing them to perform ADLs (bathing, dressing, showering) and IADLs (household management, shopping) without difficulty. However, subtle changes in limb sensation or slight discomfort might start to appear.

Stage I (Mild Stage):

- **Description**: Swelling is soft and pitting; it usually reduces with elevation. This stage is reversible with appropriate intervention.

- **Impact on ADLs/IADLs**: Some impact on ADLs. Mild swelling can cause discomfort and a feeling of heaviness in the affected limb, potentially making activities such as dressing (putting on socks or shoes) and bathing slightly more challenging. IADLs may also be affected, particularly those requiring fine motor skills or prolonged use of the affected limb, like cooking or cleaning.

Stage II (Moderate Stage):

- **Description**: Swelling becomes firmer and does not reduce significantly with elevation. The skin may start to thicken.
- **Impact on ADLs/IADLs**: Moderate impact. The increased firmness and persistent swelling can lead to significant discomfort and reduced mobility, making ADLs such as bathing, dressing, and toileting more difficult. Thickened skin and decreased flexibility can impede the ability to perform household tasks, manage finances, or engage in community activities.

Stage III (Severe Stage):

- **Description**: Also known as lymphostatic elephantiasis, this stage involves severe swelling, skin changes, and fibrosis, significantly impacting daily function and quality of life.
- **Impact on ADLs/IADLs**: Severe impact. The extensive swelling and fibrosis can lead to severe functional limitations. ADLs like bathing, dressing, and showering become extremely challenging due to the size and weight of the affected limb. IADLs such as household management, grocery shopping, and cooking can be nearly impossible without assistance. The severe physical changes can also lead to social isolation and emotional distress, further affecting quality of life.

In each stage, appropriate interventions from OTPs, such as compression garments, manual lymphatic drainage, exercise programs, and education on skin care, can help manage symptoms and improve the ability to perform ADLs and IADLs.

Occupational Therapy Interventions for Lymphedema

OTPs play a critical role in the management of lymphedema. OTPs who specialize in lymphedema management often undergo specific training courses and obtain certifications to enhance their skills. These certifications include training in manual lymphatic drainage (MLD), compression therapy, and comprehensive lymphedema management. Certified Lymphedema Therapists (CLTs) are equipped with the expertise needed to provide effective interventions for lymphedema.

OTPs without specialized training in lymphedema management can still offer valuable support by providing general strategies to manage symptoms and improve quality of life. This may include educating patients on skin care, exercise routines to enhance mobility, and techniques to reduce the risk of infection. They can also refer patients to specialists or certified therapists when more advanced interventions are needed.

Specialized Care with Training

OTPs specializing in lymphedema management undergo specific training and certification. Certified Lymphedema Therapists (CLTs) are equipped to provide advanced interventions, including:

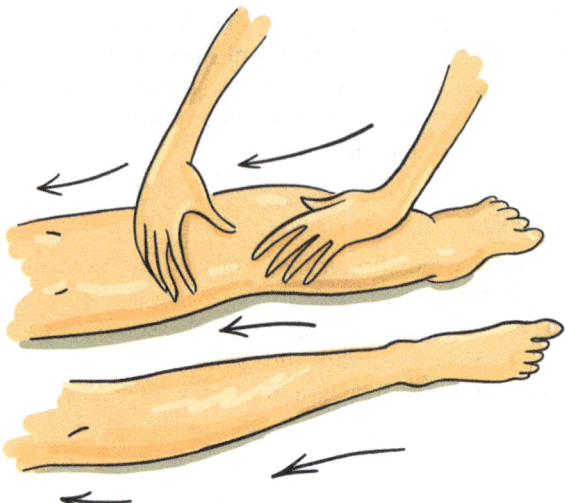

Figure 10.3 Manual lymph drainage being performed on lower extremity (LE).

Manual Lymphatic Drainage (MLD)

Manual lymphatic drainage (MLD) is a specialized, gentle massage technique designed to stimulate the lymphatic system and promote the flow of lymphatic fluid. OTPs trained in MLD perform this therapy to enhance lymphatic drainage, prevent fluid buildup, and maintain limb function. Specific examples of MLD techniques include:

- **Stationary Circles**: Gentle, circular movements applied with the hands to stimulate lymph nodes (see Figure 10.3).
- **Pump Technique**: Rhythmic, pumping motions along the extremities to encourage lymph flow.
- **Scooping**: A scooping motion with the hands to move lymph fluid toward drainage points.

General Support Strategies: Even without specialized training, OTPs can assist by:

- Educating on skin care routines to prevent infections.
- Designing exercise programs to enhance mobility and strength.
- Promoting techniques to manage symptoms and reduce complications.

Comprehensive Interventions

Compression Therapy

Compression therapy involves the use of compression garments such as sleeves or stockings, which apply graduated pressure to encourage lymph fluid movement and prevent fluid accumulation. OTPs assist in the proper fitting and use of these garments, providing education on when and how to wear them effectively. Specific examples of compression therapy include:

- **Compression Bandages**: Multi-layered bandaging applied to control swelling, often used in the initial treatment phase (see Figure 10.4).

Oncology in Women's Health 311

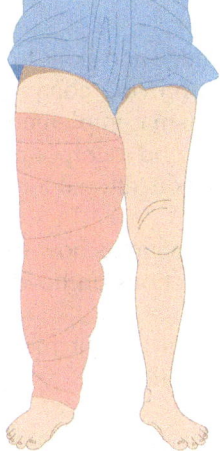

Figure 10.4 Compression bandaging on LE.

- **Compression Garments**: Custom-fitted sleeves or stockings worn daily to maintain reduction in swelling.
- **Intermittent Pneumatic Compression (IPC) Devices**: Mechanical devices that use air pressure to massage the limb and promote lymphatic drainage.

Exercise and Movement

Exercise is a critical component in the management of lymphedema. OTPs design individualized exercise programs that include breathing exercises, range of motion exercises, and light strengthening exercises. Examples of exercises include:

- **Breathing Exercises**: Deep diaphragmatic breathing to stimulate lymphatic flow.
- **Range of Motion Exercises**: Gentle stretching of the affected limb to maintain flexibility, such as arm circles or leg stretches.
- **Strengthening Exercises**: Light resistance exercises using bands or small weights to support muscle tone without overstraining the lymphatic system, such as bicep curls or seated leg lifts.

Skin Care and Hygiene

Proper skin care is vital in preventing infections and complications associated with lymphedema. OTPs educate patients on meticulous skin care routines, including:

- **Moisturizing**: Regularly applying lotion to keep the skin hydrated and prevent cracking.
- **Infection Prevention**: Keeping the skin clean and using antiseptic solutions if cuts or scrapes occur.
- **Protection**: Wearing gloves when gardening or doing household chores to avoid injuries.

Education and Self-Management

Empowering patients with the knowledge and skills to manage their condition is a cornerstone of occupational therapy. OTPs provide comprehensive education on recognizing early signs and symptoms of lymphedema, implementing daily self-massage techniques, using compression garments correctly, and incorporating lifestyle modifications to reduce the risk of exacerbation. Examples of educational topics include:

- **Self-Massage Techniques**: Teaching patients how to perform MLD on themselves.
- **Compression Garment Care**: Instructions on how to properly wear, clean, and maintain compression garments.
- **Lifestyle Modifications**: Advising on weight management, hydration, and avoiding tight clothing that can restrict lymph flow.

Psychosocial Support

Lymphedema can significantly impact a woman's emotional and psychological well-being. OTPs offer psychosocial support to help women cope with the emotional challenges of living with lymphedema. This may include:

- **Counseling**: Providing individual or group therapy to address anxiety, depression, and body image concerns.
- **Support Groups**: Facilitating connections with others experiencing similar challenges to share experiences and coping strategies.
- **Mindfulness and Relaxation Techniques**: Teaching techniques such as meditation, guided imagery, and progressive muscle relaxation to help manage stress.

Adaptive Techniques and Equipment

OTPs may recommend adaptive equipment and techniques to facilitate daily activities impacted by lymphedema. This can include ergonomic tools to reduce strain during tasks, techniques to modify activities to accommodate swelling and limited range of motion, and assistive devices to maintain independence in self-care and household tasks. Examples include:

- **Ergonomic Kitchen Tools**: Using tools with larger grips to reduce hand strain during cooking.
- **Adaptive Clothing**: Recommending clothing with easier fastenings, such as Velcro or magnetic closures.
- **Assistive Devices for Hygiene**: Long-handled sponges or shower chairs to help with bathing and self-care tasks.

Occupational therapy is integral to the effective management of lymphedema in women, providing a holistic approach that addresses physical, emotional, and functional needs. Occupational therapy integrates physical, emotional, and functional support for women with lymphedema. By providing personalized interventions and fostering self-management skills, OTPs enhance well-being and promote independence in daily living.

Case Study in Oncology in Women's Health

Background and Medical History: The client is a 45-year-old executive director of a successful business who was diagnosed with stage 2 breast cancer. Following her diagnosis, the client underwent a lumpectomy, followed by chemotherapy. During her treatment, she developed secondary lymphedema in her right arm and experienced significant cancer-related fatigue (CRF) and cognitive impairments often referred to as "chemo brain." These symptoms have impacted her ability to manage both her personal and professional responsibilities effectively.

Prior Level of Function:

- Functioned independently in all areas of occupation.
- Managed a busy work schedule as an executive director.
- Enjoyed painting in her free time.
- Managed household tasks and enjoyed cooking gourmet meals.

Household Living Arrangements and Social History:

- Lives alone in a high-rise apartment.
- Active in professional networking groups and often attended social events and business meetings.
- Enjoys spending weekends with friends and engaging in community service activities.

Change in Functional Status and Challenges: The client's recent chemotherapy and subsequent lymphedema have significantly impacted her ability to engage in daily activities across various domains of life:

- **ADLs**: Experiences difficulty with personal hygiene routines, dressing, and managing lymphedema due to swelling and pain in her right arm.
- **Work**: Struggles with concentration, memory, and stamina, affecting her ability to manage a full day of executive tasks and meetings.
- **Social Activities**: Reduced participation in professional and social events due to fatigue, physical limitations, and cognitive impairments.
- **Health Management**: Needs to adhere to a complex medication regimen and manage lymphedema care, facing challenges with time management and energy conservation.

OT Assessments:

- **Barthel Index**: The client scored 65 out of 100, indicating moderate assistance required for most ADLs due to physical limitations and fatigue.
- **Volumetric Measurement**: Used to assess the extent of edema in the client's right arm. The measurement indicated significant swelling, confirming the presence of lymphedema.
- **Dynamic Lowenstein Occupational Therapy Cognitive Assessment (DLOTCA)**: The client showed impairments in short-term memory and executive functioning, affecting her ability to perform complex tasks at work.
- **Body Image Questionnaire**: Revealed concerns about changes in appearance and self-esteem issues related to the lymphedema and cancer treatment.

- **Brief Fatigue Inventory (BFI)**: The client reported high levels of fatigue, scoring 7 out of 10, significantly impacting her daily activities and quality of life.

Occupational Therapy Plan of Care and Goals: The client will receive skilled occupational therapy services once a week for 12 weeks to improve independence in ADLs, manage anxiety and depressive symptoms, and enhance quality of life.

Goals:

1. Increase Barthel Index Score: Enhance the client's independence in personal care tasks to achieve a Barthel Index score of 80/100 within 12 weeks.
2. Implement Energy Conservation Techniques: Facilitate the client's ability to complete a full day of executive tasks using energy conservation techniques, with minimal fatigue, within 12 weeks.
3. Improve Volumetric Measurement Outcomes: Reduce arm swelling by 20% through targeted interventions, as measured by volumetric outcomes, within 12 weeks.
4. Enhance Cognitive Function: Improve cognitive functions related to complex problem-solving and administrative tasks by 30%, as measured by DLOTCA scores, within 12 weeks.
5. Address Body Image Concerns: Enhance the client's self-esteem and confidence by improving body image, aiming for a 30% improvement in body image questionnaire scores within 12 weeks.

Interventions: The following interventions will be tailored to meet the client's specific needs and address the outlined goals:

Energy Conservation Techniques:

- Educate the client on pacing activities, taking frequent breaks, and planning tasks to conserve energy throughout the day.
- Teach how to prioritize and delegate tasks both at home and work to manage fatigue effectively.

Exercise and Movement:

- Develop a graduated exercise program starting with low-impact activities like walking and gentle stretching, gradually increasing intensity to improve strength and endurance.
- Incorporate range of motion and strengthening exercises for her right arm to manage lymphedema.

ADL Retraining:

- Provide guidance on adaptive techniques and the use of assistive devices to enhance independence in personal hygiene and dressing.
- Educate the client on strategies to simplify household tasks and improve efficiency in meal preparation.

Cognitive Strategies:

- Introduce memory aids such as planners, calendars, and reminder apps to manage cognitive impairments.

- Engage in cognitive exercises like puzzles and brain games to enhance memory and executive function.

Skin Care and Hygiene:

- Educate the client on the importance of regular moisturizing to prevent skin cracking and infection.
- Teach infection prevention techniques, including keeping the skin clean and using antiseptic solutions if cuts or scrapes occur.

Psychosocial Support:

- Provide individual counseling to address anxiety and depression related to her diagnosis and treatment.
- Encourage participation in a support group for women with breast cancer to share experiences and coping strategies.
- Teach mindfulness and relaxation exercises such as meditation and progressive muscle relaxation to manage stress.

Outcomes:

Post Treatment:

- **Energy Conservation and Fatigue Management**: Demonstrated significant improvement in managing fatigue, as indicated by a 20% increase in body image questionnaire scores and a Barthel Index score improvement from 65 to 80.
- **Functional Independence**: Achieved improved independence in ADLs, allowing her to return to work and manage her professional responsibilities more effectively.
- **Emotional Well-being**: Achieved reduced anxiety and depression, reflecting improved emotional resilience and coping skills.
- **Cognitive Function**: Developed effective strategies to manage "chemo brain" symptoms, enhancing work performance and daily functioning.

Follow-Up Visits:

- Continued reinforcement of energy conservation techniques and stress management strategies to sustain progress.
- Ongoing support in managing lymphedema and cognitive function, adjusting therapy goals as needed.
- Regular monitoring of physical and emotional well-being indicators, adapting interventions to promote long-term health and functional independence.

At the conclusion of therapy, the client demonstrated marked improvements across various domains, showcasing enhanced resilience and adaptive skills in managing her condition. Significant progress was noted in fatigue management, functional independence, and emotional well-being, enabling her to engage more fully in her professional and personal life. The client's commitment to therapy and collaboration with the occupational therapy team resulted in sustainable improvements, highlighting her capacity for growth and resilience in the face of health challenges.

Further Reading

Davies, C., Levenhagen, K., Ryans, K., Perdomo, M., & Gilchrist, L. (2020). Interventions for breast cancer-related lymphedema: Clinical practice guideline from the Academy of Oncologic Physical Therapy of APTA. *Physical Therapy*, *100*(7), 1163–1179. https://doi.org/10.1093/ptj/pzaa087

He, K., Jiang, J., Chen, M., Wang, T., Huang, X., Zhu, R., Zhang, Z., Chen, J., & Zhao, L. (2023). Effects of occupational therapy on quality of life in breast cancer patients: A systematic review and meta-analysis. *Medicine*, *102*(31), e34484. https://doi.org/10.1097/MD.0000000000034484

Khan, S. (2024). The role of occupational therapy in gynecological cancer care. *OT Practice*, *29*(3), 10–14.

Kowalski, L., & Krusen, N. E. (2021). Lung cancer screening policy in Alaska and occupational therapy. *The American Journal of Occupational Therapy: Official Publication of the American Occupational Therapy Association*, *75*(3), 7503090010. https://doi.org/10.5014/ajot.2021.048231

Lattanzi, J. B., Giuliano, S., Meehan, C., Sander, B., Wootten, R., & Zimmerman, A. (2010). Recommendations for physical and occupational therapy practice from the perspective of clients undergoing therapy for breast cancer-related impairments. *Journal of Allied Health*, *39*(4), 257–264.

Monteiro, M. G. C. T., & de Morais Gouveia, G. P. (2021). Physiotherapy in the management of gynecological cancer patient: A systematic review. *Journal of Bodywork and Movement Therapies*, *28*, 354–361. https://doi.org/10.1016/j.jbmt.2021.06.027

Pergolotti, M., Bailliard, A., McCarthy, L., Farley, E., Covington, K. R., & Doll, K. M. (2020). Women's experiences after ovarian cancer surgery: Distress, uncertainty, and the need for occupational therapy. *The American Journal of Occupational Therapy: Official Publication of the American Occupational Therapy Association*, *74*(3), 7403205140p1–7403205140p9. https://doi.org/10.5014/ajot.2020.036897

Sinclair, W., McConnell, C., Clark, E., McEntire, K. B., Lewis, C., Pound, L., & Wuertz, K. (2024). The effects of cervical cancer diagnosis on occupational performance. *The Open Journal of Occupational Therapy*, *12*(2), 1–8. https://doi.org/10.15453/2168-6408.2172

Singer, S. (2018). Psychosocial impact of cancer. *Recent Results in Cancer Research. Fortschritte der Krebsforschung. Progres dans les recherches sur le cancer*, *210*, 1–11. https://doi.org/10.1007/978-3-319-64310-6_1

Stehle, L., Hoosain, M., & van Niekerk, L. (2022). A systematic review of work-related interventions for breast cancer survivors: Potential contribution of occupational therapists. *Work (Reading, Mass.)*, *72*(1), 59–73. https://doi.org/10.3233/WOR-210053

Walker, M. S., Pohl, G. M., Houts, A. C., Peltz, G., Miller, P. J. E., Schwartzberg, L. S., Stepanski, E. J., & Marciniak, M. (2017). Analysis of the psychological impact of cancer-related symptoms on patients with non-small cell lung cancer. *Psycho-Oncology*, *26*(6), 755–762. https://doi.org/10.1002/pon.4071

Welford, J., Rafferty, R., Short, D., Dewhurst, F., & Greystoke, A. (2023). Personalised assessment and rapid intervention in frail patients with lung cancer: The impact of an outpatient occupational therapy service. *Clinical Lung Cancer*, *24*(5), e164–e171. https://doi.org/10.1016/j.cllc.2023.03.009

11 Neurological Health in Women

Migraines in Women

Women's brain health presents unique challenges and considerations that differ significantly from men's, particularly in the prevalence and impact of neurological disorders. Migraines, for example, affect women three times more often than men. This disparity is largely influenced by hormonal factors unique to women, such as fluctuations in estrogen levels, which are closely linked to the menstrual cycle, pregnancy, and menopause. Understanding these differences is crucial in developing effective treatment and management strategies for conditions like migraines that disproportionately affect women.

Migraines are a significant neurological disorder that disproportionately affects women, with approximately 18% of women experiencing migraines compared to 6% of men. This condition results from a combination of genetic, environmental, and neurological factors. Hormonal changes, particularly those involving estrogen, play a major role in triggering migraines in women. These hormonal fluctuations not only contribute to the frequency and severity of migraines but also to their onset around significant life stages such as menstruation, pregnancy, and menopause. Other triggers include stress, certain foods, sleep disturbances, and sensory stimuli. Migraines can profoundly impact daily life, leading to missed workdays, reduced productivity, and diminished quality of life. Table 11.1 categorizes the

Table 11.1 Types of migraines

Type of Migraine	Characteristics	Occupations Impacted
Migraine with Aura	Visual disturbances, sensory changes, or speech difficulties occurring before or during the headache.	Work, driving, social participation, and education.
Migraine without Aura	Intense, throbbing pain usually on one side of the head, accompanied by nausea, vomiting, and sensitivity to light and sound.	Self-care, work, social participation, and rest/sleep.
Chronic Migraine	Headaches occurring on 15 or more days per month for more than three months, with migraine features on at least eight days per month.	All areas of occupation, including work, leisure, social participation, and ADLs.
Menstrual Migraine	Migraines occurring in relation to the menstrual cycle, typically starting two days before menstruation and lasting until the third day of menstruation.	ADLs, work, social participation, and rest/sleep.

different types of migraines, their characteristics, and how they impact various occupational activities.

By addressing both the physical and psychosocial aspects of migraines, OTPs can help women manage their symptoms more effectively, maintaining their roles and routines, and enhancing their quality of life.

Impact on Occupational Functioning

Migraines typically present with multiple phases, each with distinct symptoms. The **prodrome** phase may begin hours or days before the headache, with symptoms such as mood changes, fatigue, and neck stiffness. The **aura** phase can involve visual disturbances, sensory changes, or speech difficulties. The **headache** phase features intense, throbbing pain usually on one side of the head, often accompanied by nausea, vomiting, and sensitivity to light and sound. Finally, the **postdrome** phase includes fatigue, confusion, and residual head pain following the headache (see Table 11.2).

Due to their unpredictable nature and severe symptoms, migraines significantly impair a woman's ability to perform daily activities, engage in work, and participate socially, which are core areas addressed by occupational therapy. It is crucial for OTPs to screen for migraines during assessments, especially in women who report chronic headaches or related symptoms. Understanding the impact of migraines can help OTPs develop targeted interventions that accommodate the episodic nature of migraine symptoms, such as flexibility in scheduling, environmental modifications to reduce sensory triggers, and strategies for stress management and symptom relief. By incorporating migraine-specific considerations into treatment planning, OTPs can better support women in managing their symptoms and maintaining their occupational roles and quality of life.

Table 11.2 Phases of migraines, symptoms, and impacted occupations

Phase	Symptoms	Occupations Impacted
Prodrome Phase	Mood changes, fatigue, neck stiffness	**ADLs**: Reduced motivation for self-care activities (dressing, grooming). **Work**: Decreased productivity due to fatigue. **Social Participation**: Withdrawal from social activities.
Aura Phase	Visual disturbances, sensory changes, speech difficulties	**Driving**: Impaired ability to drive safely. **Work**: Difficulty with tasks requiring visual and cognitive functions. **Education**: Challenges in concentrating on studies. **Social Participation**: Communication difficulties in social interactions.
Headache Phase	Intense, throbbing pain, nausea, vomiting, sensitivity to light and sound	**Rest/Sleep**: Disrupted sleep due to pain. **Work**: Inability to perform job duties effectively. **ADLs**: Difficulty completing basic tasks like bathing, dressing, and eating. **IADLs**: Challenges with meal preparation and household management. **Social Participation**: Avoidance of social engagements due to pain and sensitivity.
Postdrome Phase	Fatigue, confusion, residual head pain	**Work**: Reduced efficiency and productivity. **Self-Care**: Continued impact on self-care activities due to lingering fatigue. **Leisure Activities**: Limited participation in leisure activities.

Occupational Therapy Approach and Intervention

Occupational therapy for women with migraines involves a comprehensive, holistic approach that addresses the unique physiological factors affecting women, such as hormonal fluctuations, as well as the multitude of roles and responsibilities they often manage. OTPs play a critical role in empowering women to identify and manage triggers, develop robust coping strategies, and modify their environments to mitigate the impacts of migraines on their daily lives. This includes addressing both physical symptoms and the psychosocial aspects of living with migraines. By enhancing their ability to maintain roles, routines, and participation in meaningful activities, OTPs help improve women's quality of life and overall well-being.

A crucial component of the occupational therapy approach is the initial screening and assessment process. OTPs should ask all female clients specific screening questions to determine if they experience migraines, which are often underreported or mistaken for less severe headaches. Questions could include:

- "Do you experience frequent headaches that affect your ability to perform daily activities?"
- "Do these headaches often come with nausea or sensitivity to light and sound?"
- "How often do these headaches occur, and do they seem to be related to your menstrual cycle or times of high stress?"

Understanding these aspects is essential because migraines can contribute to various symptoms frequently observed in rehabilitation settings, such as:

- Chronic pain.
- Fatigue and low energy.
- Cognitive impairments like difficulty concentrating.
- Emotional disturbances, including increased irritability or depression.

See Table 11.3 for a comprehensive overview of the occupational therapy interventions designed for women with migraines.

Effective management of migraines in women through occupational therapy can lead to significant improvements in quality of life. By addressing the unique triggers and symptoms associated with migraines, OTPs can help women regain control over their daily activities and enhance their overall well-being.

Occupational Therapy in Stroke Rehabilitation for Women

Stroke is a leading cause of disability in women, with women experiencing a higher lifetime risk of stroke compared to men. Approximately 55,000 more women than men have a stroke each year in the United States. The impact of stroke on women's health includes physical impairments, cognitive deficits, emotional disturbances, and challenges in performing daily activities.

Strokes occur when the blood supply to a part of the brain is interrupted or reduced, preventing brain tissue from getting oxygen and nutrients. This can result from ischemic strokes (caused by blockages) or hemorrhagic strokes (caused by bleeding) (see Table 11.4). Risk factors include hypertension, atrial fibrillation, diabetes, smoking, and hormonal factors such as the use of oral contraceptives and hormone replacement therapy.

Table 11.3 Occupational therapy interventions for women with migraines

Intervention Focus	Description	Relevance to Women's Health
Trigger Management and Lifestyle Modifications	Educating on identifying and avoiding migraine triggers such as certain foods, stress, and poor sleep hygiene. Encouraging regular exercise, a balanced diet, and maintaining a consistent sleep schedule.	Recognizing the role of hormonal fluctuations and stress management in women's health.
Stress Management Techniques	Teaching relaxation techniques such as deep breathing, progressive muscle relaxation, and mindfulness meditation.	Stress management is crucial due to the additional roles and responsibilities women often manage, such as caregiving and work-life balance.
Environmental Modifications	Recommending adjustments to the home and work environment to minimize exposure to migraine triggers. This may include ergonomic changes, controlling lighting, and reducing noise.	Tailoring home and work environments to reduce sensory overload, which is particularly relevant for women balancing multiple roles and environments.
Pain Management Strategies	Utilizing techniques such as biofeedback, cognitive-behavioural therapy (CBT), and sensory modulation to manage pain and improve overall well-being.	Addressing chronic pain through personalized pain management strategies that consider hormonal influences and lifestyle factors unique to women.
Routine Establishment	Assisting in developing structured daily routines that balance activity and rest, thereby reducing the likelihood of migraine onset.	Creating routines that incorporate self-care and rest periods, acknowledging the multitasking nature of women's daily lives and the need for balance.
ADL and IADL Retraining	Helping women adapt to and manage daily activities affected by migraines, such as dressing, grooming, meal preparation, and household management.	Providing specific strategies and tools to maintain independence in daily activities, considering the impact of migraines on physical and cognitive functioning.

Table 11.4 Types of stroke and relevance in women's health

Types of Stroke	Characteristics	Relevance in Women's Health
Ischemic Stroke	Caused by a blockage in an artery supplying blood to the brain.	More common in women than men; higher prevalence of comorbid conditions such as hypertension and atrial fibrillation.
Hemorrhagic Stroke	Caused by bleeding in or around the brain, resulting in increased pressure and damage to brain cells.	Higher mortality rate in women; women may experience more severe neurological deficits and longer recovery periods.
Transient Ischemic Attack (TIA)	Often called a mini-stroke, it involves a temporary blockage of blood flow to the brain.	Women are less likely to recognize TIA symptoms; higher risk of subsequent major stroke compared to men.

Impact on Occupational Functioning

Understanding the progression and symptoms of stroke is crucial, particularly for women, as they may experience unique challenges and symptoms that differ from men. Stroke symptoms are not only diverse but also evolve through several phases, each impacting daily living and occupational performance in distinct ways. Recognizing these phases is vital for OTPs to tailor interventions that address the specific needs of women recovering from stroke.

Table 11.5 Phases of stroke, symptoms, and changes in occupational performance

Phase	Symptoms	Changes in Occupational Performance
Acute Phase	Sudden numbness or weakness, especially on one side of the body, sudden confusion, trouble speaking, sudden trouble seeing, sudden trouble walking, dizziness, loss of balance, sudden severe headache.	**ADLs**: Difficulty with basic self-care tasks (bathing, dressing, grooming), requiring assistance with menstrual hygiene and sexual health education. **Work**: Immediate cessation of work activities, difficulty with job tasks requiring physical and cognitive abilities. **Social Participation**: Immediate withdrawal from social interactions, reduced ability to communicate. **Sleep**: Disruption due to discomfort and hospital environment. **Leisure**: Inability to engage in hobbies or activities requiring physical movement.
Subacute Phase	Continued weakness or numbness, difficulty with speech and swallowing, cognitive impairments, emotional disturbances.	**ADLs**: Ongoing challenges with self-care and mobility, requiring adaptive techniques for personal hygiene and sexual health management. **IADLs**: Inability to perform tasks like cooking, cleaning, and managing finances, necessitating assistance or adaptive strategies. **Work**: Temporary or permanent inability to return to work, need for job modifications or vocational rehabilitation. **Social Participation**: Reduced participation in social and community activities, communication barriers, need for social support networks. **Sleep**: Sleep disturbances due to pain or anxiety, requiring sleep hygiene education. **Leisure**: Reduced participation in leisure activities due to physical and cognitive limitations, need for adapted leisure activities.
Chronic Phase	Persistent motor and cognitive impairments, spasticity, chronic pain, emotional and psychological challenges.	**ADLs**: Need for long-term assistance with self-care tasks, ongoing difficulty with dressing, bathing, and grooming, including menstrual hygiene management and sexual health education. **IADLs**: Dependence on others for complex tasks like transportation, managing medications, and household chores, requiring adaptive equipment and strategies. **Work**: Long-term disability or need for job modifications, potential job loss, need for vocational rehabilitation and support. **Social Participation**: Long-term changes in social roles and relationships, isolation due to communication and mobility issues, need for community reintegration strategies. **Sleep**: Chronic sleep disturbances, need for positioning aids and sleep hygiene education. **Leisure**: Limited ability to participate in preferred leisure activities, need for adapted equipment and leisure planning.

A stroke can significantly impact a woman's ability to perform everyday tasks, affecting areas such as self-care, mobility, communication, and participation in work and social activities. Cognitive impairments, emotional changes, and physical disabilities contribute to challenges in occupational performance. Evidence-based practice indicates that tailored rehabilitation programs can help women regain function and independence, improving their ability to engage in meaningful occupations.

Occupational Therapy Approach

Occupational therapy for women recovering from a stroke involves a comprehensive and individualized approach that addresses the specific physical, cognitive, and emotional challenges they face. OTPs focus on restoring function, improving independence, and enhancing quality of life. Interventions include motor skills rehabilitation, cognitive rehabilitation, ADL and IADL training, emotional support, and home and community reintegration (see Table 11.6).

Table 11.6 Occupational therapy interventions by phase

Phase	Intervention Focus	Description	Relevance to Women's Health
Acute Phase	Motor Skills Rehabilitation	Early mobilization, positioning, and passive range of motion exercises to prevent complications.	Addressing immediate motor deficits to prevent contractures and improve bed mobility, crucial for early recovery. Unique considerations for women include addressing muscle tone and positioning to prevent pressure ulcers, which can be affected by body contours and hormonal changes.
	Cognitive Screening	Initial assessment of cognitive function to guide early intervention strategies.	Identifying cognitive impairments that may affect communication and decision-making, with specific attention to the impact of stroke on communication for women, who may experience differences in language recovery.
	Basic ADL Training	Assistance with basic self-care tasks such as bathing, dressing, and grooming.	Providing immediate support for self-care tasks to maintain personal hygiene and dignity during hospital stay, including menstrual hygiene and sexual health education. Addressing unique challenges women face in maintaining hygiene and managing menstruation during early recovery.
	Emotional Support	Counseling to address shock, fear, and anxiety following the stroke.	Offering emotional support tailored to women's unique concerns and roles, such as caregiving responsibilities and managing family dynamics. Providing resources for women to address specific fears related to body image and role changes.

(Continued)

Table 11.6 (Continued)

Phase	Intervention Focus	Description	Relevance to Women's Health
Subacute Phase	Task-Oriented Training	Engaging in functional activities to improve motor and cognitive skills.	Focusing on tasks relevant to women's daily routines, such as meal preparation and household chores. Addressing the need for adaptive equipment and strategies for safely managing these tasks, considering women's typical roles in household management.
	ADL and IADL Training	Gradual reintroduction of complex ADLs and IADLs with adaptive techniques.	Helping women adapt to changes in ability and regain independence in managing their homes and families. Incorporating adaptive strategies for menstrual hygiene, childcare responsibilities, and sexual health education to maintain roles within the family and intimate relationships.
	Emotional Support and Coping	Continued counseling and support groups to address ongoing emotional challenges.	Providing support that considers women's social roles and potential isolation from their communities. Facilitating connections with support groups and resources tailored for women to share experiences and coping strategies.
	Family Education and Training	Educating family members on how to support the patient's recovery and adapt the home environment.	Ensuring family involvement in rehabilitation to create a supportive home environment, considering women's central role in families. Educating families on the specific needs and challenges women may face, such as managing menstruation and sexual health, to promote understanding and support.
Chronic Phase	Advanced Motor Rehabilitation	Use of advanced techniques such as constraint-induced movement therapy (CIMT) and neuromuscular re-education.	Enhancing fine motor skills and functional use of the affected limbs for activities such as childcare and employment. Addressing the specific ergonomic needs and adaptations required for women's typical activities, such as lifting children and managing household tasks.
	Vocational Rehabilitation	Preparing for return to work or exploring new vocational opportunities.	Addressing specific job-related skills and exploring flexible work options to accommodate long-term disabilities. Providing support for women to manage work-life balance, childcare, and family responsibilities while returning to employment.
	Community Reintegration	Supporting participation in community activities and social roles.	Helping women reconnect with their communities and regain their social identities post-stroke. Facilitating engagement in community roles and activities that reflect women's social interests and responsibilities, including volunteer work and social groups.

(Continued)

Table 11.6 (Continued)

Phase	Intervention Focus	Description	Relevance to Women's Health
	Long-Term Emotional Support	Ongoing counseling to manage chronic emotional and psychological challenges.	Addressing long-term emotional needs, including dealing with changes in body image, self-esteem, and intimate relationships. Providing resources for women to navigate changes in sexual health and intimacy post-stroke.
	Home Modifications	Adapting the home environment for long-term safety and accessibility.	Making home modifications to support independence and accommodate physical limitations unique to women's roles at home.

Unique Considerations and Adaptive Equipment for Women with CVA

Women recovering from a stroke may face unique challenges in various aspects of their daily lives, necessitating specialized interventions from OTPs. One critical area of concern is sexual functioning. Hemiparesis, sensory difficulties, and strength deficits can significantly impact a woman's ability to engage in and enjoy sexual activities. OTPs can provide essential support through education and counseling, facilitating open discussions about sexual health to address concerns and develop strategies for maintaining intimacy. Additionally, recommending adaptive equipment such as positioning pillows, lubricants for vaginal dryness, and vibrators for sensory stimulation can help enhance comfort and satisfaction. Tailored strength and mobility training exercises can also improve overall physical condition and target specific muscles involved in sexual activity, promoting better outcomes.

Managing menstrual hygiene post-stroke can be particularly challenging due to mobility and dexterity issues. OTPs can assist by recommending adaptive equipment such as long-handled sponges, adaptive clothing, and menstrual cups, which may be easier to use than traditional tampons or pads. Providing training on effectively and safely using these tools is crucial to ensure women can maintain their hygiene independently and with dignity.

Other areas requiring specific attention include self-care, childcare, and household management. For childcare, OTPs can teach safe techniques for lifting and carrying children, using adaptive equipment like baby carriers that offer better support and reduce the risk of injury. In household management, developing strategies for meal preparation and cleaning that accommodate physical limitations is vital. This might involve using lightweight cookware, adaptive kitchen tools, and organizing the kitchen environment to minimize strain and maximize efficiency.

Occupational therapy is essential in stroke rehabilitation for women, offering tailored interventions that address the physical, cognitive, and emotional challenges resulting from a stroke. By considering unique aspects of women's health, such as sexual functioning and menstrual hygiene, OTPs can provide comprehensive care that enhances independence, functional abilities, and overall quality of life. These targeted interventions help women navigate the complexities of their recovery and support their efforts to maintain their roles within the family and community, fostering a sense of normalcy and empowerment.

Occupational Therapy and Multiple Sclerosis in Women

Multiple sclerosis (MS) is a chronic neurological condition that disproportionately affects women, with women being two to three times more likely to develop MS than men. MS is characterized by the immune system attacking the protective sheath (myelin) that covers nerve fibers, causing communication problems between the brain and the rest of the body. This condition can significantly impact daily functioning, leading to physical, cognitive, and emotional challenges that affect women's quality of life.

The exact cause of MS is unknown, but it is believed to involve a combination of genetic and environmental factors. The immune system mistakenly attacks the myelin sheath, leading to inflammation and damage to the nerve fibers. This process disrupts the transmission of nerve signals and can result in a wide range of symptoms, including motor and sensory impairments, fatigue, cognitive changes, and emotional disturbances. For a detailed overview of the different types of MS and their relevance in women's health (see Table 11.7).

Impact on Occupational Functioning

MS symptoms can vary widely and may include multiple phases, each with distinct symptoms. MS can significantly impact a woman's ability to perform everyday tasks, affecting areas such as self-care, mobility, communication, and participation in work and social activities. Cognitive impairments, emotional changes, and physical disabilities contribute to challenges in occupational performance. Fatigue is one of the most pervasive symptoms and can be influenced by the time of day. Many women with MS report feeling more fatigued in the afternoon and evening, which can disrupt their daily routines and performance patterns. Morning activities might be more manageable, while tasks later in the day could require more energy conservation strategies.

Women with MS often experience disruptions in their habits, roles, and routines. For example, a woman who is a primary caregiver may struggle to maintain her caregiving

Table 11.7 Types of multiple sclerosis and relevance in women's health

Type of MS	Characteristics	Relevance in Women's Health
Relapsing-Remitting MS (RRMS)	The most common form, characterized by clear relapses of disease activity followed by remissions.	Women are more likely to be diagnosed with RRMS; hormonal changes during menstruation, pregnancy, and menopause can influence the course of the disease.
Secondary-Progressive MS (SPMS)	Follows an initial relapsing-remitting course and then transitions to a steadily progressive form.	Women with SPMS may experience faster progression due to hormonal and lifestyle factors.
Primary-Progressive MS (PPMS)	Characterized by a steady worsening of neurologic function from the onset of symptoms, without early relapses or remissions.	PPMS is less common but can be more disabling, with women often facing unique challenges in managing daily activities and work.
Progressive-Relapsing MS (PRMS)	A rare form characterized by steadily worsening disease from the beginning with acute relapses but without remissions.	Women with PRMS may require more aggressive treatment and comprehensive support due to the severe and progressive nature of the condition.

responsibilities due to physical limitations and fatigue. Work routines can be affected by the unpredictability of symptoms, leading to absenteeism or the need for flexible working hours. Social roles and participation can also be impacted, as fatigue and physical impairments may limit the ability to engage in social activities and maintain relationships.

Evidence-based practice indicates that tailored rehabilitation programs can help women manage their symptoms, maintain function, and improve their quality of life. These programs focus on energy conservation, adaptive techniques, and personalized strategies to support the unique needs of women with MS, helping them to balance their roles and routines more effectively (see Table 11.8).

Table 11.8 Phases of MS, symptoms, and changes in occupational performance

Phase	Symptoms	Changes in Occupational Performance
Initial Phase	Visual disturbances, muscle weakness, numbness and tingling, fatigue, balance problems, bladder and bowel dysfunction.	**ADLs**: Difficulty with basic self-care tasks (bathing, dressing, grooming), managing bladder and bowel function. **Work**: Reduced productivity and challenges with job tasks requiring physical and cognitive abilities. **Social Participation**: Withdrawal from social interactions due to fatigue and physical limitations. **Sleep**: Disrupted sleep due to muscle spasms and bladder dysfunction. **Leisure**: Inability to engage in physical activities or hobbies.
Relapse Phase	Acute worsening of symptoms, new symptoms appearing, severe fatigue, increased spasticity.	**ADLs**: Increased difficulty with self-care tasks, may require assistance. **IADLs**: Inability to perform tasks like cooking, cleaning, and managing finances. **Work**: Temporary inability to work, need for job modifications or leave. **Social Participation**: Reduced participation in social activities due to symptom severity. **Sleep**: Severe sleep disturbances due to pain and discomfort. **Leisure**: Reduced participation in leisure activities, need for adapted activities.
Remission Phase	Partial or complete recovery from symptoms, periods of stability, persistent fatigue, and mild cognitive changes.	**ADLs**: Improvement in self-care abilities, but ongoing need for energy conservation strategies. **IADLs**: Gradual return to performing household tasks with modifications. **Work**: Return to work with accommodations, managing fatigue and cognitive changes. **Social Participation**: Increased ability to engage in social activities, but may require pacing and rest. **Sleep**: Improved sleep, but continued need for sleep hygiene strategies. **Leisure**: Ability to participate in leisure activities with adaptations and energy management.
Progressive Phase	Gradual worsening of symptoms, increasing disability, chronic pain, cognitive decline.	**ADLs**: Need for long-term assistance with self-care tasks, use of adaptive equipment. **IADLs**: Dependence on others for complex tasks, requiring significant adaptations. **Work**: Permanent disability, need for vocational rehabilitation or alternative employment. **Social Participation**: Significant changes in social roles, isolation due to physical and cognitive decline. **Sleep**: Chronic sleep disturbances, need for positioning aids and pain management. **Leisure**: Limited ability to participate in leisure activities, need for adapted equipment and planning.

Occupational Therapy Approach

Occupational therapy for women with MS involves a comprehensive and individualized approach that addresses the specific physical, cognitive, and emotional challenges they face. OTPs focus on maintaining function, improving independence, and enhancing quality of life. Interventions include fatigue management, cognitive rehabilitation, ADL and IADL training, emotional support, and home and community reintegration.

Table 11.9 Occupational therapy interventions by phase

Phase	Intervention Focus	Description	Relevance to Women's Health
Initial Phase	Fatigue Management	Educating on energy conservation techniques, activity pacing, and rest breaks.	Addressing unique fatigue patterns related to hormonal changes and caregiving responsibilities. Supporting women in balancing their roles and responsibilities while managing fatigue.
	Cognitive Rehabilitation	Strategies to enhance cognitive functions such as memory, attention, and executive function.	Tailoring cognitive interventions to address cognitive demands in women's daily activities, including managing family and work responsibilities.
	Basic ADL Training	Assistance with basic self-care tasks such as bathing, dressing, and grooming.	Providing immediate support for self-care tasks to maintain personal hygiene and dignity, including menstrual hygiene management and sexual health education.
	Emotional Support	Counseling to address anxiety, depression, and emotional stress.	Offering emotional support tailored to women's unique concerns and roles, such as managing family dynamics and caregiving responsibilities.
Relapse Phase	Symptom Management	Strategies to manage acute symptoms, including pain, spasticity, and sensory changes.	Providing specific interventions to manage acute symptoms, considering the impact of hormonal changes on symptom severity and management.
	ADL and IADL Training	Reintroduction of ADLs and IADLs with adaptive techniques during relapse recovery.	Helping women adapt to changes in ability and regain independence in managing their homes and families, including childcare and household management.
	Emotional Support and Coping	Continued counseling and support groups to address ongoing emotional challenges.	Providing support that considers women's social roles and potential isolation from their communities. Facilitating connections with support groups tailored for women to share experiences and coping strategies.
	Family Education and Training	Educating family members on how to support the patient's recovery and adapt the home environment.	Ensuring family involvement in rehabilitation to create a supportive home environment, considering women's central role in families. Educating families on the specific needs and challenges women may face during relapses.

(Continued)

Table 11.9 (Continued)

Phase	Intervention Focus	Description	Relevance to Women's Health
Remission Phase	Advanced Motor Rehabilitation	Use of advanced techniques such as neuromuscular re-education and task-oriented training.	Enhancing motor skills and functional use of the affected limbs for activities such as childcare and employment. Addressing specific ergonomic needs and adaptations required for women's typical activities, such as lifting children and managing household tasks.
	Vocational Rehabilitation	Preparing for return to work or exploring new vocational opportunities.	Addressing specific job-related skills and exploring flexible work options to accommodate long-term disabilities. Providing support for women to manage work-life balance, childcare, and family responsibilities while returning to employment.
	Community Reintegration	Supporting participation in community activities and social roles.	Helping women reconnect with their communities and regain their social identities post-relapse. Facilitating engagement in community roles and activities that reflect women's social interests and responsibilities, including volunteer work and social groups.
	Long-Term Emotional Support	Ongoing counseling to manage chronic emotional and psychological challenges.	Addressing long-term emotional needs, including dealing with changes in body image, self-esteem, and intimate relationships. Providing resources for women to navigate changes in sexual health and intimacy post-relapse.
Progressive Phase	Symptom Management	Advanced strategies to manage chronic symptoms, including spasticity, pain, and cognitive decline.	Providing long-term interventions to manage progressive symptoms, focusing on maintaining quality of life and adapting to increasing disabilities. Addressing the impact on caregiving roles and ensuring support for managing chronic conditions.
	ADL and IADL Adaptations	Long-term use of adaptive equipment and strategies for self-care and household management.	Ensuring women have the necessary adaptive equipment to manage self-care, household tasks, and childcare, maintaining their independence and role within the family.
	Advanced Vocational Rehabilitation	Exploring new vocational opportunities or retirement planning due to disability progression.	Providing support for transitioning out of the workforce or adapting to new roles within the community, ensuring continued engagement and purpose.
	Home Modifications	Adapting the home environment for long-term safety and accessibility.	Making extensive home modifications to accommodate significant physical limitations, ensuring a safe and supportive living environment tailored to women's specific needs.

Unique Considerations and Adaptive Equipment for Women with MS

Women with MS often face distinct challenges that require specialized interventions and adaptive equipment to manage their condition effectively. One critical area of focus is mobility. Women using wheelchairs may need tailored solutions to maintain independence and manage daily activities. OTPs can provide guidance on wheelchair selection and fitting, ensuring that the device meets the specific needs of the individual. Additionally, adaptive equipment such as transfer boards, grab bars, and shower chairs can enhance safety and ease in performing daily tasks. Training in wheelchair skills, including maneuvering in tight spaces and managing different terrains, is crucial to maintaining mobility and independence.

Managing fatigue is another significant concern for women with MS. Fatigue can be influenced by the time of day, with many women experiencing more fatigue in the afternoon and evening. This pattern can be particularly challenging for women balancing multiple roles, such as caregivers, professionals, and homemakers. OTPs can help by developing personalized energy conservation strategies, such as activity pacing, scheduled rest breaks, and the use of labor-saving devices. For example, a woman may use a lightweight vacuum cleaner or an automatic can opener to reduce physical strain. Integrating these strategies into daily routines can help women maintain their roles and responsibilities while managing fatigue effectively.

Hormonal changes related to menstruation, pregnancy, and menopause can significantly impact women with MS. Symptoms of MS, such as fatigue, muscle weakness, and cognitive changes, can worsen during menstruation or menopause due to fluctuating hormone levels. Pregnant women with MS may experience a temporary improvement in symptoms during pregnancy, but they are also at risk for postpartum relapses. OTPs can provide education and support tailored to these hormonal influences, helping women anticipate and manage symptom fluctuations. Adaptive strategies and equipment can be introduced to assist with menstrual hygiene, such as long-handled sponges and menstrual cups, ensuring women maintain their dignity and independence.

Occupational therapy is vital for women with MS, offering tailored interventions that address the physical, cognitive, and emotional challenges resulting from the condition. By considering unique aspects of women's health, such as fatigue management, menstrual hygiene, and the balance of caregiving roles, OTPs can provide comprehensive care that enhances independence, functional abilities, and overall quality of life. These targeted interventions help women navigate the complexities of their condition and support their efforts to maintain their roles within the family and community, fostering a sense of normalcy and empowerment.

Alzheimer's Disease and Cognitive Health in Women

Alzheimer's disease (AD) is a progressive neurological disorder that significantly impacts cognitive functioning, and it disproportionately affects women. Almost two-thirds of Americans living with Alzheimer's are women. Studies show that the risk of developing AD is approximately twice as high for women as for men, a disparity that profoundly influences women's health across various dimensions. While the exact reasons for this heightened risk remain unclear, hormonal differences, particularly those related to estrogen, are believed to play a crucial role. Estrogen is known to have neuroprotective effects, and its decline during menopause may contribute significantly to women's increased vulnerability to AD.

The impact of Alzheimer's on women's health extends beyond the individuals diagnosed; it also has significant implications for families and healthcare systems. Women traditionally serve as primary caregivers in the family, and the shift to becoming care recipients can strain familial relationships and existing care structures. Moreover, since women generally live longer than men, they are more likely to live with the disease for longer periods, often requiring more prolonged and intensive care. This demographic shift underscores the need for tailored healthcare strategies and supports that address the specific needs of women with AD.

Alzheimer's disease is characterized by the accumulation of amyloid plaques and tau tangles in the brain, which leads to neuronal death and brain atrophy. The pathogenesis of AD in women may be influenced by both chromosomal differences and hormonal changes across a woman's lifespan. Age remains the most significant risk factor; the likelihood of developing AD increases dramatically after age 65. Other risk factors include family history, the presence of the APOE ε4 allele, cardiovascular diseases, and lifestyle factors such as diet, exercise, and cognitive engagement. Addressing these factors through gender-specific research and public health initiatives is crucial for developing effective prevention and treatment strategies for AD in women.

Types of AD

There are several types of AD, each with its own characteristics and implications for women's health (see Table 11.10). Understanding these types can help tailor interventions and support strategies to meet the unique needs of women affected by AD.

Impact on Occupational Functioning

AD typically progresses through several stages, each with distinct symptoms and impact on daily functioning. These stages include early, middle, and late stages, with symptoms ranging from mild cognitive impairment to severe physical and mental decline (see Table 11.11). Understanding these stages helps in planning appropriate interventions and support mechanisms.

Table 11.10 Types of Alzheimer's disease and relevance in women's health

Type of Alzheimer's Disease	Characteristics	Relevance in Women's Health
Early-Onset Alzheimer's Disease	Occurs in individuals under 65, often associated with a genetic component.	Though less common, it can disrupt careers and family life significantly, especially for women balancing work and caregiving roles.
Late-Onset Alzheimer's Disease	The most common form, typically occurring after age 65, associated with a combination of genetic and lifestyle factors.	Women are more likely to develop this type due to longer life expectancy and potential cumulative effects of hormonal changes.
Familial Alzheimer's Disease	A rare form, usually affecting individuals in their 40s or 50s, caused by genetic mutations.	This type can significantly impact women who may be primary caregivers, adding to their stress and responsibilities.

Table 11.11 Stages of Alzheimer's disease, symptoms, and changes in occupational performance

Stage	Symptoms	Changes in Occupational Performance
Early Stage	Memory loss, difficulty finding words, challenges in planning and organizing, mood changes.	**ADLs**: Early difficulties with complex tasks such as managing finances and medications. **Work**: Decreased job performance and productivity, challenges in following routines. **Social Participation**: Withdrawal from social activities, difficulty maintaining relationships. **Leisure**: Reduced participation in hobbies that require cognitive effort.
Middle Stage	Increased memory loss and confusion, difficulty recognizing family and friends, trouble with spatial awareness, significant changes in behavior.	**ADLs**: Need for assistance with personal care tasks such as bathing, dressing, and grooming. **IADLs**: Dependence on others for cooking, cleaning, and managing the household. **Work**: Inability to maintain employment, need for early retirement or disability leave. **Social Participation**: Increased social withdrawal, difficulty in communication. **Sleep**: Sleep disturbances and wandering at night. **Leisure**: Limited ability to participate in previous hobbies, need for simplified activities.
Late Stage	Severe cognitive decline, loss of ability to communicate, need for full-time care, physical decline.	**ADLs**: Total dependence on caregivers for all personal care activities. **IADLs**: Complete dependence, requiring full-time caregiving support. **Work**: Long-term disability and cessation of employment. **Social Participation**: Complete withdrawal from social activities, limited interaction with others. **Sleep**: Severe sleep disturbances, need for 24-hour supervision.

AD can significantly impair a woman's ability to perform everyday tasks, disrupting areas such as self-care, mobility, communication, and participation in work and social activities. Cognitive impairments, emotional changes, and physical disabilities contribute to challenges in occupational performance. Women with AD often experience difficulties managing household tasks, finances, and personal care routines. Evidence-based practice shows that tailored rehabilitation programs can help women manage their symptoms, maintain function, and improve their quality of life by addressing their unique needs and adapting interventions accordingly.

Women with AD often struggle to maintain their roles within the family and community due to cognitive decline. For instance, managing finances, which typically involves complex decision-making and memory, becomes increasingly difficult. Personal care tasks such as bathing and dressing also become challenging as the disease progresses. The emotional burden of AD can lead to anxiety, depression, and social withdrawal, further impacting a woman's ability to engage in meaningful activities and maintain relationships.

Occupational Therapy Approach

Occupational therapy for women with AD involves a comprehensive and individualized approach that addresses the specific cognitive, physical, and emotional challenges they face. OTPs focus on maintaining function, improving independence, and enhancing quality of life. Interventions include cognitive rehabilitation, ADL and IADL training, environmental modifications, emotional support, and caregiver education (see Table 11.12).

Table 11.12 Occupational therapy interventions for women with Alzheimer's disease by stage

Stage	Intervention Focus	Description	Relevance to Women's Health
Early Stage	Cognitive Rehabilitation	Strategies to enhance memory, attention, and executive functions.	Tailoring cognitive interventions to address cognitive demands in women's daily activities, including managing family and work responsibilities.
	ADL Training	Assistance with complex self-care tasks such as managing medications and finances.	Providing support for maintaining independence in personal care and daily routines, considering the unique cognitive challenges faced by women.
	Emotional Support	Counseling to address anxiety, depression, and emotional stress.	Offering emotional support tailored to women's unique concerns and roles, such as managing family dynamics and caregiving responsibilities.
Middle Stage	Environmental Modifications	Adapting the home environment to ensure safety and ease of navigation.	Making home modifications to prevent accidents and promote independence, considering women's roles in household management.
	ADL and IADL Training	Continued support for ADLs and IADLs, incorporating adaptive techniques.	Helping women adapt to changes in cognitive and physical abilities to maintain their daily routines and independence.
	Social Participation Support	Encouraging involvement in social activities to prevent isolation.	Facilitating participation in social and community activities, tailored to the cognitive and physical abilities of women with AD. Providing support groups for women to share experiences and coping strategies.
	Caregiver Education	Training for caregivers on how to support the patient's daily activities and manage behavioural changes.	Ensuring caregivers are well-equipped to handle the specific needs of women with AD, focusing on maintaining dignity and quality of life.
Late Stage	Palliative Care	Providing comfort care and managing symptoms to improve quality of life.	Addressing the unique needs of women in the late stages of AD, focusing on comfort, dignity, and maintaining as much independence as possible.
	ADL and IADL Assistance	Full assistance with personal care and household tasks.	Ensuring comprehensive support for all daily activities, considering the severe cognitive and physical impairments.
	Emotional and Social Support	Continued emotional support for both patients and caregivers.	Offering resources and support for the emotional well-being of women with AD and their families, focusing on coping with loss and maintaining connections.

Unique Considerations and Adaptive Equipment for Women with AD

Women with AD face distinct challenges that require specialized interventions and adaptive equipment to manage their condition effectively. One critical area of focus is maintaining safety and independence at home. Women often play central roles in household management, and cognitive decline can significantly impact their ability to perform these tasks. OTPs can provide guidance on home modifications, such as installing grab bars, using automated medication dispensers, and employing simplified cooking tools to enhance safety and ease in daily activities.

Managing personal care and hygiene is another significant concern for women with AD. As the disease progresses, women may struggle with tasks such as bathing, dressing, and menstrual hygiene. OTPs can recommend adaptive equipment like long-handled sponges, shower chairs, and adaptive clothing to facilitate these activities. Training in the effective use of these tools can help women maintain their dignity and independence for as long as possible.

Emotional support and social participation are crucial for women with AD. Research shows that women are more likely than men to experience social isolation as a result of AD. The cognitive and behavioural changes associated with AD can lead to social withdrawal and isolation. OTPs can provide interventions that encourage social engagement and participation in meaningful activities. This may include facilitating connections with support groups, organizing group activities that are cognitively stimulating yet enjoyable, and providing counseling to address emotional challenges. These interventions help women maintain their social roles and improve their quality of life despite the progression of AD.

Occupational therapy plays a vital role in supporting women with AD through tailored interventions that address the cognitive, physical, and emotional challenges of the condition. By considering unique aspects of women's health, such as cognitive changes, family roles, and social participation, OTPs can provide comprehensive care that enhances independence, functional abilities, and overall quality of life. These targeted interventions help women navigate the complexities of AD and maintain their roles within the family and community, fostering a sense of normalcy and empowerment.

Case Studies in Neurological Health

CASE A: Ischemic Stroke

Background and Medical History: The client is a 52-year-old female police officer who experienced an ischemic stroke. Her stroke risk was elevated due to a combination of hypertension, a high-stress occupation, and the use of hormone replacement therapy, which are known risk factors in women, especially those over 50.

Prior Level of Function:

- **Professionally**: Actively involved in field duties requiring physical stamina and quick response capabilities, alongside administrative tasks demanding high cognitive function.
- **Socially**: Engaged in community-oriented policing programs and participated actively in sports clubs, reflecting her role as a community leader.
- **Physically**: Maintained a high level of physical activity through her job and regular workouts.

Household Living Arrangements and Social History:

- **Living Situation**: Lives in a two-story house with her husband, with grown children living independently.
- **Social Support**: Strong community ties through her role in law enforcement, though she has traditionally maintained a stoic demeanor, seldom discussing personal health issues.

Change in Functional Status and Challenges:

- **ADLs**: Experiences difficulties with tasks requiring fine motor skills and sustained physical activity, such as dressing in uniform and managing household chores, compounded by left-sided weakness.
- **Work**: Currently on medical leave due to impairments in mobility and cognitive functions critical for her safety and job performance.
- **Social Activities**: Reduced participation due to mobility issues, fatigue, and a newfound vulnerability impacting her community image.
- **Health Management**: Prioritizes blood pressure control, lifestyle modifications to reduce stress, and adjustments in hormone replacement therapy to manage stroke risk factors.

OT Assessments:

- **Barthel Index**: Scored 40 out of 100, indicating significant assistance required for daily living activities.
- **Montreal Cognitive Assessment (MoCA)**: Shows mild cognitive impairment, particularly affecting problem-solving and reaction times.
- **Fugl-Meyer Assessment**: Reveals moderate hemiparesis on the left side.
- **Women's Health Questionnaire**: Emphasizes concerns regarding hormonal management and its impact on stroke recovery, along with challenges in adapting to physical limitations in a previously active lifestyle.

Occupational Therapy Plan of Care and Goals: The client will receive skilled occupational therapy services three times a week for 12 weeks to enhance independence in daily living activities, manage neuromuscular deficits, and improve cognitive functioning.

Goals:

1. Enhance the client's independence in personal care tasks to achieve a Barthel Index score of 80/100 within 12 weeks.
2. Facilitate the client's ability to complete a full day of executive tasks using energy conservation techniques, with minimal fatigue, within 12 weeks.
3. Reduce arm swelling by 20% through targeted interventions, as measured by volumetric outcomes, within 12 weeks.
4. Improve cognitive functions related to complex problem-solving and administrative tasks by 30%, as measured by DLOTCA scores, within 12 weeks.
5. Enhance the client's self-esteem and confidence by improving body image, aiming for a 30% improvement in body image questionnaire scores within 12 weeks.

Interventions:

- **ADL Training**: Introduce adaptive devices for dressing and personal grooming to manage uniform requirements and personal hygiene.
- **Vocational Rehabilitation**: Tailor workplace adaptations for restricted duties, focusing on ergonomic adjustments and reducing physical strain.
- **Cognitive Rehabilitation**: Implement cognitive exercises and strategies to enhance decision-making and problem-solving skills critical for police work.
- **Community Reintegration**: Support gradual reintroduction to community activities, modifying participation to accommodate current physical and cognitive capacities.

Outcomes:

- **Post Treatment**: Demonstrated significant improvement in ADL independence and cognitive function, allowing part-time return to administrative police duties.
- **Follow-Up Visits**: Ongoing adaptations for workplace and community roles to maintain involvement in her professional field and social life.

This case study underscores the importance of addressing the specific physical and psychological needs of women in high-stress occupations during stroke recovery. It highlights the unique challenges faced by female law enforcement officers and the tailored occupational therapy interventions required to support their return to work and active community life.

CASE B: Early-Stage Alzheimer's Disease

Background and Medical History: The client is a 52-year-old retired police officer diagnosed with stage 1 Alzheimer's disease (AD). Her medical history is notable for hypertension and mild arthritis. The diagnosis of Alzheimer's was confirmed through a comprehensive assessment that included cognitive testing and neuroimaging techniques. MRI scans played a crucial role in her diagnosis. These scans revealed mild atrophy in the hippocampus and the entorhinal cortex—regions of the brain critically involved in memory and executive functions. Such changes are typical in the early stages of Alzheimer's and can help distinguish AD from other types of dementia. Since her diagnosis, she has experienced subtle declines in memory and executive functions, impacting her ability to manage daily activities independently.

Prior Level of Function:

- Functioned independently in all areas of occupation.
- Actively participated in her community and professional circles.
- Enjoyed socializing at her country club, gardening, and attending senior fitness classes.
- Managed her household tasks in her two-story home where she lives alone.

Household Living Arrangements and Social History:

- Lives alone in a two-story house, maintaining a high level of independence.
- Regularly attended social events at the local country club, engaging in gardening and fitness activities.

- Has a strong support network of friends and former colleagues, though she has become somewhat withdrawn since her diagnosis.

Change in Functional Status and Challenges:
- **ADLs**: Experiences slight difficulties with complex tasks such as financial management due to decreased concentration and forgetfulness.
- **Social Activities**: Reduced participation in club meetings and social gatherings, often feeling overwhelmed or disoriented in busy environments.
- **Health Management**: Struggles with medication management due to memory lapses, sometimes forgetting doses or taking them irregularly.

OT Assessments:
- **Barthel Index**: Scored 75 out of 100, indicating slight assistance needed with more complex ADLs.
- **Montreal Cognitive Assessment (MoCA)**: Demonstrated mild cognitive impairment with particular difficulties in short-term memory recall and task switching.
- **Quality of Life Scale (QOLS)**: Revealed decreased satisfaction in her current lifestyle, particularly in aspects related to social engagement and independence.
- **Health-Promoting Lifestyle Profile II (HPLP-II)**: Completed by the client and her daughter, this assessment highlighted areas for improvement in daily health-promoting behaviors such as physical activity and nutrition. The results will guide interventions aimed at enhancing her overall health and maintaining cognitive function.

Occupational Therapy Plan of Care and Goals: The client will receive skilled occupational therapy services three times a week for 12 weeks to enhance cognitive function, manage daily activities, and improve quality of life.

Goals:
1. Client will independently manage her daily medications using a pill organizer with visual and auditory reminders, achieving 100% adherence over 6 weeks.
2. Client will resume attendance at two weekly activities at her country club, using a calendar system and reminder strategies to prepare and remember events over the next 8 weeks.
3. Client will engage in tailored cognitive retraining activities focusing on memory and problem-solving skills, aiming to increase her MoCA score by 15% within 12 weeks.
4. Client will improve her Quality-of-Life Scale score by 25% through increased engagement in meaningful activities, effective stress management, and social reintegration within 12 weeks.
5. Client will participate in tailored physical activities such as senior fitness classes at least three times a week, aiming to improve her physical health and cognitive resilience within 12 weeks.
6. Client will adhere to a balanced diet plan, incorporating at least five servings of brain-healthy foods daily, as outlined by a dietitian, achieving a 90% adherence rate as tracked by a food diary over the next 12 weeks.

Interventions:

- **Cognitive Retraining**: Engage the client in memory training exercises, problem-solving tasks, and cognitive games tailored to her interests and cognitive needs to improve memory recall and executive functioning.
- **Social Reintegration**: Gradually reintroduce the client to her social activities at the country club, starting with less crowded and more familiar settings, and using reminder strategies to help her prepare and remember events.
- **Medication Management Training**: Educate the client on the use of a pill organizer, incorporating technology such as reminder apps, to enhance independence in medication management.
- **Lifestyle Modifications**: Implement structured routines that include physical exercise, social activities, and cognitive tasks to improve overall cognitive function and quality of life.
- **Quality of Life Enhancements**: Integrate stress management and relaxation techniques such as mindfulness and tailored fitness classes to improve emotional well-being and life satisfaction.
- **Dietary Planning**: Work with a dietitian to develop a personalized diet plan that includes brain-healthy foods, and use a food diary to monitor and support adherence to this diet.

Outcomes:

- **Post Treatment**: Demonstrated significant improvement in medication adherence, social engagement, cognitive function as evidenced by MoCA scores, and overall quality of life. Notable advancements in physical health and diet adherence also contribute to improved cognitive resilience.
- **Follow-Up Visits**: Continued monitoring and adaptation of interventions to support independence, cognitive health, and emotional well-being as her condition progresses. Regular reassessment of goals and strategies to ensure they remain aligned with her changing needs and preferences.

At the conclusion of therapy, the client demonstrated marked improvements across various domains, showcasing enhanced resilience and adaptive skills in managing early-stage AD. Significant progress was noted in medication management, cognitive function, social participation, physical health, and dietary habits, enabling her to engage more fully in her community and personal interests. The client's commitment to therapy and collaboration with the occupational therapy team resulted in sustainable improvements, highlighting her capacity for growth and resilience in the face of health challenges.

Further Reading

Cady, R. K. (2014). Chronic migraine in women. *The Journal of Family Practice*, 63(2 Suppl), S46–S51.

Feigin, V. L., Vos, T., Nichols, E., Owolabi, M. O., Carroll, W. M., Dichgans, M., Deuschl, G., Parmar, P., Brainin, M., & Murray, C. (2020). The global burden of neurological disorders: Translating evidence into policy. *The Lancet. Neurology*, 19(3), 255–265. https://doi.org/10.1016/S1474-4422(19)30411-9

Haki, M., Al-Biati, H. A., Al-Tameemi, Z. S., Ali, I. S., & Al-Hussaniy, H. A. (2024). Review of multiple sclerosis: Epidemiology, etiology, pathophysiology, and treatment. *Medicine, 103*(8), e37297. https://doi.org/10.1097/MD.0000000000037297

Karpova, M. I., Zariada, A. A., Dolgushina, V. F., Korotkova, D. G., Ekusheva, E. V., & Osipova, V. V. (2019). Migren' u zhenshchin: klinicheskie i terapevticheskie aspekty [Migraine in women: Clinical and therapeutical aspects]. *Zhurnal nevrologii i psikhiatrii imeni S.S. Korsakova, 119*(3), 98–107. https://doi.org/10.17116/jnevro201911903198

Kornstein, S. G., & Clayton, A. H. (2023). Women's mental health. *The Psychiatric Clinics of North America, 46*(3), xiii–xv. https://doi.org/10.1016/j.psc.2023.04.016

Kumar, A., Sidhu, J., Lui, F., & Tsao, J. W. (2024). Alzheimer disease. In *StatPearls*. StatPearls Publishing.

LaHue, S. C., Paolini, S., Waters, J. F. R., & O'Neal, M. A. (2023). Opinion and special article: The need for specialized training in women's neurology. *Neurology, 100*(1), 38–42. https://doi.org/10.1212/WNL.0000000000201451

McGinley, M. P., Goldschmidt, C. H., & Rae-Grant, A. D. (2021). Diagnosis and treatment of multiple sclerosis: A review. *JAMA, 325*(8), 765–779. https://doi.org/10.1001/jama.2020.26858

O'Neal, M. A. (2024). Women and the risk of Alzheimer's disease. *Frontiers in Global Women's Health, 4*, 1324522. https://doi.org/10.3389/fgwh.2023.1324522

Pescador Ruschel, M. A., & De Jesus, O. (2023). Migraine headache. *StatPearls [Internet]*. Medical Center Santa Rita; University of Puerto Rico, Medical Sciences Campus, Neurosurgery Section. Retrieved January 3, 2024 from https://www.statpearls.com

Ross, L., Ng, H. S., O'Mahony, J., Amato, M. P., Cohen, J. A., Harnegie, M. P., Hellwig, K., Tintore, M., Vukusic, S., & Marrie, R. A. (2022). Women's health in multiple sclerosis: A scoping review. *Frontiers in Neurology, 12*, 812147. https://doi.org/10.3389/fneur.2021.812147

Smallfield, S., Metzger, L., Green, M., Henley, L., & Rhodus, E. K. (2024). Occupational therapy practice guidelines for adults living with Alzheimer's disease and related neurocognitive disorders. *The American Journal of Occupational Therapy: Official Publication of the American Occupational Therapy Association, 78*(1), 7801397010. https://doi.org/10.5014/ajot.2024.078101

12 Women's Health Across the Lifespan

Pediatric and Adolescent Girls Health

Understanding the health of pediatric and adolescent girls is crucial for OTPs working with this population. This developmental period is marked by significant physical, emotional, and psychological changes that can have profound implications on a girl's overall health and well-being. Girls in these age groups face unique health challenges, from the onset of puberty and the menstrual cycle to dealing with issues such as obesity, mental health, substance use, and sexual health. OTPs must be equipped with the knowledge and skills to address these challenges effectively, providing holistic care that supports the girls' physical, mental, and emotional development. By doing so, OTPs can promote positive health outcomes and support girls in achieving their full potential during these critical stages of life.

Recent studies highlight the impact of these health issues on girls' occupational functioning. For example, research has shown that menstrual pain can significantly affect school attendance and participation in physical activities, with 1 in 3 adolescent girls reporting missing school due to dysmenorrhea. In one study, the prevalence of dysmenorrhea among girls was documented to be as high as 85.4%, and this was linked with poor school attendance. Furthermore, psychological issues such as anxiety and depression, which are increasingly prevalent during adolescence, can severely impact daily functioning and engagement in meaningful activities. A 2019 study revealed that nearly 30% of adolescent girls experience high levels of anxiety, which correlates with lower engagement in both school and social activities.

Puberty and Menstrual Cycle

Puberty marks a significant developmental milestone in a girl's life, typically commencing between the ages of 8 and 13. This period is characterized by a series of physical, emotional, and psychological changes driven by hormonal shifts. The primary hormones involved are estrogen and progesterone, which trigger the development of secondary sexual characteristics. Key changes during puberty include breast development (thelarche), growth of pubic and axillary hair (adrenarche), and the onset of menstruation (menarche). Additionally, girls experience a growth spurt, changes in body composition, and the development of reproductive organs. These changes can be accompanied by a range of emotional and psychological experiences, including mood swings and increased sensitivity.

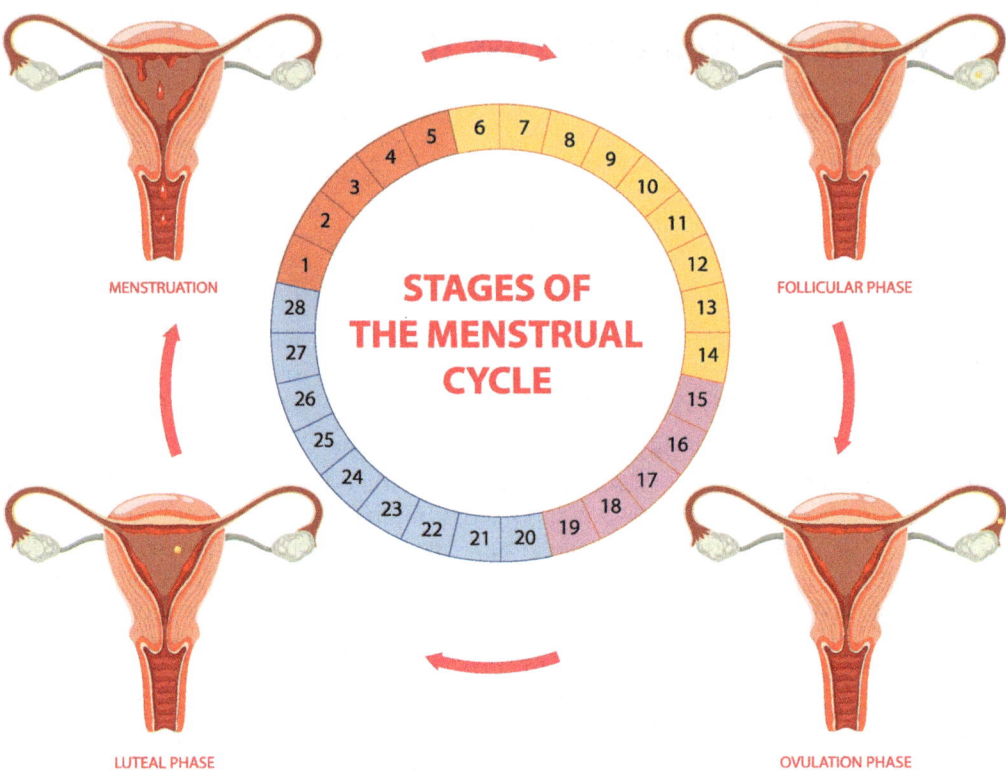

Figure 12.1 Stages of menstrual cycle.

The menstrual cycle is a monthly process that prepares the female body for pregnancy. Typically lasting about 28 days, the cycle is divided into several phases (Figure 12.1).

1. **Menstruation**: The cycle begins with menstruation, the shedding of the uterine lining, which lasts about 3–7 days. This phase is marked by bleeding and can be accompanied by symptoms such as cramps, fatigue, and mood swings.
2. **Follicular Phase**: Following menstruation, the follicular phase involves the growth and maturation of ovarian follicles under the influence of follicle-stimulating hormone (FSH). Estrogen levels rise, leading to the thickening of the uterine lining.
3. **Ovulation**: Around the midpoint of the cycle, a surge in luteinizing hormone (LH) triggers ovulation, the release of a mature egg from the ovary. This is the most fertile period of the cycle and typically occurs around day 14 in a 28-day cycle.
4. **Luteal Phase**: After ovulation, the luteal phase begins. The ruptured follicle transforms into the corpus luteum, which secretes progesterone to maintain the uterine lining. If fertilization does not occur, the corpus luteum degenerates, leading to a drop in progesterone levels and the onset of menstruation, marking the start of a new cycle.

Girls may experience various symptoms and side effects associated with the menstrual cycle, including:

- **Menstrual Cramps (Dysmenorrhea)**: Painful cramps caused by uterine contractions are common and can range from mild to severe.
- **Premenstrual Syndrome (PMS)**: Symptoms such as bloating, breast tenderness, mood swings, irritability, and fatigue may occur in the days leading up to menstruation.
- **Heavy Menstrual Bleeding (Menorrhagia)**: Excessive bleeding can lead to anemia and significant discomfort.
- **Irregular Cycles**: It is common for menstrual cycles to be irregular during the first few years after menarche as the body adjusts to hormonal changes.

Understanding the menstrual cycle and its impact on adolescent girls is crucial for OTPs. Menstrual health can significantly affect daily functioning, school attendance, participation in sports, and overall quality of life. OTPs provide valuable support by educating girls and their families about menstrual health, normalizing conversations about menstruation, and advocating for menstrual hygiene management.

Access to Menstrual Hygiene Products

Access to menstrual hygiene products is a critical issue that affects many adolescent girls. Menstrual hygiene products, such as pads, tampons, and menstrual cups, are essential for managing menstruation with dignity and maintaining hygiene. However, some girls face barriers to accessing these products due to economic constraints, lack of availability, or social stigma. This lack of access can lead to missed school days, social isolation, and increased risk of infections. OTPs can play a vital role in addressing this issue by advocating for policies that ensure access to affordable menstrual hygiene products, educating communities about the importance of menstrual hygiene, and supporting initiatives that provide free or subsidized products to those in need. By addressing this barrier, OTPs can help improve the overall health and well-being of adolescent girls, ensuring they can participate fully in their daily activities without the hindrance of menstrual health issues.

Accessibility and Management of Menstrual Hygiene Products for Girls with Disabilities

For adolescent girls with disabilities, accessing and effectively managing menstrual hygiene presents additional challenges. These may include physical barriers in handling certain products, or sensory sensitivities that make typical products uncomfortable. OTPs are uniquely positioned to assist in personalizing menstrual health management strategies that accommodate individual needs and enhance independence.

For instance, an OTP might work with a girl who has limited hand dexterity due to a physical disability, exploring alternative menstrual products such as menstrual cups with adaptive handles or pads with easier application methods. Additionally, OTPs can teach adaptive techniques for positioning and self-care that facilitate easier management of menstrual hygiene tasks. They can also advocate for the availability of adaptive menstrual products in schools and community facilities, ensuring that these essential products are accessible to all who need them.

By providing tailored support and interventions, OTPs help ensure that all girls, regardless of their physical abilities, can manage their menstrual health with dignity and independence. This support not only improves their health and hygiene but also boosts their confidence and participation in daily activities.

Adolescent Obesity

Adolescent obesity is a growing concern, with significant implications for both immediate and long-term physical and psychological health. According to the Centers for Disease Control and Prevention (CDC), about 20.6% of adolescents in the United States aged 12–19 were obese in 2017–2020, with trends showing continued increases. This condition places adolescents at a higher risk of developing chronic diseases such as type 2 diabetes, hypertension, and cardiovascular diseases—not only during their youth but extending into adulthood.

Obesity can also impact cognitive functioning; research suggests that obese adolescents may experience impairments in executive functions such as problem-solving, memory, and the ability to control impulses. These cognitive challenges can affect academic performance and social interactions, further contributing to mental health issues like depression and anxiety. Furthermore, if not adequately managed, adolescent obesity often transitions into adult obesity, perpetuating a cycle of health and social challenges.

Addressing adolescent obesity requires a multifaceted approach that includes nutritional education, promoting physical activity, and fostering a supportive environment. OTPs can play a crucial role in designing and implementing interventions that encourage healthy lifestyle choices. These interventions might include creating individualized physical activity programs that appeal to teenagers' interests, providing nutrition management alongside dietary counseling with a dietician, that teaches adolescents how to make nutritious choices, and developing group therapy sessions to improve social skills and self-esteem. By supporting adolescents in achieving and maintaining a healthy weight, OTPs help mitigate the immediate and long-term effects of obesity, enhancing overall quality of life and preventing the progression of obesity-related conditions into adulthood.

Psychological Development and Depression

Adolescence is a period of significant psychological development, characterized by the search for identity, increased independence, and the establishment of social relationships. However, this stage is also associated with heightened vulnerability to mental health issues such as depression and anxiety. According to the World Health Organization, depression is one of the leading causes of illness and disability among adolescents, and suicide is the fourth leading cause of death in people aged 15–29 years. Factors contributing to adolescent depression include academic pressures, social challenges, and hormonal changes. Depression can manifest as persistent sadness, loss of interest in activities, changes in appetite and sleep patterns, and difficulty concentrating.

Recent research highlights the importance of cognitive and executive function skills such as time management, prioritization, and addressing cognitive biases in adolescence. Studies indicate that enhancing these skills can significantly mitigate stressors that contribute to mental health issues. For example, better time management and prioritization can reduce academic stress by helping adolescents manage their workload more effectively, thereby decreasing feelings of overwhelm and anxiety. Addressing cognitive biases helps adolescents develop a more realistic and positive outlook, which is crucial in combating the negative thought patterns often associated with depression.

OTPs can support adolescents by providing coping strategies, promoting engagement in meaningful activities, and facilitating access to mental health resources. Furthermore, OTPs play a crucial role in teaching adolescents essential skills such as time management and prioritization, which are vital for academic and personal success. By helping adolescents to organize their tasks, set realistic goals, and prioritize activities, OTPs enhance their ability to cope with daily stressors, ultimately supporting their mental health and well-being. This approach not only aids in immediate stress relief but also builds resilience and adaptive skills for managing future challenges.

Substance Use in Teens

Substance use among adolescents is a significant public health concern, with potential long-term consequences for both physical and mental health. Commonly abused substances include alcohol, tobacco, and illicit drugs. Influential factors in adolescent substance use include peer pressure, family dynamics, and socioeconomic status. Substance use can impair cognitive and emotional development, leading to academic difficulties, social problems, and an increased risk of addiction. In addressing this issue, prevention and intervention efforts should focus on education, early detection, and the provision of supportive systems. OTPs play a crucial role in this area by developing prevention programs that educate and engage teens in understanding the risks and consequences of substance use. OTPs offer counseling and guidance, helping adolescents identify and replace unhealthy coping mechanisms with healthier, meaningful alternatives that align with their interests and life goals. By fostering resilience and promoting healthy lifestyle choices, OTPs support adolescents in navigating life's challenges and achieving lasting well-being.

Sexual Abuse and Teen Pregnancy

Sexual abuse and teen pregnancy are significant challenges that can deeply affect the health and well-being of adolescent girls. Sexual abuse can lead to severe physical and psychological consequences, including trauma, depression, and post-traumatic stress disorder (PTSD). Teen pregnancy complicates adolescents' lives with potential interruptions in education, economic hardships, and increased health risks for both the mother and the infant.

Research indicates that approximately 20% of adolescent girls in the United States report experiences of sexual abuse, highlighting the significance of addressing this issue through informed interventions. OTPs address these sensitive issues by applying trauma-informed care principles in their sessions ensure a safe and supportive environment where trust and safety are prioritized. This approach involves understanding the prevalence and impact of trauma and acknowledging how it can influence the individual's behavior and responses during therapy. OTPs strive to empower clients by emphasizing choice and control over their therapeutic activities, fostering resilience, and enhancing their capacities to manage daily life tasks effectively.

In sessions focusing on trauma-informed care, OTPs might engage in activities that help clients develop skills for emotional regulation, stress management, and interpersonal interactions. They might use techniques such as sensory integration therapy, mindfulness exercises, and therapeutic activities that promote relaxation and self-regulation. These activities are chosen to help mitigate the effects of trauma and support clients in regaining a sense of normalcy and control over their lives.

For adolescents facing the challenges of teen pregnancy, OTPs provide crucial support in developing essential parenting skills. This includes education on infant care, time management for balancing caregiving with personal health, and adaptive strategies for managing daily tasks. OTPs also facilitate access to community resources, such as prenatal and postnatal care, educational programs, and social support networks, which are vital for the health and well-being of both the mother and child.

Moreover, OTPs advocate for the needs of these adolescents, collaborating with schools, healthcare providers, and community organizations to ensure that pregnant teens and those recovering from trauma receive comprehensive support. This may include adjustments to educational plans, access to specialized healthcare, and connections to financial and housing assistance programs.

Sexually Transmitted Diseases (STDs)

Adolescents are at increased risk of acquiring sexually transmitted diseases (STDs) due to factors such as lack of education, risky sexual behaviors, and limited access to healthcare. Common STDs include chlamydia, gonorrhea, human papillomavirus (HPV), and herpes. STDs can have serious health consequences if left untreated, including infertility, chronic pain, and increased risk of certain cancers. Education on safe sex practices, regular screenings, and prompt treatment are crucial for preventing and managing STDs. OTPs can play a role in educating adolescents about sexual health, promoting safe behaviors, and supporting those affected by STDs through holistic interventions.

Obstetric and Gynecologic Issues in Adolescents with Chronic Illness or Disabilities

Adolescents with chronic illnesses or disabilities, particularly those with congenital conditions like spina bifida, cerebral palsy, and congenital heart defects, often encounter specific gynecological challenges that can significantly affect their health and quality of life. These conditions can lead to a range of gynecological issues, including but not limited to, menstrual irregularities such as amenorrhea or menorrhagia, and unique challenges in managing menstrual hygiene due to physical limitations or sensory impairments. Fertility can also be affected by the underlying disease or by medications used to treat it. Moreover, these adolescents might face increased risks during pregnancy, including higher rates of miscarriage, preterm labor, and complications during delivery.

The physical limitations imposed by their conditions can make the use of standard menstrual products difficult, necessitating the need for tailored solutions that accommodate mobility or dexterity constraints. For instance, a young woman with limited hand function might find traditional tampons and sanitary pads challenging to manipulate and may benefit from more accessible menstrual cups or specialized menstrual wear. Hormonal management might also be considered to regulate or suppress menstruation if it's deemed medically necessary and appropriate.

OTPs play a critical role in supporting these adolescents by offering interventions that enhance their ability to manage these gynecological issues independently. This might include:

- **Educating on adaptive techniques** for managing menstrual care, such as using modified clothing and hygiene products designed for easier use.
- **Developing personalized health care routines** that accommodate their physical and medical needs while promoting dignity and independence.

- **Advocating for appropriate medical care and support**, helping them and their families navigate health systems to access specialized gynecological services that are sensitive to their complex health profiles.

Through these interventions, OTPs ensure that these adolescents receive comprehensive care that addresses their unique needs, enhancing their well-being and enabling them to participate more fully in life activities.

Athletics in Teens as a Meaningful Occupation

Participation in athletics offers numerous benefits for adolescent girls, enhancing not only physical fitness but also mental health, self-esteem, and cognitive abilities. Recognized as a meaningful occupation, engaging in sports helps develop discipline, resilience, and teamwork—skills that contribute to healthy habits lasting a lifetime. Furthermore, involvement in sports has been linked to improved academic performance, as the discipline and time management learned on the field can translate into better focus and efficiency in schoolwork.

However, sports also pose risks such as injuries, which can range from minor sprains to severe fractures. These risks necessitate promoting safe sports practices, proper training techniques, and comprehensive injury prevention strategies.

OTPs play a crucial role in this context. As sports are considered a meaningful occupation for many adolescents, OTPs work with young athletes not only to enhance performance and prevent injuries but also to support recovery, ensuring that sports participation remains a positive and beneficial experience. Here are specific areas where OTPs can significantly contribute:

1. **Sport-Specific Training and Injury Prevention**: OTPs tailor training programs focusing on building the necessary muscle groups most used in each sport, enhancing flexibility and balance, and teaching correct techniques to prevent injuries, aligning with occupational performance needs.
2. **Pelvic Health**: Especially important for female athletes, addressing pelvic health involves educating on pelvic floor strengthening, integrating pelvic health exercises into routines, and managing issues like stress urinary incontinence through specific strategies that support daily activities and sports engagement.
3. **Menstrual Health Management**: OTPs monitor and manage the impact of athletic training on menstrual health, providing education on nutritional needs and adjusting training schedules according to menstrual cycles to optimize performance and comfort, ensuring uninterrupted participation in sports as a valued occupation.
4. **Psychosocial Considerations**: OTPs address the impact of sports on body image and mental health, provide stress management techniques, and foster the development of positive social skills through sports participation, enhancing overall well-being and social integration.
5. **Recovery and Rehabilitation**: OTPs develop personalized rehabilitation programs for injuries sustained during sports, making informed decisions about when it is safe for an athlete to return to play, crucial for maintaining engagement in this meaningful occupation.

By incorporating these tailored approaches, OTPs ensure that adolescent girls not only benefit from the physical aspects of sports participation but also receive support in managing the physiological and psychological changes they experience. These comprehensive strategies help mitigate the risks associated with sports, promote a healthy lifestyle, and support the overall development of young athletes. This holistic approach is crucial for helping adolescent girls navigate the challenges and opportunities that come with participating in athletics, ensuring they gain the maximum benefit from their sports experiences.

Occupational Therapy Interventions

OTPs play a pivotal role in addressing the unique health challenges faced by pediatric and adolescent girls. Utilizing frameworks like the Person-Environment-Occupation-Performance (PEOP) model, OTPs tailor interventions to the complex interactions between personal factors (such as hormonal changes), environmental factors (like school and social settings), and occupational engagements (such as leisure activities and schoolwork). This section delves into specialized interventions designed to support the multifaceted needs of this population during significant physical, emotional, and psychological changes. By focusing on innovative and tailored strategies, OTPs enhance the girls' ability to navigate these changes effectively. The interventions highlighted here leverage a holistic approach, integrating evidence-based practices with cutting-edge technologies to promote optimal health, well-being, and occupational engagement.

Comprehensive Health and Well-being Support:

- **Advanced Menstrual Health Management**: Targets the occupation of health management by empowering adolescent girls to maintain engagement in daily activities such as school and social interactions, even during periods of menstrual discomfort.
- **Technology-Enhanced Health Monitoring**: Supports the role of self-care manager by enabling girls to monitor and manage aspects of their physical health, sleep, and dietary habits effectively, fostering independence and informed decision-making in health-related activities.

Psychosocial and Educational Development:

- **Specialized Workshops**: These workshops contribute to the development of a healthy self-image and emotional well-being, directly impacting social participation and personal identity formation. They help adolescents navigate social roles more confidently.
- **Career and Vocational Guidance**: Prepares adolescents for the role of student and future employee by enhancing their understanding of career paths and developing necessary soft skills like teamwork and communication, crucial for professional environments.

Environmental and Community Engagement:

- **Parent and Teacher Training**: Enhances the educational and supportive roles of adults in the adolescents' environments, facilitating a better understanding of adolescent development and promoting effective support strategies in both home and school settings.
- **Environmental Modification in Schools**: Directly supports the student role by adapting educational environments to meet health and educational needs, such as providing private spaces for managing menstrual health and adjusting academic schedules to better align with students' physical states throughout the day.

By aligning these interventions with specific roles or occupations, OTPs ensure a holistic approach that not only addresses immediate health needs but also supports the overall development and integration of adolescent girls into their various social roles and environments. This structured approach not only supports individual development but also promotes a healthier transition into adulthood by instilling robust coping mechanisms and self-management skills. Furthermore, by actively involving community and educational stakeholders, OTPs facilitate a supportive ecosystem that reinforces these interventions, amplifying their impact and fostering a community-wide commitment to supporting the growth and development of young women.

Women's Health in Early Adulthood

Early adulthood, typically defined as ages 20 to 40, is a period marked by significant life transitions and responsibilities, including higher education, career establishment, marriage, and parenthood. This phase is pivotal for establishing long-term health behaviors and proactively addressing emerging health issues, which are critical for later years. According to the CDC, women in this age group face various health challenges:

- **Mental Health**: Approximately 12.8% of women aged 18–25 experience major depressive episodes.
- **Reproductive Health**: Over 50% of pregnancies in women under 30 are unplanned, which can lead to a range of health and social issues.
- **Chronic Conditions**: Around 10% of women aged 20–39 are diagnosed with hypertension, and obesity rates in women aged 20–39 are over 40%.
- **Substance Use**: About 18% of women aged 18–25 engage in binge drinking, and 11% use illicit drugs.
- **Role Transitions**: Approximately 70% of women in early adulthood experience major life transitions such as entering the workforce, pursuing higher education, marriage, and starting a family, which can significantly impact mental and physical health.

These statistics highlight the importance of targeted health interventions during early adulthood to promote long-term health and well-being.

Role Transitions

Role transitions in early adulthood, such as starting a new job, getting married, and becoming a parent, are pivotal experiences that can be both exciting and stressful. These changes frequently require significant adjustments in daily routines and responsibilities, impacting both mental and physical health. For instance, starting a new job might involve longer hours and increased stress, while becoming a parent introduces new caregiving responsibilities that can challenge sleep and self-care routines. Such transitions can lead to role strain, where balancing multiple roles becomes overwhelming. Studies indicate that during significant life transitions, about 65% of adults experience increased stress levels, highlighting the need for supportive strategies to manage these changes effectively.

Occupational Therapy Interventions

OTPs can support women during these transitions by helping them develop strategies to manage their new roles effectively and maintain occupational balance. Performance patterns in occupational therapy include roles, and addressing these through therapy is essential for reducing stress associated with transitions. For instance:

- **Time Management Training**: OTPs can provide time management training to help women balance work, family, and personal responsibilities efficiently. This includes teaching prioritization techniques and the use of tools to manage time effectively.
- **Structured Daily Routines**: Assisting in creating structured daily routines that incorporate time for self-care, leisure activities, and social participation can help women adapt to new roles without compromising their well-being.
- **Stress Management Techniques**: Techniques such as mindfulness and relaxation exercises can be critical in helping women cope with the pressures associated with new roles. OTPs can guide women in implementing these strategies into their daily routine to alleviate stress and enhance mental health.
- **Support Groups**: Facilitating support groups where women can share their experiences and strategies for managing role transitions can foster a sense of community and mutual support, crucial for emotional resilience during times of change.

By focusing on these tailored interventions, OTPs help women integrate their various roles in a way that promotes overall well-being and reduces the potential for role strain, making these transitions more manageable and less stressful. This holistic approach ensures that women can navigate these critical life stages with enhanced support and resources, aligning with long-term health and occupational satisfaction.

Reproductive Health and Family Planning

Reproductive health represents a critical aspect of well-being for women in early adulthood, encompassing a broad range of issues from contraception and family planning to fertility concerns. Research from the Guttmacher Institute reveals that approximately 45% of pregnancies in the United States are unintended, which can precipitate a variety of health and social complications. Such unplanned pregnancies can interrupt personal and professional development, leading to increased financial burdens and emotional stress. Moreover, challenges related to fertility and overall reproductive health can profoundly affect a woman's emotional state and occupational functioning, as the demands of medical appointments, treatment regimens, and the associated emotional stresses can significantly disrupt daily life and productivity.

Occupational Therapy Interventions

OTPs play a pivotal role in supporting reproductive health by offering comprehensive and personalized interventions that address complexities including:

- **Educational Workshops on Contraception**: OTPs can conduct interactive workshops on various contraception methods, providing crucial information to help women make informed decisions that align with their lifestyle and health needs. These workshops may include practical demonstrations of different contraceptive techniques, detailed discussions on their efficacy, benefits, potential side effects, and how to integrate them effectively into their daily lives.
- **Support for Fertility Challenges**: For women facing fertility issues, OTPs can provide emotional support and stress management strategies tailored to enhance coping

mechanisms during this challenging time. This might include relaxation techniques, cognitive-behavioural strategies to manage anxiety, and forming support groups to foster connections with others facing similar reproductive challenges.
- **Guidance on Prenatal and Postnatal Care**: OTPs offer guidance on prenatal care, focusing on exercises and nutrition plans tailored to the needs of pregnant women to ensure health and comfort during pregnancy. Additionally, postnatal care routines developed by OTPs can help new mothers recover physically and emotionally, enhancing bonding with the baby and facilitating a smoother transition into motherhood.
- **Personalized Health Routines**: Developing personalized health routines that accommodate prenatal and postnatal needs, addressing common discomforts during pregnancy, and supporting overall maternal health. This can include custom exercise plans that consider the individual's health status and preferences, nutritional counseling to optimize maternal and fetal health, and designing postnatal care routines that promote recovery and support the mother's role transition.

By focusing on these targeted interventions, OTPs not only address the immediate health concerns associated with reproductive challenges but also support the long-term well-being of women, empowering them to maintain occupational balance and overall health during this pivotal stage of life. These interventions ensure that women are equipped to manage the complexities of reproductive health, enabling them to pursue their personal and professional goals without compromise.

Work-Life Balance and Career Development

Balancing career demands with personal life responsibilities can be stressful. Work-related stress, job satisfaction, and work-life balance are critical for mental and physical health. According to the American Psychological Association, 66% of working adults report that work is a significant source of stress. These stressors can impact occupational functioning by reducing productivity, job satisfaction, and overall quality of life.

Occupational Therapy Interventions

OTPs can teach techniques such as prioritizing tasks, using planners, and setting realistic goals to manage work and personal responsibilities effectively. For example, OTPs might help clients create weekly schedules that balance work tasks, self-care, and leisure activities. Offering workshops on relaxation techniques, such as progressive muscle relaxation and mindfulness meditation, can help women manage work-related stress. These workshops can include guided relaxation sessions, stress relief exercises, and practical tips for integrating relaxation into daily routines. Providing vocational assessments and career planning sessions to help women navigate career transitions and advancements is also essential. OTPs can assist with resume building, interview preparation, and strategies for managing workplace challenges.

Mental Health and Emotional Well-being

Mental health issues, including anxiety and depression, are prevalent among women in early adulthood. Factors such as work stress, relationship challenges, and societal pressures can exacerbate these conditions. According to the National Institute of Mental Health, women are twice as likely as men to experience depression. Mental health issues can significantly impact occupational functioning, including the ability to perform daily activities, maintain social relationships, and achieve work goals.

Occupational Therapy Interventions

OTPs can teach cognitive-behavioural strategies to help women identify and reframe negative thoughts, managing anxiety and depression. For example, OTPs can guide clients through exercises to challenge irrational beliefs and develop healthier thought patterns. Guiding participants through mindfulness exercises, such as deep breathing and body scanning, can reduce stress and improve emotional regulation. These practices can be integrated into daily routines to help women stay grounded and present. Encouraging participation in hobbies and social activities can enhance overall well-being and reduce feelings of isolation. OTPs can help clients identify and pursue activities that bring joy and fulfillment, such as joining a book club, taking art classes, or participating in community events.

Preventive Health and Lifestyle Choices

Preventive health measures are essential to avoid chronic conditions and promote long-term health. Regular screenings, vaccinations, and healthy lifestyle choices are crucial. The CDC reports that 40% of women aged 20–39 are obese, increasing their risk for various health issues. Poor health can limit occupational functioning by reducing energy levels, increasing absenteeism, and limiting participation in social and recreational activities.

Occupational Therapy Interventions

OTPs can develop and deliver educational programs on the importance of regular health check-ups, vaccinations, and screenings. They can create informative materials and host seminars to educate women on preventive health measures. Creating personalized nutrition and exercise plans to help women achieve and maintain a healthy weight collaborating with other health professionals as needed is also vital. For example, OTPs can organize group fitness classes, provide individual consultations, and offer meal planning advice to promote healthy eating habits and regular physical activity. Providing resources and support for smoking cessation, including counseling and access to nicotine replacement therapies, is another important intervention. OTPs can facilitate support groups, offer one-on-one counseling sessions, and connect clients with community resources to help them quit smoking.

By addressing the unique health challenges faced by women in early adulthood, OTPs can support their overall well-being and help them establish healthy habits that will benefit them throughout their lives.

Women's Health in the Middle Years

The middle years, typically defined as ages 40 to 65, are characterized by significant physiological changes, including the transition to perimenopause and menopause, as well as increased risk for chronic conditions. During this period, women may also experience changes in their personal and professional lives, such as career advancements, caregiving responsibilities, and shifts in family dynamics. Addressing these changes is essential to support women's health and well-being.

According to the CDC:

- **Menopause**: Nearly 1.3 million women in the United States reach menopause each year, with symptoms that can affect occupational functioning.
- **Chronic Conditions**: Over 60% of women aged 45–65 have at least one chronic condition such as heart disease, diabetes, or cancer.
- **Mental Health**: About 23% of women aged 40–59 experience mental health issues such as anxiety and depression.
- **Caregiving Responsibilities**: Many women in this age group take on caregiving roles for aging parents, spouses, or children, which can lead to increased stress and health challenges.
- **Career Development**: This period often involves career advancements or transitions, which can impact work-life balance and overall well-being.

Perimenopause and Menopause

Perimenopause is the transitional period leading up to menopause, marked by irregular menstrual cycles and fluctuating hormone levels. Menopause marks the end of a woman's reproductive years and is characterized by a significant drop in estrogen levels. Common symptoms of both perimenopause and menopause include hot flashes, night sweats, mood swings, and sleep disturbances. These symptoms can interfere with daily activities, work productivity, and overall quality of life.

Occupational Therapy Interventions

OTPs can intervene in several meaningful ways to support women during perimenopause and menopause:

- **Bone Health and Physical Activity**: OTPs can emphasize the importance of weight-bearing exercises, which help maintain bone density and reduce the risk of osteoporosis. Tailored exercise programs can include activities like walking, dancing, or light weightlifting, which are effective in strengthening bones and improving overall physical health.
- **Cognitive Health**: To address concerns related to cognitive decline, OTPs can introduce cognitive exercises that enhance memory, focus, and executive functioning. Techniques such as brain games, new learning activities, and structured daily routines can help mitigate the impact of hormonal changes on cognitive health.
- **Dietary Guidance**: OTPs can provide nutritional management and counseling focusing on diets rich in calcium, vitamin D, and other essential nutrients that support bone health and general well-being and incorporating them into meal preparation and planning. They might collaborate with dietitians to create personalized eating plans that also help manage weight, another concern during menopause due to metabolic changes.
- **Stress Management**: Given the emotional fluctuations during this period, OTPs can offer strategies for stress reduction and emotional regulation. Techniques such as mindfulness meditation, yoga, and deep breathing exercises can be valuable in managing mood swings and improving sleep quality.
- **Hot Flash Management**: Practical advice on managing hot flashes can greatly improve daily comfort and functionality. OTPs might suggest wearing layered clothing, using

portable fans, optimizing indoor temperature settings, and identifying potential triggers for hot flashes in diet or environment.
- **Education and Advocacy**: Educating women about the physiological changes during menopause and advocating for workplace adjustments can be important. OTPs might help in developing workplace wellness programs that include flexible scheduling, stress management resources, and environments conducive to temperature control.

These interventions aim to empower women to manage the transitions of perimenopause and menopause effectively, maintaining their independence, quality of life, and engagement in valued occupations. By addressing both physical and emotional health holistically, OTPs play a crucial role in supporting women through these natural yet challenging phases of life.

Chronic Conditions

Women in the middle years are at an increased risk for chronic conditions such as heart disease, diabetes, and cancer. Chronic conditions present significant challenges for women in their middle years. According to the Centers for Disease Control and Prevention (CDC), heart disease is the leading cause of death for women in the United States, affecting approximately 1 in every 5 female deaths. Furthermore, the American Diabetes Association reports that about 13.4% of women aged 20 and older have diabetes, either diagnosed or undiagnosed. These conditions can profoundly impact occupational functioning, reducing physical activity levels, increasing fatigue, and necessitating extensive medical management.

Occupational Therapy Interventions

OTPs can work with women to manage chronic conditions through individualized exercise programs, energy conservation techniques, and self-management strategies. For example, OTPs can design tailored exercise routines that accommodate each woman's physical abilities and health status, promoting cardiovascular health and overall fitness. They can also teach energy conservation techniques, such as pacing activities and using adaptive equipment, to help women manage fatigue and maintain independence. Additionally, OTPs can provide education on self-management strategies, including medication management, dietary modifications, and stress reduction techniques, to empower women in managing their chronic conditions effectively.

Mental Health and Emotional Well-being

Mental health issues, including anxiety and depression, are prevalent among women in the middle years. Factors such as hormonal changes, caregiving responsibilities, and career-related stress can contribute to these conditions, impacting daily functioning and overall quality of life. Women may express symptoms of mental health issues differently than men, often internalizing their emotions, which can manifest as sadness, anxiety, or withdrawal. OTPs should use tailored approaches that address these specific expressions of mental health concerns. Cognitive-behavioural therapy (CBT) techniques can be adapted to challenge and modify the negative thought patterns more commonly seen in women, such as tendencies toward rumination and perfectionism.

Occupational Therapy Interventions

OTPs can provide CBT to help women identify and change negative thought patterns that contribute to anxiety and depression. For example, OTPs can guide clients through CBT exercises to develop healthier coping mechanisms and improve emotional regulation. They can also offer mindfulness-based interventions, such as guided meditation and deep breathing exercises, to help women manage stress and enhance emotional well-being. Additionally, OTPs can facilitate support groups where women can share experiences, receive social support, and learn from one another, fostering a sense of community and reducing feelings of isolation.

Caregiving Responsibilities

Many women in the middle years take on caregiving roles for aging parents, spouses, or children, which can lead to increased stress and health challenges. According to the Family Caregiver Alliance, about 60% of family caregivers are women, and they spend an average of 20 hours per week providing care. This can lead to role strain and decreased time for self-care and leisure activities.

Occupational Therapy Interventions

OTPs can support women in caregiving roles by helping them develop strategies to manage their responsibilities effectively. OTPs can teach time management and organizational skills to balance caregiving with other roles. They can also provide education on self-care techniques to prevent caregiver burnout, such as stress management, relaxation exercises, and seeking social support. Additionally, OTPs can offer training on safe caregiving techniques to prevent injury and provide resources for respite care services to give caregivers a break.

Work-Life Balance and Career Development

Many women in the middle years' experience significant transitions in both their careers and personal lives. They may be advancing in their careers, entering or returning to the workforce after child-rearing, or managing dual roles as caregivers for both children and aging parents. These responsibilities often intersect with societal expectations and personal aspirations, leading to complex challenges in achieving work-life balance.

Occupational Therapy Interventions

OTPs can provide targeted support by understanding and addressing the unique pressures faced by women. Interventions can include:

- **Customized Time Management Training**: Tailored specifically for women who balance multiple roles, this training can include strategies for effective multitasking, delegating, and setting boundaries to prioritize well-being alongside professional and familial responsibilities.
- **Stress Management Workshops**: These should address specific stressors that women face, such as gender bias in the workplace, managing "invisible" work at home, and coping with the emotional demands of caregiving. Techniques such as cognitive restructuring, stress inoculation training, and assertiveness training can be particularly beneficial.

- **Career Transition Support**: For women looking to advance in their careers or re-enter the workforce, OTPs can provide guidance on navigating gender dynamics in professional settings, enhancing leadership skills, and leveraging networks for career growth.
- **Flexible Scheduling Solutions**: Assisting women in negotiating for flexible work arrangements that accommodate their life stages and caregiving needs can significantly reduce stress and improve job satisfaction. This might include advocating for remote work opportunities, flexible hours, or job sharing.
- **Enhanced Support Networks**: Facilitating access to mentorship programs, professional women's groups, or support groups for working mothers can help women share resources, gain support, and access opportunities that can aid in their career development.

By focusing on these tailored interventions, OTPs can help women navigate the complexities of their middle years, supporting them in achieving a balanced and fulfilling professional and personal life. This holistic approach not only enhances individual well-being but also contributes to greater productivity and satisfaction at work and at home.

Women's Health in Later Life

Women's health in later life, typically defined as ages 65 and older, encompasses a range of physical, emotional, and cognitive changes. This period is not only a time for managing increased risks of chronic diseases and mobility issues but also for embracing the growth and opportunities that can arise during these years. Women in this age group often experience profound life transitions such as retirement and the loss of loved ones, which, while challenging, also offer opportunities for personal growth and deeper community engagement.

According to the CDC:

- **Chronic Conditions**: Approximately 80% of older adults have at least one chronic condition, and 50% have two or more.
- **Mobility Issues**: Nearly 25% of women aged 65 and older report some form of disability, primarily related to mobility.
- **Cognitive Decline**: About 11% of women aged 65 and older have Alzheimer's disease or other dementias.
- **Mental Health**: Depression affects around 15% of older adults, with higher rates among those with chronic health conditions.
- **Retirement Transition**: Adjusting to retirement can impact a woman's identity, social engagement, and mental health, with nearly 60% of retirees reporting a need for new routines and activities to maintain a sense of purpose and well-being.
- **Loss**: The loss of a spouse or close loved ones can lead to significant emotional distress, with 40% of widows experiencing major depression in the first year after their spouse's death, impacting overall health.

Chronic Conditions

Older women are more likely to experience chronic conditions such as heart disease, arthritis, diabetes, and osteoporosis. According to the National Council on Aging, 92% of older adults have at least one chronic disease, and 77% have two or more. Heart disease is the leading cause of death among women aged 65 and older, and nearly 50% of women aged 65 and older are living with arthritis. These conditions can significantly impact daily functioning, limiting mobility, increasing fatigue, and requiring ongoing medical management.

Occupational Therapy Interventions

OTPs can develop individualized exercise programs to help manage chronic conditions and improve physical function. For example, OTPs can create low-impact exercise routines, such as swimming or tai chi, to enhance cardiovascular health and joint mobility. They can also teach energy conservation techniques, such as pacing activities and using adaptive equipment, to help women manage fatigue and maintain independence in daily tasks. Additionally, OTPs can provide education on self-management strategies, including medication management, dietary modifications, and stress reduction techniques, empowering women to take an active role in managing their health.

Mobility Issues

Mobility issues are common among older women due to conditions such as arthritis, osteoporosis, and muscle weakness. According to the CDC, nearly 25% of women aged 65 and older report some form of disability, primarily related to mobility. Falls are a significant concern, with 1 in 4 older adults experiencing a fall each year, leading to injuries and reduced independence.

Occupational Therapy Interventions

OTPs can conduct home assessments to identify potential hazards and recommend modifications to enhance safety and accessibility. For instance, OTPs might suggest installing grab bars in the bathroom, using non-slip mats, and rearranging furniture to create clear pathways. They can also teach exercises to improve strength, balance, and coordination, reducing the risk of falls. Additionally, OTPs can provide training on the use of assistive devices, such as walkers or canes, to improve mobility and independence.

Cognitive Decline

Cognitive decline, including dementia and Alzheimer's disease, affects many older women, impacting memory, problem-solving skills, and the ability to perform daily tasks. The Alzheimer's Association reports that nearly two-thirds of Americans with Alzheimer's are women, and about 11% of women aged 65 and older have Alzheimer's disease or other dementias. This decline can lead to challenges in managing personal care, finances, and social interactions.

Occupational Therapy Interventions

OTPs can develop cognitive rehabilitation programs to help maintain cognitive function and compensate for deficits. For example, OTPs might use memory aids, such as calendars and checklists, to assist with daily planning and organization. They can also engage clients in cognitive-stimulating activities, such as puzzles, games, and hobbies, to promote mental engagement. Additionally, OTPs can provide caregiver education and support, offering strategies for managing behavioural changes and enhancing communication with loved ones.

Mental Health and Social Isolation

Older women are at risk of depression and anxiety, often exacerbated by chronic health conditions, loss of loved ones, and social isolation. According to the National Institute of Mental Health, about 15% of older adults experience depression, with higher rates among those with chronic health conditions. Social isolation can further impact mental health and overall well-being, with nearly one-quarter of community-dwelling older adults considered to be socially isolated.

Occupational Therapy Interventions

OTPs can facilitate social participation by encouraging involvement in community activities, support groups, and clubs. For instance, OTPs can help clients find and join local senior centers, volunteer organizations, or hobby groups that match their interests. They can also provide strategies for maintaining social connections through technology, such as teaching clients how to use video calling or social media to stay in touch with family and friends. Additionally, OTPs can offer mental health interventions, such as cognitive-behavioural therapy and relaxation techniques, to address depression and anxiety, promoting emotional well-being.

By addressing the unique health challenges faced by women in later life, OTPs can support their overall well-being and help them maintain independence and quality of life during this stage of life.

Retirement Transition

Adjusting to retirement can impact a woman's identity, social engagement, and mental health. According to the Transamerica Center for Retirement Studies, nearly 60% of retirees report needing to develop new routines and activities to maintain a sense of purpose and well-being. The transition from a structured work life to retirement can lead to feelings of loss, decreased social interaction, and uncertainty about the future. Establishing a new daily routine and finding meaningful activities are essential to adapting to this significant life change.

Occupational Therapy Interventions

OTPs can help women navigate the transition to retirement by assisting them in developing new routines and finding meaningful activities. For example, OTPs can guide clients in exploring hobbies, volunteer opportunities, and social groups that align with their interests and skills. They can also provide strategies for maintaining physical and mental health, such as regular exercise, continued learning, and social engagement. By supporting women in finding purpose and maintaining active lifestyles, OTPs can help enhance their overall well-being during retirement.

Loss

The loss of a spouse or close loved ones can lead to significant emotional distress, impacting overall health. According to the American Psychological Association, nearly 40% of widows experience major depression in the first year after their spouse's death. This

Women's Health Across the Lifespan 357

profound loss can lead to feelings of loneliness, depression, and anxiety, severely affecting daily functioning and quality of life. The grieving process can disrupt sleep patterns, appetite, and energy levels, making it difficult to maintain routines and engage in social activities.

Occupational Therapy Interventions

OTPs can provide crucial support to women coping with loss by offering grief counseling and facilitating support groups. These interventions help clients process their emotions and develop coping strategies to manage their grief. More uniquely, OTPs can guide women in identifying and engaging in meaningful occupations that bring joy and fulfillment. Such activities could include:

- **Creative Expressions**: Encouraging participation in arts and crafts, writing, or other creative outlets that allow for emotional expression and processing.
- **Volunteering**: Assisting women in finding volunteer opportunities that provide a sense of purpose and community connection, which can be particularly healing during times of grief.
- **Gardening/Nature Therapy**: Introducing activities that connect with nature, such as gardening or nature walks, which are not only therapeutic but also help in nurturing life and can be a metaphor for growth and healing.
- **Physical Activities**: Promoting physical activities like yoga or walking groups that not only help in maintaining physical health but also provide social interaction and support.

Additionally, OTPs can assist women in establishing new routines that accommodate their current emotional and physical state, integrating these meaningful activities into their daily lives. They can also encourage social engagement by connecting clients with community resources and support networks, helping to reduce feelings of isolation and promoting emotional healing.

Through these targeted interventions, OTPs can help women navigate their grief and rebuild a life that, while different, is still full of purpose and connection. This holistic approach not only addresses the emotional and psychological impacts of loss but also reinforces the resilience and capacity of individuals to continue engaging in life fully and meaningfully.

Physical Changes and Exercise Recommendations

As people age, they encounter several physiological changes that make common activities more challenging. These changes include a decline in maximum heart rate, meaning that older adults reach their maximum heart rate more quickly and at lower levels of exertion compared to younger individuals. Consequently, older adults often perform at a higher percentage of their maximum exercise capacity during similar activities, making those activities more demanding.

Additionally, the pulmonary system undergoes changes such as the thickening of pulmonary arteries, increased vascular resistance, and decreased pulmonary compliance. The alveolar surface area, crucial for gas exchange, also diminishes. These changes further affect the exercise capacity and overall physical endurance of older adults.

Exercise Recommendations

For deconditioned older adult women, exercise should be maintained within a range of 12–13 on the Rate of Perceived Exertion (RPE) scale and 55–64% of their maximum heart rate (HRMax). For those who are already physically active, exercise intensity can be increased to 70–85% of HRMax, with an RPE of 14–16. By tailoring exercise programs to these parameters, OTPs can help older women maintain and improve their physical health safely and effectively. The physiological changes and exercise recommendations for older adults generally apply to both women and men, though there may be some differences in how these changes manifest and are managed based on gender-specific factors. Here's a detailed gender specific comparison for consideration of older adults:

1. **Heart Rate and Exercise Capacity**
   - **Women**: Typically have a slightly higher resting heart rate and may experience a slower decrease in aerobic capacity compared to men.
   - **Men**: Often notice a steeper decline in muscle mass and strength, affecting overall exercise performance more significantly.

2. **Pulmonary System**
   - **Women**: Have smaller lung volumes and airway diameters, which can influence exercise capacity, particularly in endurance activities.
   - **Men**: Benefit from larger lung volumes, which can buffer some age-related declines in pulmonary function.

3. **Hormonal Changes**
   - **Women**: Post-menopausal hormonal changes affect bone density, muscle mass, and cardiovascular health, necessitating specific exercise considerations for bone health and cardiovascular fitness.
   - **Men**: Experience a gradual decline in testosterone impacting muscle mass and strength, emphasizing the need for resistance training.

4. **Chronic Conditions**
   - **Women**: More likely to experience osteoporosis and arthritis, requiring exercise programs that emphasize joint protection, flexibility, and strength training.
   - **Men**: More prone to heart disease and hypertension, necessitating aerobic exercises and resistance training to manage these conditions effectively.

Understanding and addressing the unique health challenges faced by older women is crucial for promoting their overall well-being and independence. The physical, emotional, and cognitive changes that occur in later life, including chronic conditions, mobility issues, cognitive decline, and mental health concerns, necessitate targeted and individualized interventions. OTPs play a vital role in managing these challenges by developing personalized exercise programs, ensuring home safety, providing cognitive rehabilitation, and supporting mental health. Additionally, recognizing gender-specific differences in physiological changes and exercise needs allows for more effective therapeutic strategies. By addressing these needs comprehensively, OTPs can significantly enhance the quality of life for older women, helping them navigate life transitions, maintain social connections, and continue to engage in meaningful activities.

Women's Health Across the Lifespan 359

Case Studies in Women's Health Across the Lifespan

CASE A: Managing Adolescent Dysmenorrhea and Enhancing Daily Functioning

Background and Medical History: The client is a 16-year-old high-school student who has been experiencing dysmenorrhea since her menarche at the age of 12. Initially, the symptoms were mild, but they have progressively intensified over the past four years, significantly worsening in the last year. Her medical chart includes a history of multiple consultations with a pediatrician regarding severe menstrual cramps. These consultations have ruled out underlying reproductive conditions but noted a persistent increase in symptom severity, impacting her daily activities and quality of life.

Prior Level of Function:

- **Academic**: Consistently maintained above-average grades and participated actively in school.
- **Extracurricular**: Engaged in sports and various school clubs.
- **Social**: Enjoyed a vibrant social life with a wide circle of friends.

Household Living Arrangements and Social History:

- **Living Situation: Resides** with parents and a younger brother in a suburban private one-level home.
- **Family and Social Support**: Comes from a supportive family environment; has a strong social network, though her participation has been limited recently due to pain.

Change in Functional Status and Challenges:

- **Academic Impact**: Increased absenteeism, particularly during menstrual periods, negatively impacting her academic performance.
- **Physical Activities**: Has withdrawn from sports due to pain.
- **Social Interaction**: Experiences decreased social interactions due to anxiety and discomfort related to her symptoms.

OT Assessments:

- **Pain Assessment Scale**: Reports severe pain during menstrual periods, scoring 8 out of 10, which significantly restricts her participation in daily and recreational activities.
- **Occupational Performance Inventory**: Noted a decline in engagement in both school attendance and extracurricular activities.
- **Pelvic Floor Impact Questionnaire (PFIQ)**: Indicates significant impact on social, physical, and emotional aspects due to pelvic floor symptoms.
- **Menstrual Cycle Tracking**: Over the past three months, the client tracked her menstrual cycle, noting that her pain peaks during the first two days of menstruation, with moderate pain persisting for up to five days. This information allows for better planning and management of academic and social engagements.
- **Coping Strategies Inventory (CSI)**: Evaluated her coping mechanisms, indicating a reliance on avoidance behaviors.

Occupational Therapy Plan of Care and Goals: The client will receive skilled occupational therapy services three times a week for a duration of 12 weeks. The focus of therapy will be to improve independence in daily living activities, manage symptoms associated with dysmenorrhea, and enhance overall quality of life.

Goals:

1. Client will achieve at least a 50% reduction in pain intensity using non-pharmacological methods within three months, enabling her to participate in daily activities without significant discomfort.
2. Client will attain at least 90% attendance during the upcoming school semester, allowing her to maintain academic performance and progress.
3. Client will re-engage in at least two extracurricular activities by the next school term, improving her social participation and physical health.
4. Client will achieve a 50% improvement in the Pelvic Floor Impact Questionnaire (PFIQ) score, enhancing pelvic floor function and decreasing the impact on daily activities within three months.

Interventions:

1. **Pain Management Education**
    - **Relaxation Techniques**: Teach deep breathing, progressive muscle relaxation, and guided imagery.
    - **Dietary Adjustments**: Collaborate with a dietitian to develop a diet plan that reduces inflammation and supports menstrual health.
    - **Physical Exercises**: Introduce gentle yoga and stretching exercises focusing on pelvic floor relaxation and overall body relaxation.

2. **Activity Pacing**
    - **Energy Management**: Educate on scheduling high-demand activities during low-symptom days and incorporating regular rest breaks.
    - **Time Management**: Assist in developing a weekly planner to balance schoolwork, rest, and leisure activities.

3. **Social Skills Training**
    - **Confidence Building**: Conduct role-playing sessions to enhance social interactions and reduce anxiety related to her symptoms.
    - **Support Groups**: Facilitate connections with peer support groups for adolescents experiencing similar challenges.

4. **Pelvic Floor Therapy**
    - **Pelvic Floor Exercises**: Introduce Kegel exercises and biofeedback to strengthen and relax the pelvic floor muscles.
    - **Manual Therapy**: Perform gentle manual therapy techniques to alleviate pelvic tension and discomfort.

5. **Menstrual Cycle Education**
    - **Cycle Tracking**: Continue to track menstrual cycles and identify pain exacerbation phases to better plan major assignments and training.
    - **Self-Care Strategies**: Educate on the use of heat pads and appropriate positioning during menstrual periods to alleviate pain.

Outcomes:

- **Post Treatment**: Demonstrated significant reduction in pain, improved school attendance, and increased engagement in social and physical activities.
- **Follow-Up Visits**: Continue monthly follow-up sessions to adjust intervention strategies and provide ongoing support.

With dedicated occupational therapy interventions focused on pain management, menstrual cycle education, activity pacing, and pelvic floor health, the client has shown considerable improvement in managing her dysmenorrhea. These improvements have positively impacted her academic performance, physical engagement, and social interactions, highlighting the role of occupational therapy in enhancing the quality of life for adolescents facing similar challenges.

CASE B: Teen Pregnancy

Background and Medical History: The client is a 17-year-old high-school student who is currently 6 months pregnant with her first child. She has been experiencing high levels of stress due to the challenges of balancing her pregnancy, schoolwork, and preparing for motherhood. The client has a history of anxiety, which has been exacerbated by her current situation. She lives with her single mother and has limited social support from friends and family.

Prior Level of Function:

- Attended high school full-time, maintaining average grades.
- Participated in extracurricular activities such as the school choir and volunteer work.
- Managed all ADLs and IADLs independently.
- Socially active with friends and involved in community events.

Household Living Arrangements and Social History:

- Lives with her single mother in a small apartment.
- Limited support system, primarily relying on her mother for emotional and financial support.
- Few close friends due to the stigma of teen pregnancy.

Change in Functional Status and Challenges: The client reports significant stress and anxiety related to her pregnancy, school responsibilities, and future planning. Specific areas affected include:

ADLs:

- Difficulty with personal care tasks due to fatigue and pregnancy-related discomfort.
- Challenges with maintaining a healthy diet and regular prenatal care appointments due to time constraints and lack of transportation.

IADLs:

- Struggles with meal preparation and grocery shopping, relying heavily on her mother for assistance.
- Difficulty managing school assignments and studying due to stress and fatigue.

Schoolwork:

- Increased absenteeism and difficulty concentrating in class, impacting her academic performance.
- High levels of stress related to keeping up with assignments and preparing for exams.

Social Activities:

- Reduced participation in extracurricular activities and social gatherings due to fatigue and feelings of isolation.
- Difficulty maintaining friendships and engaging in community events.

Occupational Therapy Assessments:

- **Canadian Occupational Performance Measure (COPM):** Identified issues in managing self-care, productivity, and leisure activities.
- **Beck Anxiety Inventory (BAI):** Scores reflecting moderate to severe anxiety symptoms.
- **Prenatal Psychosocial Profile (PPP):** Assessed psychosocial stressors, indicating significant emotional and social challenges.
- **Adolescent Stress Questionnaire:** The client's responses indicated elevated stress levels in several domains. Key findings include:
  - **School Pressure**: High stress related to keeping up with academic demands, reporting difficulty concentrating, frequent absenteeism, and fear of failing exams.
  - **Social Relationships**: Moderate to high stress due to social isolation, loss of friendships, and perceived stigma associated with teen pregnancy.
  - **Personal Concerns**: Elevated stress from pregnancy-related changes, including concerns about future planning, parenting responsibilities, and managing physical discomforts.
  - **Home Life**: Mild stress related to relying heavily on her mother for support, with feelings of guilt and worry about burdening her with additional responsibilities.

Occupational Therapy Plan of Care and Goals: The client will receive skilled occupational therapy services twice a week for 12 weeks to improve her independence in ADLs, manage stress, and enhance her ability to balance schoolwork and pregnancy. Goals include:

1. **Client will independently manage personal care tasks** with minimal fatigue, using energy conservation techniques, achieving a 30% improvement in COPM scores within 12 weeks.
2. **Client will attend all prenatal care appointments** and maintain a healthy diet, with assistance in scheduling and transportation, achieving a 50% improvement in adherence to prenatal care within 12 weeks.
3. **Client will complete school assignments on time** using stress management techniques and a structured study schedule, improving academic performance as measured by teacher reports and self-reported stress levels within 12 weeks.
4. **Client will reduce anxiety symptoms**, with BAI scores decreasing to below 15 within 12 weeks through targeted psychosocial interventions.
5. **Client will increase participation in social activities**, re-engaging in at least one extracurricular activity or social event per week, as measured by self-reported participation and satisfaction within 12 weeks.

6. **Client will develop a support network** by connecting with peer support groups and community resources for teen mothers, improving her Prenatal Psychosocial Profile scores by 40% within 12 weeks.

Occupational Therapy Interventions:

The following interventions will be tailored to meet the client's specific needs and address the outlined goals:

Stress Management Strategies:

- Teach relaxation techniques such as deep breathing, progressive muscle relaxation, and guided imagery to manage anxiety.
- Implement mindfulness practices and cognitive-behavioural techniques to improve emotional regulation and reduce stress.

Activity Modification and Energy Conservation:

- Educate the client on energy conservation techniques, such as pacing activities and incorporating frequent rest breaks.
- Advise on modifying activities to reduce fatigue, such as breaking tasks into smaller, manageable steps.

ADL and IADL Training:

- Conduct specialized training on the use of adaptive equipment tailored for individuals experiencing fatigue, incorporating ergonomic tools and techniques to enhance efficiency and independence in personal care tasks.
- Develop and instruct on advanced meal preparation strategies that emphasize quick, nutritious recipes and efficient kitchen management, ensuring the client maintains a balanced and healthy diet during pregnancy.
- Provide guidance on safe lifting techniques and body mechanics to reduce strain and discomfort during household chores and childcare activities.
- Assist in creating a personalized plan for managing prenatal appointments, medication schedules, and self-care routines, integrating these tasks seamlessly into her daily life.

Schoolwork Management:

- Develop a comprehensive and adaptable study schedule that integrates schoolwork with necessary rest periods and prenatal care, ensuring a balanced approach to academic responsibilities.
- Implement advanced organizational strategies and tools to optimize task management, enabling the client to efficiently track and prioritize assignments and deadlines.

Social and Emotional Support:

- Facilitate connections with peer support groups for teen mothers to provide emotional support, reduce feelings of isolation, and share experiences and coping strategies.
- Offer psychosocial counseling sessions to address anxiety and stress, employing cognitive-behavioural techniques to enhance emotional regulation and resilience.
- Provide training and strategies for effective communication skills to improve interactions with teachers, parents, and significant others, fostering supportive relationships and reducing conflicts.

- Guide the client in managing relationships with teachers by developing proactive communication plans, ensuring academic needs are met, and accommodations are understood and implemented.
- Assist in enhancing communication skills to better navigate relationships with parents and significant others, promoting understanding and support.
- Address and mitigate the impact of cognitive biases in adolescence, such as negative self-perception and social comparison, through targeted interventions and reflective practices.

Transportation and Scheduling Assistance:

- Assist the client in coordinating transportation for prenatal care appointments.
- Develop a calendar system to help the client manage her schedule effectively.

Outcomes:

Post Treatment:

- **Stress Management**: Significant reduction in anxiety symptoms, evidenced by a decrease in BAI scores to below 15, with the client reporting improved emotional regulation and reduced daily stress.
- **ADL and IADL Independence**: Improved engagement in personal care and household tasks, with the client achieving a Barthel Index score increase from 60 to 85, reflecting increased independence and reduced need for assistance.
- **School Performance**: Improved academic performance, with the client maintaining consistent attendance and completing assignments on time, as reported by teachers and reflected in improved grades.
- **Social Engagement**: Increased participation in social activities and re-engagement in extracurricular activities, enhancing the client's sense of community and support.
- **Support Network**: Establishment of a strong support network through peer groups and community resources, improving the client's Prenatal Psychosocial Profile scores by 40%.

Follow-Up Visits:

- Continuously reinforce stress management techniques and activity modifications to ensure the sustainability of the client's improvements in daily activities and school performance.
- Provide ongoing support and adjust the client's treatment plan based on her feedback, changes in her symptoms, and any new challenges that arise in managing her pregnancy and school responsibilities.

The client demonstrated significant improvement in managing her pregnancy, schoolwork, and stress, enhancing her overall functionality and independence. She is now capable of performing daily tasks and school activities with greater efficiency and less anxiety. The tailored occupational therapy interventions enabled her to balance her roles as a student and an expectant mother effectively. Through the collaborative and holistic approach of occupational therapy, the client has regained a better quality of life and improved her capacity to engage in meaningful activities.

CASE C: Middle Adulthood Role Transition, Divorce, and Stress

Background and Medical History: The client is a 42-year-old woman who recently went through a divorce. She has one 10-year-old child and is experiencing significant stress related to the role transition, managing single parenthood, and balancing work responsibilities. The client has a history of mild hypertension and is currently managing it with lifestyle modifications and medication. She reports feeling overwhelmed, anxious, and fatigued due to the recent changes in her life.

Prior Level of Function:

- **Work**: Worked full-time as a business manager, efficiently managing professional responsibilities.
- **Community Involvement**: Actively participated in her child's school activities and community events.
- **ADLs and IADLs**: Managed all ADLs and IADLs independently.
- **Physical Activity**: Engaged in regular physical exercise, including running and yoga.

Household Living Arrangements and Social History:

- **Living Situation**: Recently moved to a new apartment with her child post-divorce.
- **Family and Social Support**: Limited support system, primarily relying on friends and distant family for emotional support.
- **Social Network**: Active in her community and social circles before the divorce.

Change in Functional Status and Challenges: The client reports significant stress and anxiety related to her divorce, single parenthood, and work responsibilities. Specific areas affected include:

ADLs:

- Difficulty with personal care tasks due to fatigue and stress, including reduced frequency of showering and grooming.
- Challenges with maintaining a healthy diet and regular exercise routine due to time constraints and emotional distress.

IADLs:

- Struggles with managing household chores such as cleaning, cooking, and grocery shopping due to increased responsibilities.
- Difficulty coordinating her child's school activities and managing her own work schedule.

Work:

- Increased absenteeism and difficulty concentrating at work, impacting her job performance.
- High levels of stress related to balancing work and personal life.

Social Activities:

- Reduced participation in social gatherings due to fatigue and feelings of isolation.
- Difficulty maintaining friendships and engaging in community events.

Occupational Therapy Assessments:

- **Canadian Occupational Performance Measure (COPM)**: Identified issues in managing self-care, productivity, and leisure activities, with the client reporting significant difficulties in balancing her roles as a single parent and professional. The COPM scores indicated a low satisfaction and performance in these areas.
- **Beck Anxiety Inventory (BAI)**: Scores reflecting moderate to severe anxiety symptoms, with the client scoring 28, indicating a high level of anxiety impacting her daily functioning and overall well-being.
- **Parenting Stress Index (PSI)**: Assessed the level of stress associated with parenting, indicating high levels of stress and emotional strain. The client scored in the 85th percentile, highlighting significant challenges in managing single parenthood.
- **Work Role Functioning Questionnaire (WRFQ)**: Evaluated the impact of stress on work performance, highlighting difficulties in maintaining focus and meeting job demands. The client reported a significant decline in work productivity and increased absenteeism, with a total score reflecting moderate to severe impact on work performance.
- **Role Checklist**: Assessed the client's roles and satisfaction with these roles, identifying areas of role transition stress. The client reported a high level of dissatisfaction with her current roles and the challenges of adjusting to single parenthood and work responsibilities.
- **Occupational Balance Questionnaire (OBQ)**: Evaluated the client's balance between work, leisure, and self-care activities, indicating significant imbalance. The client's scores reflected a lack of engagement in leisure and self-care activities, contributing to her overall stress and fatigue.

Occupational Therapy Plan of Care and Goals: The client will receive skilled occupational therapy services twice a week for 12 weeks to improve her independence in ADLs, manage stress, and enhance her ability to balance her roles as a single parent and professional.

Goals:

1. Client will independently manage personal care tasks with minimal fatigue, using energy conservation techniques, achieving a 30% improvement in COPM scores within 12 weeks.
2. Client will establish a consistent meal preparation routine using stress management and organizational strategies, improving adherence to a healthy diet within 12 weeks.
3. Client will manage household chores efficiently, using time management and energy conservation techniques, achieving a 40% improvement in IADL performance as measured by self-report within 12 weeks.
4. Client will improve work performance and attendance, reducing absenteeism and enhancing focus, as measured by WRFQ scores and employer feedback within 12 weeks.
5. Client will reduce anxiety symptoms, with BAI scores decreasing to below 15 within 12 weeks through targeted psychosocial interventions.
6. Client will increase participation in social activities, re-engaging in at least one community event or social gathering per week, as measured by self-reported participation and satisfaction within 12 weeks.
7. Client will reduce parenting stress, improving PSI scores by 30% through the implementation of stress management techniques and support strategies within 12 weeks.

Interventions:

1. **Stress Management Strategies**

    - **Relaxation Techniques**: Teach deep breathing, progressive muscle relaxation, and guided imagery to manage anxiety.
    - **Mindfulness Practices**: Implement mindfulness practices and cognitive-behavioural techniques to improve emotional regulation and reduce stress.
    - **Cognitive-Behavioural Therapy (CBT)**: Use CBT techniques to help the client identify and reframe negative thought patterns, replacing them with more positive and realistic thoughts. This will aid in reducing symptoms of depression and anxiety.
    - **Motivational Interviewing**: Employ motivational interviewing to enhance the client's motivation to engage in therapeutic activities, set goals, and make positive changes.

2. **Activity Modification and Energy Conservation**

    - **Energy Conservation**: Educate the client on energy conservation techniques, such as pacing activities and incorporating frequent rest breaks.
    - **Activity Modification**: Advise on modifying activities to reduce fatigue, such as breaking tasks into smaller, manageable steps.

3. **ADL and IADL Training**

    - **Adaptive Equipment**: Provide training on the use of adaptive equipment designed for individuals with limited energy, such as ergonomic tools for personal care tasks.
    - **Meal Preparation**: Teach meal preparation techniques that are quick and nutritious, supporting a healthy diet during stress.
    - **Household Management**: Develop strategies for efficient household management, including time-saving techniques and organizational tools.
    - **Personal Care Routine**: Create a structured personal care routine to ensure regular showering and grooming, incorporating relaxation techniques to reduce stress-related avoidance behaviors.

4. **Work-Life Balance**

    - **Structured Schedule**: Develop a structured schedule that balances work, parenting, and self-care activities.
    - **Organizational Tools**: Provide advanced organizational tools and strategies to help the client keep track of work tasks, deadlines, and personal responsibilities.

5. **Parenting Support**

    - **Support Groups**: Facilitate connections with parenting support groups to provide emotional support and reduce feelings of isolation.
    - **Counseling Sessions**: Offer psychosocial counseling sessions to address parenting stress and anxiety, employing cognitive-behavioural techniques.

6. **Social and Emotional Support**

    - **Peer Support**: Facilitate connections with peer support groups and community resources to provide emotional support and reduce feelings of isolation.
    - **Stress Management**: Implement stress management strategies to help stabilize mood and enhance overall mental well-being.

Outcomes:

Post Treatment:

- **Stress Management**: Significant reduction in anxiety symptoms, evidenced by a decrease in BAI scores to below 15, with the client reporting improved emotional regulation and reduced daily stress.
- **ADL and IADL Independence**: Improved engagement in personal care and household tasks, with the client achieving a COPM score increase, reflecting increased independence and reduced need for assistance.
- **Work Performance**: Improved work performance and attendance, with the client maintaining consistent attendance and meeting job demands, as reported by employer feedback.
- **Social Engagement**: Increased participation in social activities and re-engagement in community events, enhancing the client's sense of community and support.
- **Parenting Stress**: Reduced parenting stress, with improved PSI scores by 30%, reflecting better emotional regulation and reduced strain.

Follow-Up Visits:

- Continuously reinforce stress management techniques and activity modifications to ensure the sustainability of the client's improvements in daily activities and work tasks.
- Provide ongoing support and adjust the client's treatment plan based on her feedback, changes in her symptoms, and any new challenges that arise in managing her role transition and parenting responsibilities.

The client demonstrated significant improvement in managing her role transition, stress, and parenting responsibilities, enhancing her overall functionality and independence. She is now capable of performing daily tasks and work activities with greater efficiency and less anxiety. The tailored occupational therapy interventions enabled her to balance her roles as a single parent and professional effectively. Through the collaborative and holistic approach of occupational therapy, the client has regained a better quality of life and improved her capacity to engage in meaningful activities.

Further Reading

Al-Qahtani, M. A., Allajhar, M. A., Alzahrani, A. A., Asiri, M. A., Alsalem, A. F., Alshahrani, S. A., & Alqahtani, N. M. (2023). Sports-related injuries in adolescent athletes: A systematic review. *Cureus, 15*(11), e49392. https://doi.org/10.7759/cureus.49392

Centers for Disease Control and Prevention. (n.d.). Obesity and overweight. National Center for Health Statistics. Retrieved March 1, 2024, from https://www.cdc.gov/nchs/fastats/obesity-overweight.htm.

Cherenack, E. M., & Sikkema, K. J. (2022). Puberty- and menstruation-related stressors are associated with depression, anxiety, and reproductive tract infection symptoms among adolescent girls in Tanzania. *International Journal of Behavioral Medicine, 29*(2), 160–174. https://doi.org/10.1007/s12529-021-10005-1

Desbrow, B. (2021). Youth athlete development and nutrition. *Sports Medicine (Auckland, N.Z.), 51*(Suppl 1), 3–12. https://doi.org/10.1007/s40279-021-01534-6

El Khoudary, S. R., Greendale, G., Crawford, S. L., Avis, N. E., Brooks, M. M., Thurston, R. C., Karvonen-Gutierrez, C., Waetjen, L. E., & Matthews, K. (2019). The emenopause transition and women's health at midlife: A progress report from the Study of Women's Health Across the Nation (SWAN). *Menopause (New York, N.Y.), 26*(10), 1213–1227. https://doi.org/10.1097/GME.0000000000001424

Femi-Agboola, D. M., Sekoni, O. O., & Goodman, O. O. (2017). Dysmenorrhea and its effects on school Absenteeism and school activities among adolescents in selected secondary schools in Ibadan, Nigeria. *Nigerian Medical Journal: Journal of the Nigeria Medical Association, 58*(4), 143–148. https://doi.org/10.4103/nmj.NMJ_47_17

Flynn, T. A., Jones, B. A., & Ausderau, K. K. (2016). Guided imagery and stress in pregnant adolescents. *The American Journal of Occupational Therapy: Official Publication of the American Occupational Therapy Association, 70*(5), 7005220020p1–7005220020p7. https://doi.org/10.5014/ajot.2016.019315

Hill, J., Vogler, J., & Gullo, H. (2023). Occupational therapists' understanding of supporting physical activity participation when working with children and adolescents: A national survey. *Australian Occupational Therapy Journal, 70*(3), 303–313. https://doi.org/10.1111/1440-1630.12854

Morgan, N., & McEvoy, J. (2014). Exploring the bereavement experiences of older women with intellectual disabilities in long-term residential care: A staff perspective. *Omega, 69*(2), 117–135. https://doi.org/10.2190/OM.69.2.b

Mughal, S., Azhar, Y., Mahon, M. M., & Siddiqui, W. J. (2023). Grief reaction and prolonged grief disorder. In *StatPearls*. StatPearls Publishing.

Nagy, C., Jones, P., & Bernard, M. A. (2021). Aging and women's health: An update from the National Institute on Aging. *Clinics in Geriatric Medicine, 37*(4), 533–541. https://doi.org/10.1016/j.cger.2021.05.002

O'Neill, E. A., Ramseyer Winter, V., & Pevehouse, D. (2018). Exploring body appreciation and women's health-related quality of life: The moderating role of age. *Journal of Health Psychology, 23*(14), 1810–1819. https://doi.org/10.1177/1359105316675212

Phipps, M. G., Son, S., Zahn, C., O'Reilly, N., Cantor, A., Frost, J., Gregory, K. D., Jones, M., Kendig, S. M., Nelson, H. D., Pappas, M., Qaseem, A., Ramos, D., Salganicoff, A., Taylor, G., Conry, J., & Women's Preventive Services Initiative (2019). Women's Preventive Services Initiative's well-woman chart: A summary of preventive health recommendations for women. *Obstetrics and Gynecology, 134*(3), 465–469. https://doi.org/10.1097/AOG.0000000000003368

Temelturk, R. D., Ilcioglu Ekici, G., Beberoglu, M., Siklar, Z., & Kilic, B. G. (2021). Managing precocious puberty: A necessity for psychiatric evaluation. *Asian Journal of Psychiatry, 58*, 102617. https://doi.org/10.1016/j.ajp.2021.102617

13 Inter-Partner Violence and Trauma-Informed Care

Chapter Objectives

Upon completion of this chapter, the reader will be able to:

1. Describe the impact of inter-partner violence (IPV) on the occupational performance and daily lives of women.
2. Identify common physical, emotional, and psychosocial challenges faced by women experiencing IPV.
3. Implement trauma-informed care (TIC) principles in occupational therapy practice to support IPV survivors.
4. Apply evidence-based occupational therapy interventions tailored to the needs of women recovering from IPV.
5. Develop culturally competent and inclusive care plans for women affected by IPV.
6. Advocate for the integration of occupational therapy services in IPV support networks and multidisciplinary teams to ensure comprehensive care and support for women throughout their recovery journey.

Inter-Partner Violence

Inter-partner violence (IPV) is a pervasive issue affecting millions of women worldwide, with significant implications for their physical, emotional, and psychological well-being. According to the World Health Organization (WHO), approximately 30% of women globally have experienced physical or sexual violence by an intimate partner. In the United States, the National Intimate Partner and Sexual Violence Survey (NISVS) reports that nearly 1 in 4 women (24.3%) have experienced severe physical violence by an intimate partner in their lifetime, compared to about 1 in 7 men (13.8%).

IPV can result in a range of health issues, including injuries, chronic pain, mental health disorders such as depression and anxiety, and increased risk for substance abuse. Women who experience IPV are more likely to suffer from PTSD, suicidal behavior, and other psychological conditions. They are also more likely to have poorer overall health and higher healthcare costs compared to those who have not experienced IPV. The Centers for Disease Control and Prevention (CDC) estimates that the lifetime economic cost of IPV for women is $103,767 per victim, including medical services, lost productivity, and criminal justice costs.

Impact of IPV on Occupational Performance in Women's Health

IPV significantly disrupts the lives of millions of women globally, influencing their ability to function effectively in personal, social, and professional roles. While IPV affects individuals of all genders, women often face unique and severe challenges due to a complex interplay of social, cultural, and biological factors. These factors not only shape the nature and severity of the violence experienced but also impact the occupational performance and overall well-being of the victims. Recognizing and addressing these nuances is crucial for OTPs to provide effective, empathetic, and empowering care.

1. **Nature and Severity of Violence**: Women are more likely to experience severe forms of IPV, including sexual violence, strangulation, and stalking. Men may more often experience less severe physical violence and psychological aggression. OTPs may need to focus on TIC approaches, ensuring that therapy settings are safe and supportive, and possibly working on assertiveness training to help these women regain control over their personal boundaries and interactions. For instance, OTPs might use role-playing exercises to help women practice setting boundaries and expressing their needs clearly.
2. **Power Dynamics**: IPV against women often occurs within a context of power and control, where the abuser exerts dominance over various aspects of the woman's life. This control can be financial, emotional, or social, making it difficult for women to leave abusive relationships. OTPs must be adept at recognizing these dynamics and may need to employ strategies that empower women within the therapeutic relationship and support them in regaining control over their lives and decisions. For example, introducing goal-setting activities that promote personal decision-making can help restore a sense of autonomy and self-efficacy.
3. **Societal Norms and Gender Roles**: Cultural expectations and gender roles can exacerbate IPV's impact on women. Societal norms that promote male dominance and female submissiveness can perpetuate abuse and make it harder for women to seek help or be believed when they do. OTPs need to be culturally sensitive and may need to work closely with clients to challenge these internalized roles and norms, fostering a more empowering environment for rehabilitation. For instance, OTPs might facilitate group therapy sessions where women can share experiences and support each other in overcoming societal expectations and personal hurdles.
4. **Reproductive Coercion and Sexual Violence**: Women are more likely to experience reproductive coercion, including birth control sabotage and forced pregnancies. Sexual violence and coercion are also more common, leading to significant physical and psychological trauma. OTPs might focus on interventions that address body autonomy and provide education about sexual and reproductive health, alongside therapeutic interventions to manage the trauma associated with such abuse. OTPs might employ body mapping techniques to help women reclaim bodily autonomy after reproductive coercion, paired with educational sessions on sexual health rights and contraception to empower informed personal decisions.
5. **Economic Dependency**: Women, particularly those with children, may face greater economic dependency on their partners, making it more challenging to leave abusive relationships. This dependency can be compounded by unequal access to education and employment opportunities. OTPs can assist by providing support in developing life skills that increase employability and financial independence, such as vocational training and budgeting skills, thereby addressing one of the root causes of their vulnerability to IPV.

6. **Health Consequences**: The health impact of IPV on women is extensive, including injuries, chronic pain, mental health disorders such as depression and anxiety, and an increased risk for substance abuse. Women who experience IPV are also more likely to suffer from PTSD, suicidal behavior, and other psychological conditions. The CDC estimates that the lifetime economic cost of IPV for women is $103,767 per victim, which includes medical services, lost productivity, and criminal justice costs. This might include direct interventions like pain management and mental health therapy, as well as coordination with other health professionals to ensure a holistic approach to healthcare and recovery.

Understanding and addressing the impact of IPV on occupational performance is essential for OTPs. This comprehensive approach helps tailor interventions to meet the specific needs of women recovering from IPV, enhancing their ability to manage daily activities, work, and social interactions effectively.

Types of Trauma Resulting from IPV

The trauma resulting from IPV is multifaceted, affecting various aspects of a victim's life. Understanding the different types of trauma can help in providing targeted and effective interventions. IPV can lead to various types of trauma, including:

- **Physical Trauma**: Injuries, chronic pain, and disabilities resulting from physical violence.
- **Emotional Trauma**: Long-term emotional distress, low self-esteem, and feelings of worthlessness due to emotional abuse.
- **Psychological Trauma**: Mental health disorders such as depression, anxiety, and PTSD.
- **Sexual Trauma**: Physical and emotional consequences of sexual violence and coercion.

It is essential to recognize how individuals respond to trauma, which can vary dramatically (see Figure 13.1). Common trauma responses include:

- **Fight**: Confrontational behavior that might appear in situations where the individual feels trapped or threatened.
- **Flight**: Avoidance behaviors, where the individual may leave or attempt to escape situations that feel unsafe.
- **Freeze**: Inability to act or respond during confrontations or stressful events, often leading to immobilization even in necessary daily activities.
- **Fawn**: Appeasing behavior, where the individual tries to please or placate others to avoid conflict.
- **Flop**: Physical collapse or fainting, which may occur in intensely traumatic situations.

These responses can manifest distinctly in ADLs and occupations, impacting the ability to perform routine tasks, engage socially, and manage personal care. For example, a "freeze" response may cause a person to become non-responsive and unable to complete basic household tasks during a trigger event or unable to drive once in a vehicle, whereas a "fawn" response might lead to overexertion in caregiving roles at the expense of personal well-being.

Understanding these trauma responses within the context of IPV is crucial for OTPs. It allows them to tailor interventions that not only address the physical and emotional

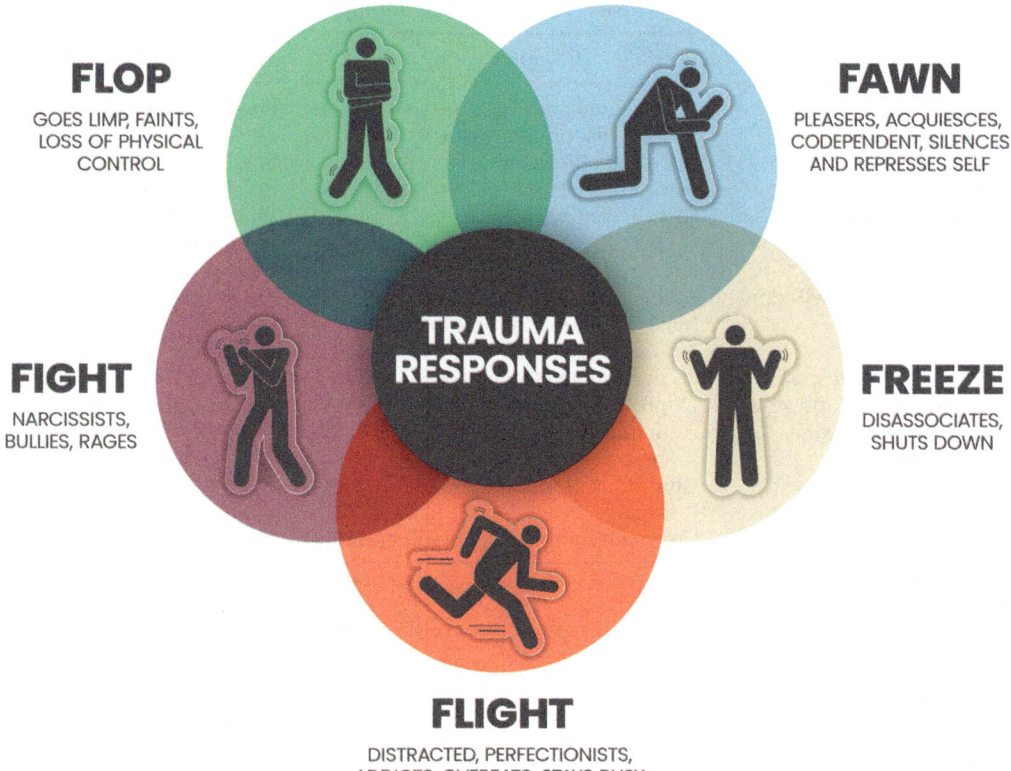

Figure 13.1 Trauma response.

aspects of trauma but also help individuals develop healthier coping mechanisms to manage their daily lives effectively.

It is important to note that not all individuals who experience IPV will be traumatized to the same extent. The impact of IPV can vary significantly based on a range of factors, including the severity and duration of the abuse, the individual's psychological resilience, previous trauma history, and available social support. Two people experiencing the same event may respond differently, with one showing significant signs of trauma while the other may not. Understanding these nuances is crucial for providing effective and personalized care.

Assessments in Occupational Therapy for IPV

OTPs conduct comprehensive assessments to understand the full impact of IPV on a woman's life. These assessments typically include evaluating physical injuries, psychological state, and the effects on daily living and occupational performance. In addition to standardized assessment tools, OTPs also rely on their observations and the information gathered during client interviews. They assess non-verbal communication and body language for signs of distress or discomfort that may not be verbally expressed. Questions are framed carefully to avoid triggering the client while gathering essential information about their experiences and needs.

Table 13.1 Common non-verbal cues indicative of trauma during an interview

Non-Verbal Cue	Possible Indication	Type of Trauma
Flinching	Fear, anxiety, anticipation of harm	Physical, emotional
Avoiding eye contact	Shame, discomfort, distrust	Emotional, psychological
Crossed arms/legs	Self-protection, defensiveness	Emotional, psychological
Fidgeting/hyperactivity	Nervousness, anxiety, discomfort	Psychological
Trembling or shaking	Fear, severe anxiety	Physical, emotional, psychological
Sighing, deep breaths	Stress, attempts to self-calm	Emotional, psychological
Sudden silence or withdrawal	Feeling overwhelmed, dissociation	Psychological, emotional
Inconsistent facial expressions	Masking true emotions, confusion	Psychological, emotional
Increased startle response	Hypervigilance, heightened sensitivity	Physical, Psychological
Reduced physical movements	Depression, resignation, helplessness	Psychological, emotional
Guarding movements	Anticipation of pain, protecting injured areas	Physical
Tense posture	Chronic stress, readiness to react to threats	Emotional, Psychological
Tearfulness	Overwhelming sadness, vulnerability	Emotional, Psychological

Non-Verbal Communication and Body Language

During client interviews, OTPs pay close attention to non-verbal cues such as body language, eye contact, and facial expressions. Signs such as flinching, avoiding eye contact, or displaying signs of anxiety can indicate trauma. These observations are critical in understanding the client's current emotional state and tailoring the assessment process to be as supportive and non-threatening as possible. Table 13.1 highlights common non-verbal cues indicative of trauma during an interview and the types of trauma they may indicate.

Sensitive Questioning Techniques

OTPs should use sensitive questioning techniques to gather information without causing further distress. Questions are open-ended and framed to give the client control over the information they share. Examples of sensitive questions include:

1. "Can you tell me about a typical day in your life?"
2. "What are some activities you find challenging to do?"
3. "Are there any situations or places that make you feel unsafe or uncomfortable?"

These questions help gather relevant information about the client's daily life and challenges without directly probing into traumatic experiences.

Standardized Assessment Tools

Relevant assessment tools include:

- **Canadian Occupational Performance Measure (COPM)**: This tool is relevant to IPV as it helps assess perceived performance and satisfaction in daily activities, which can be

significantly disrupted by the physical and psychological effects of IPV. By identifying specific areas where the woman feels challenged, OTPs can prioritize interventions that enhance her daily functioning and well-being.
- **PTSD Checklist (PCL)**: IPV often leads to post-traumatic stress disorder (PTSD), which can severely impact a woman's mental health and ability to engage in daily activities. The PCL screens for PTSD symptoms, allowing OTPs to tailor interventions that address trauma-related challenges and improve occupational performance.
- **Trauma Symptom Inventory (TSI)**: The TSI assesses the severity of trauma-related symptoms, including anxiety, depression, dissociation, and anger. This comprehensive understanding of trauma symptoms is essential for developing therapeutic approaches that address the multifaceted impact of IPV on a woman's life.
- **Life Events Checklist (LEC)**: Identifying potentially traumatic events experienced by the client provides context for their current psychological state and needs. The LEC helps OTPs understand the broader context of the client's trauma history, enabling them to create more personalized and effective intervention plans.
- **State-Trait Anxiety Inventory (STAI)**: Anxiety is frequently experienced by women who have suffered IPV, impacting their ability to participate in daily activities and maintain social relationships. The STAI assesses both the current state of anxiety and the more enduring trait anxiety, helping OTPs design interventions that reduce anxiety and promote a sense of security and calm.
- **Beck Depression Inventory (BDI)**: Depression is a common consequence of IPV, affecting motivation, energy levels, and overall mental health. The BDI measures the severity of depression, providing critical insights into the emotional state of the client and guiding the development of effective therapeutic strategies.
- **Safety Assessment**: Evaluating immediate and long-term safety needs is crucial for women experiencing IPV. This assessment helps identify the risk of ongoing violence and the need for emergency resources or safe housing, ensuring that interventions prioritize the client's safety and stability.

By utilizing these assessment tools and techniques, OTPs can develop a personalized intervention plan that addresses the specific needs of women affected by IPV, ensuring a holistic and effective approach to recovery and empowerment.

Occupational Therapy Approaches in Trauma Healing for Women

Trauma healing in the context of IPV requires a holistic and client-centered approach. Implementing TIC in occupational therapy involves recognizing the widespread impact of trauma and integrating this understanding into all aspects of practice. This section delves into the essential components and principles of TIC, highlighting the significant role of occupational therapy in addressing the multifaceted challenges faced by women experiencing IPV. By understanding and applying these principles, OTPs can create a supportive and empowering environment for trauma survivors. Contextualizing occupational performance and functioning within TIC is critical, as it allows for a deeper understanding of how trauma affects daily life and activities.

The Three "E's" of Trauma: Event(s), Experience of Event(s), and Effect

According to the Substance Abuse and Mental Health Services Administration (SAMHSA), trauma involves three critical components:

- **Event(s)**: Trauma can result from single or repeated events involving extreme threats of physical or psychological harm (e.g., natural disasters, violence) or severe neglect that imperils healthy development.
- **Experience of Event(s)**: How an individual experiences and interprets the event(s) is crucial. This can be influenced by cultural beliefs, social supports, and developmental stage. One person may find an event traumatic while another may not.
- **Effect**: The long-lasting adverse effects of the event(s) on an individual's mental, physical, emotional, and social well-being. These effects can be immediate or delayed, short-term or long-term, and can include difficulties in coping, trust, cognitive processes, behavior regulation, and emotional expression.

These components emphasize the importance of viewing trauma through a personalized lens, recognizing that each individual's response to trauma is unique and multifaceted.

Principles of TIC

SAMHSA outlines six key principles that guide a trauma-informed approach. These principles are designed to create a supportive environment that promotes healing and empowerment for trauma survivors:

1. **Safety**: Ensuring the physical and emotional safety of clients is paramount. This involves creating a welcoming environment and establishing clear boundaries.
2. **Trustworthiness and Transparency**: Building trust through consistent and open communication.
3. **Peer Support**: Encouraging connections with others who have experienced similar trauma.
4. **Collaboration and Mutuality**: Empowering clients by involving them in the decision-making process.
5. **Empowerment, Voice, and Choice**: Focusing on strengths and fostering resilience.
6. **Cultural, Historical, and Gender Issues**: Being sensitive to and addressing cultural, historical, and gender-specific factors that influence the client's experience.

By adhering to these principles, OTPs can foster a therapeutic alliance that respects and validates the client's experiences and promotes recovery.

Impact on ADLs

IPV can significantly disrupt a woman's ability to perform daily activities. This disruption can manifest in various ways, affecting self-care, household management, work productivity, and social participation. Recognizing these impacts is crucial for providing comprehensive and effective occupational therapy interventions:

- **Self-Care**: Physical injuries or psychological distress can make basic self-care tasks, such as bathing, dressing, and grooming, challenging. Research indicates that approximately 45% of women experiencing IPV report difficulties in performing self-care activities due to physical injuries and mental health issues.
- **Household Management**: Managing household responsibilities, including cooking, cleaning, and childcare, can become overwhelming due to physical limitations, emotional exhaustion, or controlling behaviors from the abuser. Studies show that nearly 38% of women facing IPV have reported challenges in maintaining household tasks and managing childcare responsibilities effectively.

- **Work and Productivity**: Maintaining employment or academic responsibilities may be difficult due to frequent absences, decreased concentration, and the impact of trauma on cognitive functions. Data from the Bureau of Labor Statistics reveal that women experiencing IPV are more likely to miss work, with 25% reporting job loss due to the abuse.
- **Social Participation**: Victims of IPV often experience social isolation, either imposed by the abuser or self-imposed to avoid shame and potential triggers. This isolation can lead to a decline in social and recreational activities, further impacting mental health. According to the CDC, about 50% of women who have experienced IPV report significant reductions in their social interactions and community participation.

Understanding these impacts allows OTPs to develop targeted interventions that address both the physical and psychological barriers to daily functioning, ultimately promoting a more holistic recovery process for women affected by IPV.

Occupational Therapy Interventions for Trauma Healing

OTPs can utilize various therapeutic modalities to address the complex needs of women recovering from trauma. It is important to note that some interventions may require specialized training and OTPs should abide by the laws within their state and regulatory body/regulations.

- **Cognitive-Behavioural Therapy (CBT)**: CBT can help clients reframe negative thought patterns and develop healthier coping mechanisms. OTPs can integrate CBT techniques to address issues such as anxiety, depression, and PTSD.
- **Sensory Integration Therapy**: This approach can assist in regulating sensory processing issues often exacerbated by trauma, improving overall emotional regulation. Techniques may include the use of sensory diets, therapeutic use of pressure, and controlled sensory experiences to enhance sensory modulation and coping skills.
- **Expressive Therapies**: Art, music, and dance therapies can provide non-verbal outlets for expressing and processing trauma. These therapies can be particularly useful for clients who find it difficult to articulate their experiences verbally. Activities might include painting, drawing, playing musical instruments, or movement exercises that facilitate emotional release and self-expression.
- **Occupational Engagement**: Encouraging participation in meaningful activities can foster a sense of purpose and normalcy, aiding in the recovery process. Activities can range from hobbies and crafts to volunteer work and community involvement. This approach helps clients rebuild their identities and develop new routines that support their well-being.
- **Emotional Support and Coping Strategies**: Providing emotional support through counseling and teaching coping strategies such as mindfulness and relaxation techniques can help manage anxiety and depression. Techniques may include guided imagery, progressive muscle relaxation, and breathing exercises. Additionally, teaching clients grounding techniques can help them stay present and manage flashbacks or dissociation.
- **Mindfulness-Based Stress Reduction (MBSR)**: Incorporating mindfulness practices can help clients increase their awareness of the present moment, reduce stress, and enhance emotional regulation. Techniques include mindful breathing, body scans, and mindful movement (e.g., yoga).

- **Dialectical Behavior Therapy (DBT)**: DBT can be effective for clients experiencing intense emotions and self-destructive behaviors. It combines CBT techniques with mindfulness and distress tolerance strategies. OTPs may need specialized training to integrate DBT skills training, including emotion regulation, distress tolerance, interpersonal effectiveness, and mindfulness.
- **Narrative Therapy**: This approach involves helping clients reframe and reconstruct their personal narratives to make sense of their experiences and develop a more empowering story. Techniques include life story work, journaling, and therapeutic writing.
- **Psychoeducation**: Educating clients about trauma and its effects can empower them to understand their responses and engage actively in their healing process. Topics may include understanding PTSD, the impact of trauma on the brain and body, and strategies for self-care and resilience.
- **Physical Activity and Exercise**: Engaging in regular physical activity can help reduce symptoms of depression and anxiety, improve mood, and enhance overall physical health. Tailored exercise programs can include walking, yoga, swimming, or strength training, depending on the client's preferences and physical abilities.
- **Social Skills Training**: Rebuilding social connections and improving communication skills are crucial for clients who have experienced social isolation due to trauma. Activities might include role-playing, group therapy, and social outings designed to enhance interpersonal skills and build supportive relationships.
- **Life Skills Training**: Teaching practical skills that enhance independence and daily functioning can be particularly empowering for clients. This may include time management, financial management, job readiness, and problem-solving skills.
- **Relaxation and Stress Management Techniques**: Techniques such as deep breathing exercises, progressive muscle relaxation, and biofeedback can help clients manage stress and reduce physiological arousal associated with trauma.
- **Peer Support and Group Therapy**: Facilitating or connecting clients to support groups and group therapy sessions can provide a sense of community and shared experience. Peer support can be a powerful tool in the healing process, offering validation, mutual support, and practical advice from others who have experienced similar challenges.

By integrating these diverse interventions, OTPs can provide holistic and effective support to women recovering from trauma, enhancing their overall well-being and enabling them to reclaim their daily lives.

Specific OT Interventions for IPV

Given the unique challenges faced by women experiencing IPV, certain occupational therapy interventions can be particularly beneficial:

- **Safety Planning**: Assisting clients in developing a safety plan is crucial. This involves identifying safe spaces, understanding how to seek help, and creating an emergency kit with essential items.
- **Empowerment through Skill Building**: Teaching skills that enhance independence and self-efficacy, such as budgeting, time management, and assertiveness training, can empower women to regain control over their lives.

- **Support Groups**: Facilitating or connecting clients to support groups can provide a sense of community and shared experience. Peer support can be a powerful tool in the healing process.
- **Advocacy and Resource Navigation**: Helping clients navigate available resources, including legal assistance, housing services, and healthcare, ensures they receive comprehensive support. OTPs can act as advocates, coordinating care and connecting clients with necessary services.
- **Trauma-Informed Occupational Engagement**: Tailoring occupational activities to be trauma-sensitive, ensuring that they are paced appropriately and that the client feels safe and in control throughout the process.

By integrating these interventions, OTPs can provide holistic and effective support to women recovering from the trauma of IPV, enhancing their overall well-being and enabling them to reclaim their daily lives.

Implementing Trauma-Informed Practice in OT settings

Implementing trauma-informed practice in OT settings involves integrating key principles into every aspect of care to support the healing and recovery of women who have experienced IPV. This approach ensures that the care provided is sensitive to the needs and experiences of these women, fostering a safe and supportive environment for their rehabilitation. Below, we discuss practical strategies for applying these principles in various OT settings and detail specific assessment and intervention techniques.

Key Principles of Trauma-Informed Practice in OT Settings

1. **Safety**: Ensuring physical and emotional safety for clients is paramount in OT settings. Therapists can create a safe environment by ensuring privacy, reducing environmental triggers (e.g., loud noises, harsh lighting), and establishing clear boundaries and routines that help clients feel secure and supported.
2. **Trustworthiness and Transparency**: Building trust through consistent and open communication is essential. Therapists should explain the purpose of each intervention, provide clear information about the therapy process, and involve clients in setting goals and making decisions about their treatment.
3. **Peer Support**: Encouraging connections with others who have experienced similar trauma can be a powerful tool for healing. In OT settings, therapists can facilitate support groups or connect clients with peer mentors, fostering a sense of community and shared understanding.
4. **Collaboration and Mutuality**: Promoting a sense of partnership between therapist and client enhances the therapeutic relationship. Therapists should actively involve clients in the treatment planning process, respect their input, and work together to identify and achieve therapy goals, reinforcing the client's role as an active participant in their recovery.

5. **Empowerment, Voice, and Choice**: Providing opportunities for clients to make choices about their treatment empowers them and helps build self-efficacy. Therapists can offer various intervention options and encourage clients to select activities that they find meaningful and relevant, thereby promoting autonomy and self-confidence.
6. **Cultural, Historical, and Gender Sensitivity**: Understanding and respecting the cultural, historical, and gender contexts of each client's experiences is crucial. Therapists should educate themselves on the client's background, incorporate culturally relevant practices into therapy, and address any specific needs related to the client's identity and experiences of trauma.

Practical Strategies for Trauma-Informed Assessment and Evaluation

Effective trauma-informed assessment and evaluation involve using tools and techniques that are sensitive to the impacts of trauma, minimizing re-traumatization, and gathering comprehensive information to inform intervention planning.

- **Use Trauma-Sensitive Assessment Tools**: Employ tools that consider the physical, emotional, and psychological impacts of trauma.
- **Gentle, Open-Ended Questioning**: Frame questions to avoid triggering the client, ensuring they feel safe and in control.
- **Observe Non-Verbal Cues**: Pay close attention to body language, eye contact, and facial expressions to gain insights into the client's emotional state.

To integrate these principles into various OT settings, specific interventions and strategies must be tailored to the unique needs of each practice area. Table 13.2 lists how trauma-informed practices can be implemented across different OT settings, highlighting assessment and intervention techniques specific to women experiencing IPV.

By tailoring trauma-informed practices to each specific setting, OTPs can create supportive environments that facilitate the recovery and empowerment of women experiencing IPV, addressing their unique needs and challenges effectively.

Implications for OTPs

Incorporating trauma-informed practices into occupational therapy settings is essential, as trauma is not always evident in a client's medical history. Therefore, it is best practice for OTPs to utilize these principles universally with all clients, particularly women, to ensure a sensitive and supportive approach. This comprehensive application helps in recognizing and addressing potential trauma, fostering resilience, and enhancing overall well-being. By adopting TIC, OTPs can better support the healing journey of their clients, ultimately leading to more effective and meaningful therapeutic outcomes.

Community Engagement and Cultural Competence in Trauma Recovery

Community engagement and cultural competence are crucial elements in the recovery process for women who have experienced IPV. Effective community engagement and culturally competent care can significantly enhance the recovery process by addressing the unique needs of women from diverse backgrounds. Research shows that when

Table 13.2 Implementing trauma-informed practices in various OT settings

Setting	Assessment/Evaluation	Intervention
Neurorehabilitation	– Use COPM to identify specific challenges in daily activities affected by neurological conditions and trauma.	– Integrate CBT techniques to address trauma-related cognitive and emotional challenges. – Use sensory integration therapy to help regulate sensory processing issues exacerbated by trauma.
Orthopedic Rehabilitation	– Assess physical injuries using TSI to understand the impact of trauma on recovery. – Evaluate pain levels and functional limitations with standardized tools like the Visual Analog Scale (VAS) and the Disabilities of the Arm, Shoulder, and Hand (DASH).	– Develop personalized exercise programs that consider physical limitations and trauma history. – Use mindfulness-based stress reduction (MBSR) techniques to manage chronic pain and emotional stress.
Community Health	– Conduct safety assessments to identify immediate and long-term safety needs. – Use the Life Events Checklist (LEC) to understand the broader context of the client's trauma history.	– Facilitate support groups and connect clients with community resources for legal and housing assistance. – Implement community-based activities that promote social engagement and empowerment, such as community gardening or art projects.
Inpatient/Outpatient	– Use the PTSD Checklist (PCL) to screen for PTSD symptoms and tailor interventions accordingly. – Assess anxiety and depression levels using the State-Trait Anxiety Inventory (STAI) and the Beck Depression Inventory (BDI).	– Implement mindfulness practices, such as mindful breathing and body scans, to enhance emotional regulation. – Offer expressive therapies, including art and music therapy, to provide non-verbal outlets for expressing and processing trauma.
Psychiatric Units	– Use the Trauma Symptom Inventory (TSI) to assess the severity of trauma-related symptoms. – Conduct detailed interviews to understand the client's psychological state and daily challenges.	– Provide psychoeducation about trauma and its effects to empower clients with knowledge. – Use dialectical behavior therapy (DBT) skills training to help clients manage intense emotions and develop healthier coping strategies.
School-Based Practice	– Assess the impact of trauma on academic performance and social participation using standardized tools and observations. – Use tools like the Child Occupational Self-Assessment (COSA) to gather student perspectives.	– Collaborate with school counselors to provide a safe and supportive learning environment. – Implement trauma-sensitive classroom strategies, such as providing quiet spaces and using consistent routines. – Facilitate social skills groups to enhance peer interactions and build supportive relationships.

(Continued)

Table 13.2 (Continued)

Setting	Assessment/Evaluation	Intervention
Intensive Care Unit (ICU)	– Monitor for signs of acute stress and trauma using real-time observations and brief assessment tools. – Evaluate the impact of ICU stay on mental health with tools like the Intensive Care Psychological Assessment Tool (ICPAT).	– Provide family-centered care to reduce stress and trauma, including regular updates and involving family in care planning. – Use relaxation techniques and sensory modulation (e.g., music therapy) to reduce anxiety and promote a sense of control.
Pediatric Settings	– Use child-friendly assessment tools to gauge the impact of trauma on play and daily activities. – Observe play behavior for signs of distress or trauma (e.g., withdrawal, aggression, repetitive play themes).	– Implement play therapy techniques to help children express and process trauma. – Engage in family therapy sessions to support the child and family in understanding and coping with trauma.
Home Health	– Conduct home safety assessments to identify potential triggers and ensure a safe environment. – Use the COPM to understand the client's challenges in their home context (e.g., difficulty managing household tasks, interacting with family members, engaging in leisure activities)	– Provide home-based interventions that promote a sense of safety and stability, such as creating a calming routine. – Use mindfulness and relaxation techniques to manage stress and anxiety in the home setting.

healthcare providers, including OTPs, engage with the community and apply culturally competent practices, the outcomes for trauma recovery improve substantially.

The Importance of Community Engagement

Community engagement involves working collaboratively with individuals, groups, and organizations within the community to address the needs and challenges faced by women recovering from IPV. This approach promotes a sense of belonging, empowerment, and support, which are essential for healing and recovery.

Benefits of Community Engagement

1. **Enhanced Support Networks**: Building strong support networks within the community can provide women with essential resources, emotional support, and a sense of solidarity. A study published in the *American Journal of Community Psychology* found that social support from the community significantly reduces PTSD symptoms and promotes psychological well-being among survivors of trauma.
2. **Access to Resources**: Engaging with community organizations can help women access resources such as legal assistance, housing, healthcare, and job training. The *Journal of Social Service Research* reports that women who are connected with community

resources are more likely to find stable housing and employment, which are critical factors in long-term recovery and independence.
3. **Empowerment and Advocacy**: Community engagement empowers women to advocate for their rights and participate actively in their recovery process. Empowered women are more likely to regain control over their lives and make decisions that promote their well-being. Research indicates that community-based advocacy programs increase self-efficacy and confidence among survivors, leading to better mental health outcomes and reduced symptoms of depression and anxiety.
4. **Cultural Relevance**: Collaborating with community members ensures that interventions are culturally relevant and respectful of the diverse backgrounds of the women being served. A study in the *Journal of Cultural Diversity and Ethnic Minority Psychology* shows that culturally tailored interventions are more effective in engaging clients and improving health outcomes. Women who receive culturally competent care report higher satisfaction and better adherence to treatment plans.

OTPs play a vital role in facilitating community engagement for women recovering from IPV. By building strong partnerships with local organizations, providing culturally sensitive care, empowering clients through education and advocacy, and conducting thorough cultural assessments, OTPs can significantly enhance the effectiveness of recovery programs. These actions ensure that the care provided is comprehensive, culturally relevant, and supportive, fostering a healing environment that addresses the complex needs of women affected by IPV.

The Role of Cultural Competence

Cultural competence is the ability of healthcare providers to understand, respect, and effectively respond to the cultural and linguistic needs of patients from diverse backgrounds. In the context of IPV and trauma recovery, cultural competence involves recognizing and addressing the unique cultural factors that influence a woman's experience of violence and her path to recovery.

Key Aspects of Cultural Competence

1. **Cultural Awareness**: Being aware of one's own cultural beliefs and biases and understanding how these may impact interactions with clients.
   - **OTPs' Role**: OTPs engage in self-reflection and training to recognize their biases and how these might affect their professional interactions. They seek to understand the cultural backgrounds of their clients and how these influence their experiences and needs.
2. **Cultural Knowledge**: Gaining knowledge about different cultural practices, beliefs, and values, particularly those related to health, healing, and interpersonal relationships.
   - **OTPs' Role**: OTPs educate themselves about the cultural backgrounds of the communities they serve. They attend cultural competence training and actively seek information about cultural practices that may influence their clients' health and well-being.
3. **Cultural Skills**: Developing the skills to communicate effectively and provide culturally sensitive care.
   - **OTPs' Role**: OTPs learn to use culturally appropriate communication techniques, including language and non-verbal cues, and may utilize interpreters when

necessary. They adapt their therapeutic approaches to align with the cultural values and practices of their clients.
- **Cultural Encounters**: Engaging in interactions with clients from diverse backgrounds to build cultural competence and improve service delivery.
- **OTPs' Role**: OTPs actively engage with clients from various cultural backgrounds, seeking to understand their unique needs and preferences. This engagement helps build trust and rapport, making clients feel more comfortable and supported in their recovery journey.

Developing cultural competence is a dynamic and ongoing process that requires commitment and effort from OTPs. By continuously engaging in self-reflection, seeking education and training, honing communication skills, and building meaningful relationships with clients from diverse backgrounds, OTPs can provide more effective and compassionate care. This not only enhances the therapeutic outcomes for women recovering from IPV but also fosters an inclusive and supportive healthcare environment that respects and values diversity.

Actionable Steps for Enhancing Cultural Competence

As OTPs continue to serve increasingly diverse populations, it is imperative to cultivate and enhance cultural competence. Doing so not only enriches the therapeutic relationship but also ensures that interventions are effectively tailored to meet the unique cultural needs of each client. The following table, Table 13.3, provides a structured guide on how

Table 13.3 Actionable steps for OTPs to enhance cultural competence

Key Aspect	Actionable Steps for OTPs
Cultural Awareness	Engage in self-reflection exercises to identify personal biases and assumptions.
	Participate in workshops and training sessions focused on cultural competence and self-awareness.
	Seek feedback from colleagues and clients about potential cultural insensitivities and areas for improvement.
	Maintain an open and non-judgmental attitude when learning about different cultures.
Cultural Knowledge	Educate yourself about the cultural backgrounds of the clients you serve through reading, online courses, and cultural events.
	Attend cultural competence training programs and seminars.
	Engage with cultural liaisons or consultants to gain insights into specific cultural practices and health beliefs.
	Develop resource materials that include culturally relevant information for clients.
Cultural Skills	Learn and practice culturally appropriate communication techniques, including the use of respectful language and gestures.
	Utilize professional interpreters when necessary to ensure accurate communication.
	Adapt therapeutic interventions to align with the cultural values and practices of your clients.
	Incorporate cultural rituals and practices into therapy sessions when appropriate.
Cultural Encounters	Actively seek opportunities to work with clients from diverse cultural backgrounds.
	Participate in community events and activities to better understand the cultural context of your clients.
	Build relationships with cultural leaders and community organizations to foster trust and collaboration.
	Reflect on and document your experiences with culturally diverse clients to improve future interactions.

OTPs can develop and apply cultural competence in their practice, spanning cultural awareness, knowledge, skills, and encounters.

By taking these specific steps, OTPs can significantly enhance their cultural competence, leading to more effective, respectful, and relevant care for women recovering from IPV. This comprehensive approach not only improves therapeutic outcomes but also ensures that care is holistic and inclusive, effectively addressing the diverse needs of all clients. In the context of women's health, such practices are essential for fostering a supportive environment that promotes healing, empowerment, and long-term well-being.

Case Study in IPV and TIC

Background and Medical History: The client, a 34-year-old woman, has been enduring IPV for over five years. Initially, she sought medical attention for anxiety and sleep disturbances but later revealed recurring physical and emotional abuse by her partner. Medical records include multiple visits for injuries such as bruises, a fractured wrist, and chronic lower back pain initially attributed to accidents. Psychological evaluations show symptoms of severe depression and post-traumatic stress disorder (PTSD). Her medical history includes chronic migraines and gastrointestinal issues, which have been exacerbated by the ongoing stress and trauma.

Prior Level of Function:

- **Professional**: Employed as a school teacher, well-respected by peers and students.
- **Social**: Actively participated in community groups and had a vibrant social life.
- **Physical**: Engaged regularly in yoga and jogging.
- **Living Situation**: Previously lived with her partner in a shared apartment.

Household Living Arrangements and Social History:

- **Current Living Situation**: Now residing with her sister in a different town, several towns away from her previous residence.
- **Family and Social Support**: Mother of two children, ages 7 and 9; her social support was limited due to her partner's controlling behavior.

Change in Functional Status and Challenges:

- **ADLs**: Experiences difficulties in managing daily tasks due to physical injuries and emotional exhaustion.
- **Work**: Frequent leaves of absence have put her job at risk.
- **Social Activities**: Greatly reduced involvement in community activities, leading to social isolation.

OT Assessments:

- **Trauma Symptom Inventory (TSI)**: High scores indicate severe distress and PTSD symptoms.
- **Life Event Checklist (LEC)**: Confirms multiple traumatic events related to ongoing IPV.
- **Observational assessment during interviews**: Noted guarded body language, such as crossed arms and avoidance of eye contact, indicative of a heightened state of alertness and anxiety. The client displayed signs of hypervigilance, frequently scanning the environment and exhibiting a startle response to sudden noises. These behaviors suggest ongoing trauma and fear, impacting her ability to engage fully in therapeutic activities.

- **Canadian Occupational Performance Measure (COPM)**: Scored 3/10 in performance and satisfaction, indicating significant difficulties in occupational performance and satisfaction with current abilities.
- **Numeric Pain Rating Scale**: Reports a pain level of 7/10 in the lower back and 5/10 in the wrist, affecting daily activities.

Occupational Therapy Plan of Care and Goals: The client will receive skilled occupational therapy services three times a week for 12 weeks to improve independence in ADLs, manage anxiety and depressive symptoms, and enhance quality of life.

Goals:

- Target a 30% reduction in TSI scores within three months through focused therapy, including the use of grounding techniques to manage triggers, to improve her ability to manage daily tasks and engage in social activities.
- Increase COPM performance and satisfaction scores to 7/10 within three months to enable the client to perform daily activities with minimal assistance and improve her work attendance.
- Re-establish connections with family and participate in community activities monthly to reduce social isolation and increase emotional support.
- Achieve a 50% reduction in pain levels in both the lower back and wrist within three months through targeted therapeutic interventions to improve her ability to engage in daily activities and maintain employment.

Interventions:

- **Trauma-Informed Care**: Implement cognitive-behavioural therapy to manage PTSD and anxiety, focusing on coping strategies, emotional regulation, and the use of grounding techniques when triggered.
- **Safety Planning and Advocacy**: Develop a safety plan and connect with local services for support, ensuring the client's immediate safety and providing resources for long-term stability.
- **Social Skills Training**: Encourage social interactions and confidence rebuilding through supported community activities, helping the client re-engage with her social network and community.
- **Grounding Techniques Education**: Teach and practice grounding techniques to help the client manage and reduce symptoms of anxiety and PTSD, particularly during moments of high stress or triggers.
- **Pelvic Floor Therapy**: Introduce exercises and techniques to strengthen the pelvic floor and reduce symptoms, incorporating education on menstrual cycle tracking to identify phases with exacerbated pain for better activity planning.
- **Physical Therapy for Pain Management**: Utilize modalities such as heat therapy, TENS units, and gentle stretching exercises to manage lower back pain. Introduce wrist exercises to improve strength and flexibility, and use splinting techniques if necessary to support the healing process.

Outcomes:

- **Post Treatment**: Showed significant improvement in managing PTSD, with a 35% reduction in TSI scores, and improved functional independence with COPM scores of 7/10.

- **Functional Independence**: Achieved improved independence in daily tasks, allowing her to maintain her job and perform her professional duties effectively.
- **Social Reintegration**: Successfully reconnected with family and regularly attended community support groups, enhancing her social support system and emotional well-being.
- **Pain Reduction**: Reported a 50% reduction in pain levels in both the lower back and wrist, significantly improving her ability to perform daily activities and maintain employment.

At the conclusion of therapy, the client demonstrated marked improvements across various domains, showcasing enhanced resilience and adaptive skills in managing the impacts of IPV. Significant progress was noted in PTSD management, functional independence, social reintegration, and pain reduction, enabling her to engage more fully in her professional and personal life. The client's commitment to therapy and collaboration with the occupational therapy team resulted in sustainable improvements, highlighting her capacity for growth and resilience in the face of adversity.

Further Reading

American Occupational Therapy Association. (2020). Occupational therapy practice framework: Domain and process (4th ed.). *American Journal of Occupational Therapy, 74*(Supplement_2), 7412410010. https://doi.org/10.5014/ajot.2020.74S2001

Ballan, M., Freyer, M., & Romanelli, M. (2022). Occupational functioning among intimate partner violence survivors with disabilities: A retrospective analysis. *Occupational Therapy in Health Care, 36*(4), 368–390. https://doi.org/10.1080/07380577.2021.1994684

Colantonio, A., & Valera, E. M. (2022). Brain injury and intimate partner violence. *The Journal of Head Trauma Rehabilitation, 37*(1), 2–4. https://doi.org/10.1097/HTR.0000000000000763

Grossman, S., Cooper, Z., Buxton, H., Hendrickson, S., Lewis-O'Connor, A., Stevens, J., Wong, L. Y., & Bonne, S. (2021). Trauma-informed care: Recognizing and resisting re-traumatization in health care. *Trauma Surgery & Acute Care Open, 6*(1), e000815. https://doi.org/10.1136/tsaco-2021-000815

Javaherian-Dysinger, H., Krpalek, D., Huecker, E., Hewitt, L., Cabrera, M., Brown, C., Francis, J., Rogers, K., & Server, S. (2016). Occupational needs and goals of survivors of domestic violence. *Occupational Therapy in Health Care, 30*(2), 175–186. https://doi.org/10.3109/07380577.2015.1109741

Kyle, J. (2023). Intimate partner violence. *The Medical Clinics of North America, 107*(2), 385–395. https://doi.org/10.1016/j.mcna.2022.10.012

Mason, J., & Stagnitti, K. (2023). Occupational therapists' practice with complex trauma: A profile. *Australian Occupational Therapy Journal, 70*(2), 190–201. https://doi.org/10.1111/1440-1630.12846

Sorrentino, A. E., Iverson, K. M., Tuepker, A., True, G., Cusack, M., Newell, S., & Dichter, M. E. (2021). Mental health care in the context of intimate partner violence: Survivor perspectives. *Psychological Services, 18*(4), 512–522. https://doi.org/10.1037/ser0000427

Toccalino, D., Asare, G., Fleming, J., Yin, J., Kieftenburg, A., Moore, A., Haag, H. L., Chan, V., Babineau, J., MacGregor, N., & Colantonio, A. (2024). Exploring the relationships between rehabilitation and survivors of intimate partner violence: A scoping review. *Trauma, Violence & Abuse, 25*(2), 1638–1660. https://doi.org/10.1177/15248380231196807

14 Special Topics

Chapter Objectives

Upon completion of this chapter, the reader will be able to:

1. Identify emerging technologies in women's health ("FemTech") and their applications in occupational therapy to enhance client care and independence.
2. Discuss the unique physiological and psychological challenges faced by female athletes and the role of occupational therapy in addressing these challenges to optimize performance and prevent injuries.
3. Describe the impact of long-term disabilities on women's health and daily functioning, and implement evidence-based occupational therapy interventions to support these clients.
4. Integrate nutrition management strategies into occupational therapy practice to support overall health and specific conditions like osteoporosis and hormonal imbalances.
5. Incorporate alternative medicine practices into occupational therapy care plans in a way that aligns with client preferences and enhances therapeutic outcomes.
6. Advocate for policies and practices that promote women's health, emphasizing the role of occupational therapy in addressing health disparities and supporting

Women's Health and Technology

Historically, women's health has seen insufficient investment in research and development. Emerging technologies aimed at enhancing women's health ("FemTech") have the potential to significantly improve this area. Assistive technology plays a pivotal role in addressing women's unique health challenges, promoting independence and quality of life in various domains. These technologies are tailored to women's diverse physiological, social, and psychological needs, empowering them to overcome health-related barriers. For OTPs, integrating assistive technology offers opportunities to deliver client-centered care and enhance independence. Considerations such as cultural sensitivity, educational levels, language barriers, and disabilities are essential in utilizing modern technology effectively. The National Centers of Excellence in Women's Health (CoEs) aim to increase the use of information technology to improve women's care, highlighting the importance of adapting technology to meet individual patient needs. From personal hygiene to mobility and clothing management, specialized devices cater to women's specific needs, fostering autonomy and comfort in daily occupations.

Assistive Technology for Breast Health

Devices for breast health cater to the unique needs of women, supporting early detection and management of breast conditions. OTPs play a critical role in recommending and integrating these technologies to support clients in maintaining personal hygiene and monitoring breast health independently.

- **Breast Self-Examination Aids**: These aids assist women in performing thorough and accurate self-examinations of their breasts. They typically include guides or markers to ensure comprehensive coverage during examinations, empowering women in proactive breast health monitoring. These aids are particularly helpful for women with limited mobility or those needing assistance in maintaining a consistent examination technique. By promoting regular self-examinations, OTPs empower women to take proactive steps in their health care, promoting occupational engagement through self-care practices. See Table 14.1 for techniques for breast self-examination (BSE) for women with limited mobility.
- **Breast Pumps**: Breast pumps aid in expressing and storing breast milk, supporting breastfeeding mothers who may face challenges with latching, milk production, or scheduling feedings. They offer convenience and flexibility for nursing mothers, enabling them to continue breastfeeding while managing other responsibilities or when direct breastfeeding is not possible. OTPs educate and assist clients in using breast pumps effectively, ensuring that mothers can maintain their occupational roles and routines while supporting infant feeding needs.

Table 14.1 OT techniques and assistive devices for performing breast self-examination (BSE) with limited mobility

Technique	Description
Seated BSE	Instruct the woman to perform BSE while seated, using her opposite hand to examine each breast thoroughly.
Wall-Mounted Mirror	Recommend using a wall-mounted mirror to aid in visual inspection of the breasts, adjusting for angles.
Long-Handle Mirror	Extendable mirrors with handles for better reach and visibility during self-examination.
Tactile Markers	Raised or textured markers applied to breasts to ensure complete coverage during examination.
Bra Aids	Adaptive hooks or fasteners for easier bra removal and examination access.
Adaptive Breast Self-Examination	Teach the use of adaptive devices with handles or grips to facilitate thorough and accurate breast examination.
Guided Self-Examination Technique	Provide a step-by-step guide or checklist to ensure comprehensive coverage during self-examination.

- **Nipple Shields**: Used to protect sore or cracked nipples during breastfeeding, nipple shields provide a barrier between the baby's mouth and the breast. They can alleviate discomfort and encourage continued breastfeeding, particularly benefiting women experiencing pain or difficulty with latching. OTPs may recommend nipple shields to enhance comfort during breastfeeding, promoting sustained breastfeeding practices that support maternal and infant occupational roles.

Assistive Technology for Reproductive Health

In the realm of reproductive health, assistive technology encompasses solutions tailored to women's needs. OTPs are instrumental in educating and guiding clients on the use of these technologies to optimize reproductive health and support occupational engagement:

- **Fertility Monitors**: These devices track hormonal changes in urine or saliva to predict ovulation and identify fertile days. They assist women in natural family planning or when trying to conceive, offering insights into reproductive health cycles and optimizing the timing of conception attempts. OTPs empower women by providing tools for informed family planning decisions, supporting occupational engagement through proactive health management.
- **Ovulation Prediction Devices**: Similar to fertility monitors, ovulation prediction devices use various methods, such as basal body temperature tracking or hormone analysis, to pinpoint the most fertile days in a woman's cycle. They provide valuable information for women aiming to conceive or understand their menstrual cycle patterns. OTPs guide clients in using ovulation prediction devices to optimize fertility awareness, supporting occupational roles and life planning goals.
- **Pregnancy Support Belts**: Designed to provide abdominal and back support, pregnancy support belts alleviate discomfort and strain on the lower back and pelvis during pregnancy. They help maintain posture and mobility as the body changes, supporting women in carrying out daily activities comfortably. OTPs recommend and fit pregnancy support belts to enhance comfort and mobility during pregnancy, enabling women to sustain occupational roles and activities throughout gestation.
- **Maternity Supports**: These devices offer compression and stability for abdominal muscles and ligaments, reducing discomfort associated with pregnancy. They promote comfort and assist women in maintaining an active lifestyle throughout pregnancy, supporting occupational roles and activities during this transformative period. OTPs prescribe maternity supports to optimize comfort and mobility, enabling women to engage in daily occupations with reduced physical strain.
  - **Maternity Belly Bands**: These bands provide gentle support to the lower abdomen and back, helping to alleviate discomfort and distribute weight more evenly.
  - **Maternity Compression Leggings**: Designed to support the lower body, these leggings reduce swelling and provide compression to improve circulation during pregnancy.
  - **Maternity Support Pillows**: These pillows are specially shaped to support the body during sleep, promoting better alignment and reducing discomfort during the occupation of sleep.
  - **Maternity Back Braces**: These braces provide additional support to the lumbar spine, reducing strain and promoting better posture.

Special Topics   391

- **Maternity Support Panties**: These panties provide gentle support to the abdomen and pelvis, helping to alleviate discomfort and support pelvic floor muscles.
- **Breastfeeding Technology**: Devices such as breast pumps and nipple shields can support breastfeeding mothers by facilitating milk expression and reducing discomfort during feeding. OTPs can educate mothers on the proper use of these devices to ensure effective breastfeeding practices that support maternal and infant health:
  - **Breast Pumps**: Assist in expressing and storing breast milk, offering convenience and flexibility for nursing mothers who may face challenges with latching, milk production, or scheduling feedings.
  - **Nipple Shields**: Used to protect sore or cracked nipples during breastfeeding, providing a barrier between the baby's mouth and the breast, which can alleviate discomfort and encourage continued breastfeeding.
- **Pelvic Floor Trainers**: These devices help women strengthen their pelvic floor muscles, which can be particularly beneficial during pregnancy and postpartum. OTPs can guide clients in using these trainers to improve pelvic floor health, supporting activities such as continence and sexual health:
  - **Kegel Trainers**: These devices provide biofeedback to help women perform pelvic floor exercises correctly, enhancing muscle strength and function.
  - **Perineal Massagers**: Used to prepare the perineum for childbirth, reducing the risk of tearing and improving postpartum recovery.

By integrating these technologies into their practice, OTPs can provide comprehensive support that addresses the unique reproductive health needs of women. This not only enhances physical comfort and health but also promotes greater engagement in daily activities and occupational roles during various stages of reproductive health.

Devices for Dressing

Assistive technology for dressing addresses the specific challenges women face with various articles of clothing, promoting independence and ease in daily routines. OTPs play a critical role in recommending and integrating these technologies to support clients in maintaining personal hygiene and dressing independently:

- **Ergonomic Hooks and Fasteners**: These devices assist in the donning of bras by providing easier grip and leverage, crucial for individuals with dexterity limitations or reduced hand mobility. OTPs can incorporate these into interventions to facilitate clients in maintaining personal hygiene and dressing independently.
- **Front-Closure Bras**: Adaptive bras with front-closure designs eliminate the need for reaching behind the back, making them easier to put on and take off. They are ideal for women with shoulder mobility issues or those recovering from surgeries that restrict arm movement, supporting occupational roles that require dressing and undressing without assistance.
- **Adaptive Bra Aids**: These aids include specialized dressing sticks or hooks designed specifically for managing straps or adjusting bra closures. They simplify the process of securing straps or making adjustments, ensuring comfort and proper fit without relying on intricate maneuvers, facilitating occupational performance in dressing tasks.

- **Skirt Pullers and Elastic Waistband Extenders**: Designed to aid in independent dressing, skirt pullers allow users to pull up skirts without excessive bending or reaching. Elastic waistband extenders accommodate fluctuations in waist size, providing comfort and flexibility, promoting ease in dressing for daily activities.
- **Button Aids and Hooks**: These tools streamline the fastening process for shirts and pants. Button aids feature extended grips or loops that facilitate buttoning, ideal for individuals with limited grip strength or fine motor control. OTPs can recommend these devices to enhance clients' ability to dress independently, supporting occupational engagement in various environments.
- **Zipper Pulls**: Extended zipper pulls with larger grips make zipping up dresses and pants easier for those with limited finger dexterity or strength, facilitating occupational participation in dressing tasks.

By integrating these assistive technologies, OTPs can significantly enhance the independence and self-efficacy of women facing challenges with dressing. These interventions not only support daily functioning and personal hygiene but also contribute to a greater sense of autonomy and confidence. This holistic approach ensures that women can continue to engage in their desired occupations and maintain their quality of life.

Menstrual Management Assistive Technology

Assistive technology for menstrual management offers practical solutions to enhance comfort and efficiency during menstruation, supporting women in their daily occupations. OTPs are instrumental in educating and guiding clients on the use of these technologies to manage menstrual hygiene independently:

- **Menstrual Cups**: These reusable silicone cups provide an eco-friendly alternative to traditional menstrual products. They are inserted into the vaginal canal to collect menstrual flow and can be emptied, cleaned, and reused. Women with environmental concerns or sensitivities to traditional pads and tampons find menstrual cups particularly beneficial. OTPs can educate clients on using menstrual cups to manage menstruation independently, promoting comfort and participation in daily activities.
- **Ergonomic Applicators**: Designed for ease of use, ergonomic applicators facilitate the insertion of tampons or menstrual cups, ensuring comfortable and hygienic menstrual care. They are especially helpful for women with limited dexterity or motor control, making insertion and removal easier and more manageable. OTPs can recommend these tools to enhance clients' ability to manage menstrual hygiene independently, supporting occupational engagement without reliance on external assistance.
- **Period-Tracking Apps**: Mobile applications equipped with menstrual calendars allow users to track their menstrual cycles, predicting periods and fertile windows. Some apps also log symptoms and moods, offering insights into reproductive health patterns. Women who struggle with irregular cycles or need to monitor fertility find these apps invaluable for planning and managing their reproductive health. OTPs can guide clients in using these apps to monitor and understand their menstrual health, facilitating informed decision-making and promoting occupational engagement.
- **Disposable and Reusable Pads**: Modern pads incorporate ergonomic designs and advanced materials for enhanced comfort and absorption, catering to diverse preferences and needs. They are suitable for women seeking reliable and comfortable

menstrual protection, accommodating varying flow levels and sensitivities. OTPs can recommend appropriate pads based on individual needs, promoting comfort during menstruation and supporting ongoing participation in daily occupations.
- **Heating Pads**: Used for menstrual cramp relief, heating pads provide localized warmth to soothe abdominal discomfort associated with menstruation. They are ideal for women experiencing menstrual pain or conditions like endometriosis, providing non-invasive pain relief that supports occupational performance by alleviating discomfort and promoting comfort during daily activities.

By incorporating these advanced technologies, OTPs empower women to overcome challenges associated with menstrual hygiene and pain management. This approach enhances their ability to engage fully in their daily activities and occupational roles, ensuring they can participate in life with minimal disruption and greater comfort. Practitioners should stay informed about the latest assistive technologies and incorporate them into personalized care plans, thereby improving client outcomes and promoting overall well-being. By doing so, they can provide comprehensive support that addresses the unique needs of each client, fostering independence and confidence in managing their health.

The Female Athlete

In occupational therapy, sports and athletics are recognized as essential occupations that contribute significantly to individuals' health, well-being, and identity. This section explores specialized considerations and interventions crucial for supporting female athletes in their occupational engagement. OTPs play a pivotal role in enhancing performance, preventing injuries, and promoting holistic well-being across various sports and competitive levels. The section discusses physiological differences, injury prevention strategies, performance enhancement techniques, and rehabilitation approaches tailored to optimize occupational engagement in sports and physical activities among female athletes. By addressing these unique needs, OTPs empower female athletes to achieve their occupational goals, whether professional, collegiate, or recreational, fostering lifelong participation in sports and athletic endeavors.

Physiological Considerations

Female athletes face unique physiological challenges that impact their performance and overall health outcomes. OTPs are well-positioned to address these differences comprehensively, considering factors such as hormonal fluctuations, bone density concerns, and cardiovascular health. By understanding these physiological variations, OTPs can develop personalized interventions that optimize training adaptations and support menstrual health. Table 14.2 highlights the key physiological differences between women and men that impact sports performance, emphasizing the need for gender-specific considerations in occupational therapy interventions for athletes:

- **Client Factors**: OTPs collaborate with healthcare professionals like radiologists or physicians to assess individual physiological profiles and tailor interventions. For example, collaborating with a radiologist, an OTP may review bone density scan results and assess hormone levels through blood tests for a female athlete experiencing recurrent stress fractures. Based on these assessments, the OTP and healthcare team including a

394 Occupational Therapy and Women's Health

Table 14.2 Physiological differences impacting sports performance between women and men

Aspect	Women	Men
Heart Rate and Exercise Capacity	- Higher resting heart rate (average 70–80 bpm) - Aerobic capacity declines at 1% per year after age 30	- Lower resting heart rate (average 60–70 bpm) - Aerobic capacity declines at 0.8–1% per year after age 30
Pulmonary System	- Smaller lung volumes (10–12% less than men) - Smaller airway diameters	- Larger lung volumes - Greater pulmonary reserve
Hormonal Changes	- Significant hormonal changes post-menopause affecting bone density and muscle mass	- Gradual decline in testosterone (1–2% per year after age 30), impacting muscle mass and strength
Chronic Conditions	- Higher risk of osteoporosis (1 in 2 women over 50 will break a bone due to osteoporosis) - Higher prevalence of arthritis (26% in women vs. 18% in men)	- Higher risk of heart disease (leading cause of death) - Higher prevalence of hypertension (about 49% of men over 45)

dietician may develop a customized exercise regimen focusing on weight-bearing activities and nutritional recommendations to improve bone health and prevent injuries.
- **Performance Skills**: OTPs work on enhancing specific physiological capacities like endurance, strength, and flexibility through targeted therapeutic exercises, activities and training protocols. For instance, collaborating with the healthcare team, an OTP may design a strength training program that includes resistance exercises and plyometrics to improve muscular endurance and power for a female sprinter aiming to enhance her performance in track competitions.
- **Performance Patterns**: OTPs establish routines and strategies to manage physiological fluctuations effectively, integrating training cycles that align with menstrual cycles to optimize performance and recovery.

Female athletes face unique physiological challenges that impact their performance and overall health outcomes. OTPs are well-positioned to address these differences comprehensively, considering factors such as hormonal fluctuations, bone density concerns, and cardiovascular health. By understanding these physiological variations, OTPs can develop personalized interventions that optimize training adaptations and support menstrual health, empowering female athletes to achieve their occupational goals with resilience and confidence.

Injury Prevention and Rehabilitation

Effective injury prevention strategies are crucial for sustaining long-term athletic participation. OTPs utilize evidence-based approaches such as biomechanical analysis, strength and conditioning programs, and ergonomic assessments to mitigate injury risks and promote safe participation in sports.

- **Client Factors**: OTPs conduct biomechanical assessments to identify movement patterns and muscle imbalances that contribute to injury risk. They also assess joint

stability and flexibility to customize injury prevention strategies. For female athletes, this may include addressing specific concerns such as the higher prevalence of anterior cruciate ligament (ACL) injuries in women by incorporating neuromuscular training programs designed to improve knee stability and reduce the risk of such injuries.
- **Performance Skills**: OTPs focus on improving movement mechanics and proprioception through targeted exercises and corrective techniques, enhancing athletes' ability to perform skills safely. For example, they might design balance and proprioceptive exercises to reduce the risk of ankle sprains, which are more common in female athletes due to differences in ligament laxity.
- **Performance Patterns**: OTPs implement injury prevention protocols as part of athletes' daily routines, emphasizing warm-up strategies, cool-down exercises, and recovery practices to maintain optimal performance levels and prevent overuse injuries. For female athletes, these routines might be adapted to account for menstrual cycle phases, which can affect ligament laxity and injury risk.

Effective injury prevention strategies are crucial for sustaining long-term athletic participation. OTPs utilize evidence-based approaches such as biomechanical analysis, strength and conditioning programs, and ergonomic assessments to mitigate injury risks and promote safe participation in sports. By integrating these strategies into athletes' routines, OTPs foster a proactive approach to injury management that supports continuous occupational engagement, ensuring athletes can perform at their best while minimizing the impact of injuries on their overall well-being.

Performance Enhancement

OTPs collaborate closely with coaches, trainers, and athletes to optimize athletic performance beyond injury management. This includes enhancing biomechanical efficiency, functional movement patterns, and sport-specific skills through comprehensive assessments and tailored interventions.

- **Client Factors**: OTPs assess physical strengths and weaknesses, identifying areas for improvement in coordination, agility, and sport-specific techniques. For female athletes, this might include focusing on lower body strength and power, considering that women generally have less lower body muscle mass compared to men.
- **Performance Skills**: OTPs design performance enhancement programs that incorporate skill development, strength training, and conditioning exercises to improve athletic performance metrics. For instance, they might include plyometric exercises to enhance explosive power in female volleyball players, which is crucial for activities such as spiking and blocking.
- **Performance Patterns**: OTPs integrate performance-enhancing strategies into athletes' training schedules, focusing on consistency in practice and competition preparation to enhance skill execution and competitive readiness. For female athletes, this might involve periodizing training loads to optimize performance while minimizing the impact of hormonal fluctuations throughout the menstrual cycle.

OTPs collaborate closely with coaches, trainers, and athletes to optimize athletic performance beyond injury management. This includes enhancing biomechanical efficiency, functional movement patterns, and sport-specific skills through comprehensive assessments and tailored interventions. By focusing on individual strengths and areas for improvement, OTPs empower athletes to reach their full potential in training and competition, promoting lifelong participation and achievement in sports.

Psychosocial Well-being

Psychosocial factors significantly impact athletes' overall well-being and occupational satisfaction. OTPs address psychological aspects such as stress management, performance anxiety, and coping skills development to promote resilience and positive occupational engagement.

- **Client Factors**: OTPs conduct psychosocial assessments to identify stressors, anxiety triggers, and coping mechanisms among athletes. For female athletes, this might include addressing body image concerns and pressures that can be more prevalent due to societal expectations and media portrayals.
- **Performance Skills**: OTPs teach cognitive-behavioural strategies, mindfulness techniques, and visualization exercises to enhance mental resilience and focus during training and competition. For example, they might use mindfulness-based stress reduction techniques to help female athletes manage pre-competition anxiety.
- **Performance Patterns**: OTPs integrate psychosocial support into athletes' routines, emphasizing mental health check-ins, team-building activities, and peer support networks to foster a supportive athletic environment and enhance overall well-being. For female athletes, creating a supportive community that addresses gender-specific challenges can be particularly beneficial in maintaining motivation and mental health.

Psychosocial factors significantly impact athletes' overall well-being and occupational satisfaction. OTPs address psychological aspects such as stress management, performance anxiety, and coping skills development to promote resilience and positive occupational engagement. Through psychosocial assessments and targeted interventions, OTPs empower athletes to manage mental health challenges effectively, enhancing their ability to navigate competitive pressures and maintain a healthy relationship with their sport.

Holistic Approach to Women's Health in Athletics

OTPs advocate for a comprehensive approach to women's health in athletics, recognizing the intricate interplay of physical, psychological, and social factors crucial for optimizing performance and promoting health and wellness. OTPs collaborate with athletes to develop strategies that promote overall health and well-being, including effective sleep hygiene, which plays a critical role in performance optimization and recovery.

Furthermore, OTPs prioritize injury prevention through biomechanical assessments and personalized training regimens, ensuring athletes can safely pursue their athletic endeavors over the long term. By fostering a holistic understanding of women's health needs in sports, OTPs empower athletes to achieve their occupational goals while promoting sustainable participation and lifelong health benefits. This approach not only enhances athletic performance but also supports athletes in cultivating resilience, managing stress, and maintaining a positive relationship with their sport, contributing to their overall occupational satisfaction and well-being.

OT for Females with Long-Term Disabilities

Millions of women live with long-term disabilities, significantly impacting their daily lives and overall well-being. According to the Centers for Disease Control and Prevention (CDC), approximately 27% of women in the United States have a disability, with many experiencing limitations in physical functioning, cognition, and social participation. The Disablement Model, which outlines the progression from pathology to impairment, functional limitation, and disability, is particularly relevant in occupational therapy as it provides a framework for understanding and addressing the multifaceted needs of women with long-term disabilities. This model emphasizes the importance of considering the environmental and personal factors that influence an individual's ability to perform daily activities and participate in meaningful occupations.

Categories of Long-Term Disabilities

Women can experience various types of long-term disabilities, each with unique challenges and implications for occupational performance:

- **Physical Disabilities**: Conditions such as spinal cord injuries, multiple sclerosis, and arthritis, which primarily affect physical mobility and function.
- **Cognitive Disabilities**: Includes impairments such as traumatic brain injury, stroke, and neurodegenerative diseases that affect memory, problem-solving, and other cognitive functions.
- **Sensory Disabilities**: Encompasses hearing loss, vision impairments, and other conditions that affect sensory processing.
- **Psychiatric Disabilities**: Includes mental health conditions such as severe depression, bipolar disorder, and schizophrenia, which can affect emotional regulation and social interactions.

Psychosocial Considerations for Long-Term Disabilities

The psychosocial impact of long-term disabilities can vary significantly depending on whether the disability was present from birth or acquired later in life. Women who have grown up with long-term disabilities often face different challenges compared to those who acquire disabilities as adults. Women who acquire disabilities as adults may struggle with the sudden loss of function and independence, leading to feelings of grief, loss, and identity crises. They may need to adjust to new limitations and navigate changes in their roles and relationships. On the other hand, women who have lived with disabilities from a young age often develop adaptive skills and coping mechanisms early on but may face ongoing social and environmental barriers that impact their participation in various life activities. Table 14.3 presents a comparison of women with long-term disabilities at birth and acquired.

Table 14.3 Comparison of women with disabilities from birth vs. acquired disabilities

Aspect	Women with Disabilities at Birth	Women with Acquired Disabilities
Adaptive Skills	Develop strong adaptive skills early, but may need to learn new techniques for milestones such as motherhood, breastfeeding, ergonomic adaptations for infant care, career transitions, managing household tasks, and recreational activities.	Need to learn new adaptive skills for daily tasks and milestones such as returning to work, household management, parenting, and social integration.
Psychosocial Impact	Face ongoing social and environmental barriers, potentially leading to chronic stress and anxiety.	Experience grief, loss, and identity crises due to sudden changes, which can lead to depression and anxiety.
Coping Mechanisms	Develop coping strategies early, which can be robust but may require adaptation for new life stages or challenges.	Need to develop new coping strategies to adjust to the sudden changes and new limitations.
Role Adjustment	Consistent role adaptations over time, with gradual adjustments to new roles and responsibilities.	Gradual adjustments to new roles and responsibilities. Sudden and significant role changes, requiring rapid adjustment to new realities.
Support Systems	Often have established long-term support networks, including family, friends, and community resources.	May need to build new support networks, which can be challenging and time-consuming.
Identity and Self-Perception	Strong sense of identity shaped by disability, with a focus on capabilities and strengths.	May experience identity crises and struggle with self-perception due to the sudden loss of abilities.

Occupational Therapy Approaches and Interventions

OTPs play a critical role in supporting women with long-term disabilities through various evidence-based interventions. These interventions are designed to enhance occupational functioning by addressing the physical, cognitive, and psychosocial challenges associated with long-term disabilities. By adopting a holistic and individualized approach, OTPs can significantly enhance the quality of life for women with long-term disabilities, empowering them to achieve their goals and participate fully in their chosen activities.

Client-Centered Assessment

OTPs begin with a thorough client-centered assessment to understand the unique needs and challenges faced by women with long-term disabilities. Activity analysis involves a detailed examination of daily activities to identify barriers and facilitators to participation. By understanding the specific tasks that are difficult or impossible for the client, therapists can tailor interventions that enhance functional performance and independence. Additionally, environmental modifications are crucial for creating accessible and safe living, working, and community spaces. This might involve recommending home adaptations like installing grab bars or wheelchair ramps to improve mobility and safety. For example, a therapist might suggest rearranging kitchen storage to ensure that frequently used items are within easy reach for a client with limited upper body strength.

Adaptive Skills Training

Adaptive skills training is essential for enhancing the independence of women with long-term disabilities. This training includes the use of assistive technology, such as wheelchairs, communication aids, and adaptive tools, which can significantly improve the client's ability to perform daily tasks. Self-management techniques are also vital, teaching strategies for managing symptoms, conserving energy, and effectively managing time. These techniques empower clients to handle their conditions proactively and maintain a higher quality of life. For instance, a therapist might teach a client with multiple sclerosis how to use a planner to manage fatigue by scheduling rest periods throughout the day.

Psychosocial Interventions

Psychosocial interventions address the emotional and mental health needs of women with long-term disabilities. Cognitive-behavioural therapy (CBT) helps clients reframe negative thought patterns and develop healthier coping mechanisms, which can significantly improve their mental health. Peer support groups facilitate connections with others who have similar experiences, providing mutual support and shared coping strategies. These groups create a sense of community and reduce feelings of isolation. For example, a therapist might organize a support group for women with spinal cord injuries to share their experiences and strategies for coping with daily challenges.

Vocational Rehabilitation

Vocational rehabilitation helps women with long-term disabilities find and maintain meaningful employment. This includes job training and placement services that accommodate the client's abilities and interests, ensuring they find suitable and fulfilling work. Workplace modifications are also recommended to support job performance and prevent injury, such as ergonomic adjustments to workstations or providing specialized equipment. For example, a therapist might work with an employer to modify a workstation for a woman with carpal tunnel syndrome, including ergonomic keyboards and adjustable desks.

Health and Wellness Promotion

Promoting health and wellness is a key aspect of supporting women with long-term disabilities. OTPs design individualized exercise programs to help maintain physical health and prevent secondary conditions such as obesity or cardiovascular disease. Nutrition counseling provides guidance on healthy eating habits to support overall well-being and manage specific health conditions. These programs are tailored to the client's needs and abilities, promoting long-term health and wellness. For instance, a therapist might develop a low-impact exercise routine for a woman with arthritis to help maintain joint flexibility and reduce pain.

Storytelling and Expressive Therapies

Storytelling and expressive therapies offer powerful tools for healing and self-expression. Narrative therapy encourages women to share their stories and experiences, helping them reframe their identities and promote healing. Art, music, and dance therapies provide creative outlets for expressing emotions, reducing stress, and improving mental health.

These therapies help clients process their experiences and find new ways to express themselves. For example, a therapist might use art therapy with a woman who has experienced a traumatic brain injury, allowing her to express her feelings and experiences through painting or drawing.

By adopting a holistic and individualized approach, OTPs can significantly enhance the quality of life for women with long-term disabilities, empowering them to achieve their goals and participate fully in their chosen activities.

Nutrition Considerations in Women's Health

Nutrition plays a fundamental role in women's health across the lifespan. Proper nutrition is essential for maintaining physical and psychosocial health, preventing chronic diseases, and supporting overall well-being. Women have unique nutritional needs that vary throughout different life stages, including adolescence, reproductive years, pregnancy, lactation, menopause, and older adulthood. Understanding and addressing these needs is crucial for promoting optimal health outcomes in occupational therapy.

The nutritional needs of women change significantly throughout different life stages, influenced by physiological, hormonal, and lifestyle factors. Women and men have distinct nutritional needs due to physiological and hormonal differences. Women generally require higher iron intake due to menstruation and higher calcium intake to prevent osteoporosis, particularly during and after menopause. Women also need more folic acid during reproductive years to support pregnancy and fetal development. Conversely, men typically have higher calorie requirements due to greater muscle mass and higher basal metabolic rates. Table 14.4 summarizes key nutritional changes and requirements for various age groups and conditions, highlighting how these needs can impact overall health and occupational engagement.

OTPs should consider these differences when assisting with nutrition management, educating clients on healthy eating, especially for those with chronic conditions, and all meal preparation interventions. For example, an OTP working with a female client with osteoporosis should emphasize calcium and vitamin D-rich foods, while an OTP working with a male athlete might focus on adequate protein intake to support muscle repair and growth. By tailoring nutritional advice and interventions to the unique needs of women, OTPs can better support their clients' health, promote effective recovery from illness or injury, and enhance overall well-being.

Role of OTPs in Nutrition Management

OTPs are uniquely positioned to integrate nutrition management into their practice. By collaborating with dietitians and other healthcare professionals, OTPs can provide holistic care that addresses the nutritional needs of their clients. This interdisciplinary approach enhances the overall health and well-being of women, allowing them to participate fully in their daily activities and occupations. OTPs can play a significant role in nutrition management through the following activities:

- **Assessment and Education**: Conducting assessments to identify nutritional deficits and educating clients about the importance of balanced nutrition. For example, OTPs use tools like the Mini Nutritional Assessment (MNA) to screen for malnutrition, especially in older adults. By understanding a client's nutritional status, OTPs can develop

Table 14.4 Nutritional needs and considerations across different life stages and conditions for women compared to men

Life Stage/ Condition	Nutritional Needs	Changes and Considerations	Differences in Women Compared to Men
Adolescents/ Teenagers	Increased need for protein, iron, calcium, and vitamin D	Support for menstrual health; prevention of bone density loss; focus on balanced diet	Higher iron needs due to menstruation; typically, lower calorie needs than male counterparts
Young Adults	Balanced intake of macronutrients and micronutrients	Maintenance of overall health; support for reproductive health; prevention of chronic diseases	Similar macronutrient needs; women may need more iron and folic acid
Middle Age	Increased need for calcium, vitamin D, and antioxidants	Management of menopausal symptoms; prevention of osteoporosis; maintenance of muscle mass	Lower calorie needs; higher risk of osteoporosis requiring more calcium and vitamin D
Older Adults	Higher protein intake, increased need for calcium and vitamin B12	Support for muscle mass maintenance; prevention of sarcopenia and bone fractures	Similar needs for protein and vitamin D; women may need more calcium due to higher osteoporosis risk
Recovering from Injury/ Illness	Higher protein and calorie intake, increased vitamins and minerals	Support for tissue repair and immune function; management of inflammation; promoting faster recovery	Similar needs for recovery, but women may need specific nutrients based on the injury/illness
Sedentary Individuals	Balanced diet with appropriate calorie intake, focus on fiber	Prevention of weight gain and chronic diseases; support for digestive health	Similar needs; overall lower calorie intake
Athletes	Increased protein, carbohydrates, and electrolyte intake	Support for high energy expenditure; maintenance of muscle mass and repair; hydration management	Similar macronutrient needs; women may need more iron and calcium to support bone health

personalized intervention plans that consider both physical and psychosocial health needs. Educating clients about nutrition empowers them to make informed choices that support their overall health and ability to engage in meaningful activities.
- **Meal Preparation and Planning**: Assisting clients in developing meal plans and teaching skills for meal preparation and safe food handling. OTPs help clients integrate healthy eating into their daily routines, which is crucial for maintaining independence and managing chronic conditions. By teaching meal planning and preparation, OTPs enable clients to perform these tasks safely and efficiently, enhancing their ability to participate in daily activities and reducing the risk of malnutrition and related health issues.
- **Adaptive Equipment and Techniques**: Recommending adaptive equipment and techniques to facilitate independent meal preparation and consumption for women with physical or cognitive limitations. Adaptive equipment, such as easy-grip utensils, cutting boards with stabilizers, and lightweight pots, can make meal preparation more accessible for clients with physical disabilities or limitations. OTPs assess each client's specific needs and recommend appropriate tools to promote independence and safety in the kitchen, thereby supporting their ability to engage in meaningful occupations related to cooking and eating.

- **Behavioural Interventions**: Implementing behavioural interventions to promote healthy eating habits and address issues such as emotional eating or eating disorders. Behavioural interventions, including cognitive-behavioural strategies and mindfulness practices, help clients develop healthier relationships with food. OTPs work with clients to identify triggers for unhealthy eating patterns and develop strategies to manage them. These interventions support clients' overall mental health and well-being, enabling them to maintain balanced nutrition and participate fully in their daily lives.

By integrating these activities into their practice, OTPs provide comprehensive support that addresses the multifaceted aspects of nutrition management. This holistic approach is particularly important in women's health, where nutritional needs can vary widely due to factors such as hormonal changes, pregnancy, and menopause. Ensuring that clients have the knowledge, skills, and resources to manage their nutrition effectively allows OTPs to enhance their clients' physical and psychosocial well-being. This support is crucial for enabling women to maintain independence, manage chronic conditions, and recover from illness or injury, ultimately promoting their full participation in all areas of life.

Impact of Nutrition on Women Receiving OT Services

Nutrition directly affects recovery and function while an individual is under an OTP's care. OTPs should be concerned with and address the nutritional intake and eating patterns of their patients and clients, as proper nutrition can significantly influence rehabilitation outcomes. Women receiving OT services, particularly those recovering from injury and illness, benefit greatly from comprehensive nutrition management. Nutrition can impact these clients in many ways:

- **Recovery from Injury**: Adequate nutrition is crucial for tissue repair, muscle strength, and overall recovery. Nutrients like protein, vitamins, and minerals support the body's healing processes, reduce inflammation, and improve immune function.
- **Psychosocial Health**: Proper nutrition also plays a vital role in mental health. Nutrient-rich diets can help manage stress, anxiety, and depression, which are often associated with chronic illness and injury. For instance, omega-3 fatty acids have been shown to improve mood and cognitive function, while deficiencies in vitamins such as B12 and folate can lead to mood disturbances.
- **Energy Levels**: Good nutrition helps maintain energy levels, which is essential for participating in therapy sessions and daily activities. Carbohydrates, proteins, and fats provide the necessary energy to support physical and mental exertion.
- **Functional Performance**: Nutrition influences overall functional performance, enabling clients to engage in meaningful activities. Proper dietary intake ensures that clients have the strength, endurance, and cognitive function needed to perform daily tasks and participate in their roles and responsibilities effectively.

Nutrition and Meal Preparation Activities

Effective nutrition management encompasses more than just choosing the right foods; it involves practical aspects of meal preparation tailored to the individual's lifestyle and health needs. OTPs can play a crucial role in helping women navigate these activities by integrating nutritional strategies into their daily routines. This approach not only promotes physical and psychosocial health but also ensures that nutritional needs are met in a way that supports overall occupational engagement.

Assessing Nutritional Needs

OTPs can collaborate with dietitians to conduct thorough nutritional assessments, considering the client's occupational activities and lifestyle. This partnership ensures that nutritional plans are not only medically appropriate but also practical and tailored to the individual's daily life.

- **Mini Nutritional Assessment (MNA)**: This screening tool is particularly useful for older adults at risk for malnutrition. It helps identify individuals who may require more comprehensive nutritional intervention and supports the development of tailored nutritional plans.
- **Comprehensive Nutritional Assessment**: Using additional tools like the Subjective Global Assessment (SGA) or the Malnutrition Universal Screening Tool (MUST) to provide a more in-depth evaluation of nutritional status.
- **Life Stage Considerations**: Understanding the specific nutritional needs of women at different life stages, such as increased iron requirements during menstruation or calcium needs during menopause. Tailoring nutritional plans to these life stages can help manage symptoms and promote overall well-being.
- **Chronic Conditions**: Addressing nutritional needs related to chronic conditions common in women, such as osteoporosis, cardiovascular diseases, and diabetes. Nutritional strategies should be adapted to the individual's level of physical activity, work demands, and lifestyle.

Education on Healthy Eating for Women

OTPs can educate clients on the components of a balanced diet, emphasizing the importance of macronutrients (carbohydrates, proteins, and fats) and micronutrients (vitamins and minerals). This education can help clients make informed choices that support their health and well-being.

- **Balanced Diet**: Educating clients on how to achieve a balanced diet that supports their overall health and specific nutritional needs.
- **Dietary Restrictions**: Helping clients navigate dietary restrictions due to allergies, intolerances, or health conditions by providing practical advice and alternative food options that fits into daily routine in conjunction with a dietician.

Meal Preparation and Planning

To support recovery, it's important to emphasize whole, nutrient-dense foods while minimizing processed foods:

- **Balanced Diet**: Educating clients on the components of a balanced diet, including macronutrients (carbohydrates, proteins, and fats) and micronutrients (vitamins and minerals).
- **Dietary Restrictions**: Helping clients navigate dietary restrictions due to allergies, intolerances, or health conditions.

Table 14.5 Nutritional needs and considerations across different life stages and conditions for women compared to men

Category	Recommended Foods (Aid in Recovery)	Foods to Limit/Avoid (Hinder Recovery)
Proteins	Lean meats (chicken, turkey), fish, eggs, legumes, nuts, seeds	Processed meats (sausages, hot dogs), fried foods
Carbohydrates	Whole grains (brown rice, quinoa, oats), sweet potatoes, fruits, vegetables	Refined grains (white bread, pastries), sugary snacks
Fats	Healthy fats (avocado, olive oil, nuts, seeds)	Trans fats (margarine, fried foods), high-fat processed snacks
Vegetables	Leafy greens (spinach, kale), cruciferous vegetables (broccoli, cauliflower), colorful vegetables (bell peppers, carrots)	Canned vegetables with added sodium or preservatives
Fruits	Fresh fruits (berries, oranges, apples), frozen fruits without added sugar	Canned fruits in syrup, fruit juices with added sugars
Dairy	Low-fat or fat-free dairy (milk, yogurt, cheese)	Full-fat dairy, flavored yogurts with added sugars
Hydration	Water, herbal teas, hydrating foods (cucumbers, oranges, melons)	Sugary drinks (sodas, sweetened teas), excessive caffeine
Snacks	Healthy snacks (nuts, seeds, fresh fruit, vegetable sticks with hummus)	Processed snacks (chips, candy, cookies)

- **Safety and Hygiene**: Teaching safe food handling and hygiene practices to prevent foodborne illnesses.
- **Time Management**: Developing strategies for efficient meal preparation, including batch cooking and using time-saving appliances.

Table 14.5 provides a simple guide to help women incorporate healthier foods into their meal preparation and planning.

When helping women incorporate healthier foods and less processed options into their diets, several considerations should be taken into account. These include energy conservation techniques to reduce fatigue, purchasing healthy food on a budget, such as using frozen vegetables, and planning meals to ensure balanced nutrition:

1. **Batch Cooking**: Prepare larger portions of meals and freeze individual servings. This ensures you have healthy, homemade meals readily available, reducing reliance on processed foods.
2. **Fresh Ingredients**: Emphasize the use of fresh vegetables and fruits. Aim to fill half of your plate with vegetables and fruits at each meal.
3. **Minimize Processed Foods**: Choose whole foods over processed options. For example, opt for whole grain bread instead of white bread, and fresh fruit instead of fruit juice.
4. **Healthy Cooking Methods**: Use healthier cooking methods such as baking, grilling, steaming, or sautéing with minimal oil instead of frying.
5. **Meal Planning**: Plan your meals ahead of time to ensure a balanced intake of all essential nutrients. Include a variety of foods to cover all nutritional needs.
6. **Reading Labels**: Learn to read food labels to avoid added sugars, unhealthy fats, and excessive sodium. Look for items with minimal ingredients and those you can easily recognize.

7. **Portion Control**: Be mindful of portion sizes to maintain a balanced diet and avoid overeating.
8. **Energy Conservation**: Use energy-saving techniques such as sitting while preparing food, using lightweight utensils, and planning meals that require less preparation time.

By following these guidelines and using the table above, women can effectively incorporate healthier foods into their diet, which supports faster recovery and promotes overall well-being. These strategies, when combined with the comprehensive support provided by OTPs, can help women return to their daily activities and occupations more effectively.

Adaptive Equipment and Techniques

Adaptive equipment and techniques can greatly enhance the ability of women with physical or cognitive limitations to prepare meals independently. These tools and strategies are designed to reduce physical strain and improve safety in the kitchen, enabling more efficient and enjoyable meal preparation:

- **Ergonomic Tools**: Recommending ergonomic kitchen tools that reduce strain and improve safety, such as lightweight pots, easy-grip utensils, and adaptive cutting boards.
- **Energy Conservation**: Teaching energy conservation techniques to women with fatigue or limited endurance, such as sitting while preparing food or using pre-cut vegetables.

By incorporating adaptive equipment and energy conservation strategies, OTPs can help women maintain their independence and confidence in the kitchen. These tools and techniques not only support physical health but also contribute to a greater sense of self-efficacy and well-being.

Behavioural Interventions

Behavioural interventions can play a crucial role in promoting healthy eating habits and addressing issues such as emotional eating or eating disorders. By focusing on mindfulness and support systems, OTPs can help women develop a positive relationship with food and make sustainable changes to their dietary habits:

- **Mindful Eating**: Promoting mindful eating practices to help women develop a healthy relationship with food and recognize hunger and satiety cues.
- **Support Systems**: Encouraging the use of support systems, such as family involvement in meal preparation or participation in community cooking classes.

These behavioural interventions are essential for supporting women's overall mental health and well-being. By fostering mindful eating and strong support networks, OTPs can help women maintain balanced nutrition and achieve their health goals more effectively.

By incorporating healthy eating pattern interventions, meal preparation and management strategies, and nutrition management with healthy food options, OTPs can significantly improve functional outcomes for women. By ensuring that clients have the knowledge, skills, and resources to manage their nutrition effectively, OTPs enhance their clients' ability to participate fully in meaningful activities and roles, ultimately promoting a higher quality of life and overall well-being.

Alternative Medicine

Alternative medicine encompasses a variety of therapies and practices that are used alongside or instead of conventional medical treatments. For women, these therapies can play a significant role in managing health conditions, promoting wellness, and enhancing overall quality of life. More than half of adults in the United States say they use some form of alternative medicine, with women being more likely to use these therapies than men. OTPs can integrate alternative medicine practices into their care plans to provide a holistic approach that addresses the physical, emotional, and psychosocial needs of women.

OTPs can help clients explore and incorporate alternative medicine practices that complement traditional healthcare. By understanding the benefits and limitations of various alternative therapies, OTPs can guide women in making informed decisions about their health and wellness. Research indicates that CAM can effectively manage symptoms such as chronic pain, anxiety, and stress, which are prevalent among women.

Common Alternative Medicine Practices

Alternative medicine encompasses a wide range of therapies that can complement traditional medical treatments. These practices focus on holistic approaches to health, often addressing the physical, emotional, and spiritual aspects of well-being. Common alternative medicine practices that OTPs can incorporate into their care plans include:

- **Acupuncture**: This ancient Chinese practice involves inserting thin needles into specific points on the body to balance energy flow. Acupuncture is used to treat a variety of conditions, including chronic pain, menstrual disorders, and menopausal symptoms. Approximately 6.5% of adults in the United States have used acupuncture, with women being more likely to use this therapy than men.
- **Herbal Medicine**: The use of plants and plant extracts for medicinal purposes. Herbal remedies can help manage symptoms of conditions such as PMS, menopause, and urinary tract infections. Globally, about 80% of the population in some countries use herbal medicine as a part of primary healthcare, with a significant portion being women.
- **Yoga and Tai Chi**: These mind-body practices combine physical movement, meditation, and breathing exercises to promote mental and physical well-being. They are beneficial for stress reduction, improving flexibility and balance, and managing chronic pain. In the United States, around 21 million adults practice yoga, with women making up approximately 72% of practitioners.
- **Massage Therapy**: This practice involves manipulating the body's soft tissues to relieve pain, reduce stress, and improve circulation. Massage therapy can be particularly beneficial for women dealing with muscle tension, chronic pain, or the physical changes associated with pregnancy. Approximately 19% of women in the United States use massage therapy for health reasons.
- **Aromatherapy**: The use of essential oils for therapeutic purposes. Aromatherapy can help manage stress, improve sleep, and alleviate symptoms of depression and anxiety. In the United States, about 5% of adults use aromatherapy, with women being the predominant users of this practice.
- **Chiropractic Therapy**: This practice focuses on diagnosing and treating musculoskeletal disorders, particularly those related to the spine. Chiropractic adjustments aim to improve spinal alignment, relieve pain, and enhance overall health. Studies have

shown chiropractic care to be effective for conditions such as back pain, neck pain, and headaches. Approximately 10% of adults in the United States visit a chiropractor annually, with a significant number being women.
- **Reiki**: A form of energy healing that involves the practitioner placing their hands lightly on or over the body to promote healing by channeling universal life energy. Reiki is used to reduce stress, promote relaxation, and enhance overall well-being. Although scientific evidence is limited, many people report positive experiences with Reiki for managing stress and improving mental health.
- **Reflexology**: This practice involves applying pressure to specific points on the feet, hands, or ears that correspond to different organs and systems in the body. Reflexology is believed to promote healing and improve health by stimulating these points. Research indicates that reflexology can help reduce pain, improve relaxation, and enhance overall well-being. Approximately 6% of adults in the United States use reflexology, with women being the predominant users.

By understanding these common practices and their prevalence, OTPs can better guide their clients in integrating alternative medicine into their overall health management strategies.

Considerations for Alternative Medicine

When integrating alternative medicine into occupational therapy, OTPs should consider several important factors to ensure the safety and efficacy of these practices. By addressing these considerations, OTPs can enhance the therapeutic process and provide a more holistic approach to women's health:

- **Safety and Efficacy**: Ensure that the alternative therapies used are safe and supported by evidence for their effectiveness. OTPs should stay informed about current research and best practices in alternative medicine.
- **Client Preferences and Beliefs**: Respect the client's cultural beliefs and personal preferences regarding alternative medicine. Collaborate with clients to develop personalized care plans that align with their values and goals.
- **Interdisciplinary Collaboration**: Work with other healthcare providers, including physicians, herbalists, acupuncturists, and massage therapists, to provide comprehensive care that incorporates both conventional and alternative treatments.

By integrating alternative medicine practices, OTPs can enhance the therapeutic process and provide a more holistic approach to women's health.

Contraindications for Common Alternative Medicine Practices

When considering alternative medicine practices, it is crucial to be aware of potential contraindications to ensure client safety. Table 14.6 provides a summary of contraindications for common alternative medicine practices.

By considering safety, client preferences, and collaborating with other healthcare professionals, OTPs can effectively integrate alternative medicine practices into their care plans. This approach not only supports the physical and psychosocial well-being of women but also aligns with a holistic view of health. Being mindful of contraindications

Table 14.6 Contraindications for common alternative medicine practices

Alternative Medicine Practice	Contraindications
Acupuncture	Bleeding disorders, use of blood thinners, pregnancy (certain points), severe skin conditions, infection at needle site
Herbal Medicine	Allergies to specific herbs, interactions with prescribed medications, pregnancy, breastfeeding, certain medical conditions (e.g., hypertension, liver disease)
Yoga and Tai Chi	Severe balance disorders, recent surgery, acute musculoskeletal injuries, severe cardiovascular conditions
Massage Therapy	Severe osteoporosis, deep vein thrombosis (DVT), open wounds or skin infections, recent surgery, severe varicose veins
Aromatherapy	Allergies to specific essential oils, asthma, pregnancy, epilepsy (certain oils), young children (certain oils)
Chiropractic Therapy	Severe osteoporosis, spinal cord compression, severe arthritis, bleeding disorders, conditions requiring surgery, acute fractures
Reiki	No specific contraindications, but it should not be used as a replacement for medical treatment, and caution is advised for individuals with severe mental health issues
Reflexology	Foot fractures, unhealed wounds, severe circulatory problems, severe osteoporosis, infections, pregnancy (certain points)

ensures that alternative therapies are used safely, maximizing their therapeutic benefits and enhancing the overall quality of care.

Incorporating Client Values into Care Plans

According to the OTPF, incorporating client values is essential in providing client-centered care. If a client values alternative medicine, OTPs can include these practices in the plan of care to ensure it aligns with the client's preferences and beliefs. Here's how OTPs can incorporate alternative medicine into the care plan:

- **Assessment of Client Values**: During the initial assessment, inquire about the client's beliefs and experiences with alternative medicine. Document their preferences and any specific therapies they are interested in.
- **Education and Informed Decision-Making**: Provide clients with information on the benefits, limitations, and contraindications of the alternative therapies they are interested in. Encourage clients to ask questions and express their concerns to make informed decisions.
- **Collaborative Goal Setting**: Work with clients to set realistic and achievable goals that incorporate alternative medicine practices. Ensure that these goals align with the overall therapeutic objectives.
- **Integration into Intervention Plans**: Develop intervention plans that seamlessly integrate alternative medicine practices with conventional treatments. For example, combine yoga sessions with physical therapy exercises or include aromatherapy during relaxation techniques.
- **Monitoring and Evaluation**: Regularly monitor the client's progress and response to the integrated care plan. Adjust the plan as needed based on the client's feedback and therapeutic outcomes.

- **Interdisciplinary Coordination**: Collaborate with other healthcare providers to ensure a coordinated approach to care. This may include referrals to certified practitioners of alternative medicine when necessary.

By incorporating alternative medicine practices that are valued by the client, OTPs can enhance engagement, satisfaction, and overall therapeutic outcomes. This client-centered approach respects individual preferences and promotes holistic well-being.

Women's Health Advocacy and Policy

Advocacy and policy play a critical role in advancing women's health by addressing systemic issues, influencing legislation, and promoting equitable access to healthcare services. OTPs have the opportunity to be strong advocates for women's health, ensuring that their voices are heard and their needs are met. This section explores the importance of advocacy and policy in women's health and provides strategies for OTPs to engage in advocacy efforts effectively.

Advocacy in women's health is essential for several reasons:

1. **Addressing Health Disparities**:
   - Women, particularly those from marginalized communities, often face significant health disparities. Advocacy efforts can highlight these disparities and push for changes that promote equity in healthcare access and outcomes.

2. **Influencing Policy and Legislation**:
   - Effective advocacy can lead to the development and implementation of policies that protect and enhance women's health. This includes advocating for reproductive rights, maternal health services, and funding for women's health research.

3. **Promoting Public Awareness**:
   - Advocacy raises public awareness about critical women's health issues, helping to educate the community and reduce stigma associated with certain health conditions.

4. **Empowering Women**:
   - By advocating for policies that support women's health, OTPs can empower women to take control of their health and well-being, providing them with the resources and support they need to thrive.

By actively engaging in advocacy, OTPs can influence positive change and ensure that women's health issues receive the attention and resources they deserve. This includes leveraging their expertise to educate policymakers, collaborating with advocacy groups to amplify their impact, and participating in community outreach to raise awareness. Effective advocacy requires a commitment to staying informed about current health issues and policies affecting women, as well as actively participating in efforts to promote health equity. The following strategies provide a roadmap for OTPs to effectively advocate for women's health at various levels, from local communities to national platforms.

Strategies for OTPs in Women's Health Advocacy

OTPs can engage in various advocacy efforts to promote women's health. Here are some strategies to consider:

1. **Educate and Inform**:
   - Staying informed about current issues in women's health and sharing this knowledge with clients, colleagues, and the community is fundamental. Education serves as a powerful tool for advocacy, helping to spread awareness and understanding.
   - Utilize evidence-based information to inform policymakers and stakeholders about the importance of addressing women's health issues. Providing accurate data and compelling narratives can influence policy decisions and resource allocation.

2. **Collaborate with Advocacy Groups**:
   - Partnering with local, national, and international organizations dedicated to women's health can significantly amplify advocacy efforts. Collaboration allows for shared resources, expertise, and a unified voice.
   - Engage in joint initiatives, campaigns, and events that focus on women's health advocacy. These collaborative efforts can raise awareness, drive policy changes, and provide comprehensive support to women.

3. **Engage in Policy Making**:
   - Participation in public hearings, forums, and discussions related to women's health policy is crucial. Providing expert testimony and contributing to the development of policies that support women's health ensures that professional insights are considered in decision-making processes.
   - Write letters to legislators, submit op-eds to newspapers, and use social media platforms to advocate for women's health issues. These actions can help to influence public opinion and legislative agendas.

4. **Support Grassroots Movements**:
   - Getting involved in grassroots movements that aim to improve women's health at the community level can have a profound impact. This includes organizing community health fairs, support groups, and educational workshops.
   - Encourage and support clients and community members to participate in advocacy efforts. Empowering individuals to take part in grassroots advocacy helps to build a stronger, more engaged community.

5. **Advocate for Research Funding**:
   - Push for increased funding for research on women's health issues. Highlight the need for studies that address the unique health challenges faced by women, emphasizing the gaps in current research.
   - Support initiatives that promote the inclusion of women in clinical trials and research studies. Ensuring that research reflects the diverse experiences and needs of women is essential for developing effective health interventions.

6. **Promote Inclusive Health Policies**:
   - Advocate for health policies that are inclusive of all women, regardless of race, ethnicity, socioeconomic status, or sexual orientation. Ensuring that policies address the needs of diverse populations is crucial for achieving health equity.

- Support policies that provide comprehensive healthcare coverage, including reproductive health services, mental health care, and preventative care. Comprehensive coverage ensures that all women have access to the care they need to maintain their health and well-being.

By actively engaging in these strategies, OTPs can influence positive change and ensure that women's health issues receive the attention and resources they deserve. Advocacy efforts must be sustained and multifaceted, addressing immediate needs while also working toward long-term systemic change.

Key Areas of Focus for Women's Health Advocacy

To be effective advocates, OTPs should focus on key areas that have a significant impact on women's health. Addressing these areas can help to reduce disparities, improve health outcomes, and empower women to take control of their health and well-being. Key areas of focus include reproductive health, maternal health, mental health, chronic conditions, and violence against women. Each of these areas requires targeted advocacy efforts to ensure that women receive the comprehensive care and support they need.

Reproductive Health

Advocate for access to comprehensive reproductive health services, including contraception, prenatal care, and safe abortion services. Support policies that protect reproductive rights and provide education on reproductive health. Ensuring women have access to these services is crucial for their overall well-being and autonomy.

Maternal Health

Promote policies that ensure access to quality maternal health care, reduce maternal mortality rates, and support postpartum care. Advocate for programs that provide support for high-risk pregnancies and address the needs of pregnant teens and women of color. These efforts are essential to improve maternal health outcomes and support women through the critical stages of pregnancy and postpartum.

Mental Health

Push for policies that improve access to mental health services for women, particularly those dealing with postpartum depression, anxiety, and trauma. Advocate for the integration of mental health care into primary healthcare settings. Addressing mental health is vital for the holistic well-being of women, as it impacts their ability to function and thrive in various aspects of life.

Chronic Conditions

Support policies that address the prevention and management of chronic conditions such as cardiovascular disease, diabetes, and osteoporosis in women. Advocate for research and education on the gender-specific aspects of these conditions. By focusing on chronic conditions, we can help reduce long-term health complications and improve the quality of life for women.

Violence Against Women

Advocate for policies that protect women from domestic violence, sexual assault, and other forms of gender-based violence. Support programs that provide resources and support for survivors of violence. Ensuring safety and providing support for survivors are critical steps in promoting the overall health and empowerment of women.

Women's health advocacy is a vital aspect of promoting equitable healthcare and addressing the unique needs of women. OTPs have numerous ways to participate in advocacy efforts and make a meaningful impact. Engaging in hill days to meet with legislators, signing petitions to support women's health initiatives, and emailing house representatives to voice concerns and support for relevant policies are all effective methods of advocacy. Additionally, OTPs can join professional organizations that focus on women's health, participate in public awareness campaigns, and collaborate with advocacy groups to amplify their efforts. By actively engaging in these activities, OTPs can help shape a healthcare system that is responsive to the needs of all women, ensuring they receive the comprehensive and compassionate care they deserve.

Case Studies in Special Topics in Women's Health

CASE A: Athlete

Background and Medical History: The client is a 25-year-old woman, a professional athlete, experiencing recurring stress fractures and hormonal imbalances. She reports a history of disordered eating during her teenage years, which she believes has contributed to her current bone density issues. Recently, she has been struggling with menstrual irregularities, which have impacted her athletic performance and overall well-being. Her medical history includes a diagnosis of osteoporosis and a history of multiple stress fractures in her lower extremities. Additionally, she has a family history of osteoporosis and cardiovascular disease. She has consulted with her endocrinologist, who conducted a comprehensive hormonal profile assessment, including estrogen, progesterone, FSH, LH, cortisol, and thyroid function tests. These assessments indicated hormonal imbalances contributing to her menstrual irregularities and bone health issues. The bone density scan conducted confirms osteoporosis with significant reduction in bone density.

Prior Level of Function:

- **Professional**: Competes at a national level in long-distance running, well-respected in the athletic community.
- **Social**: Active in her local running club and participates in community events.
- **Physical**: Engages in rigorous training schedules, including running, strength training, and flexibility exercises.
- **Living Situation**: Lives independently in a two-bedroom apartment close to her training facilities.

Household Living Arrangements and Social History:

- **Current Living Situation**: Continues to live independently, but has limited her training due to recurring injuries.
- **Family and Social Support**: Strong support network from her family and running community; regularly receives encouragement and assistance from her coach and teammates.

Change in Functional Status and Challenges:

- **ADLs**: Manages daily tasks but experiences pain and fatigue that limit her ability to train and perform at peak levels.
- **Work**: Reduced training time and frequent breaks have led to concerns about maintaining her competitive edge.
- **Social Activities**: Continued participation in social activities, though with modifications to accommodate her physical limitations.

OT Assessments:

- **Canadian Occupational Performance Measure (COPM)**: Scored 4/10 in performance and satisfaction, indicating moderate difficulties in occupational performance and satisfaction with current abilities.
- **Numeric Pain Rating Scale**: Reports a pain level of 6/10 in her lower extremities, affecting daily activities and training.
- **Functional Performance Test (FPT)**: Assessed to determine functional performance in sport-specific activities. Results indicated deficiencies in:
  - **Strength and Power**: Below average for her competitive level.
  - **Speed**: Noticeably reduced compared to her baseline.
  - **Endurance**: Decreased stamina impacting long-distance running.
  - **ROM and Flexibility**: Limited range of motion in lower extremities.
  - **Balance and Proprioception**: Compromised, affecting running form.
  - **Agility**: Slower response times in agility drills.
  - **Functional and Safe Movement Patterns**: Identified compensatory patterns contributing to stress injuries.
- **Psychosocial Assessment**: Assessed mental health and stress levels using the Depression, Anxiety, and Stress Scale (DASS-21). Results indicated moderate levels of anxiety and high levels of stress, significantly impacting her daily life and athletic performance.

Occupational Therapy Plan of Care and Goals:

The client will receive skilled occupational therapy services twice a week for 16 weeks to improve bone health, manage hormonal imbalances (in collaboration with her endocrinologist), and enhance athletic performance and overall well-being.

Goals:

1. Achieve a 10% increase in bone density within four months through focused nutrition and weight-bearing exercises to improve participation in sports and daily physical activities.
2. Achieve regular menstrual cycles within four months through dietary modifications and stress management techniques to enhance overall health and well-being, impacting daily routines and athletic performance.
3. Increase COPM performance and satisfaction scores to 7/10 within three months, enabling the client to perform daily activities (ADLs) and training with reduced pain and fatigue.
4. Achieve a 50% reduction in pain levels in the lower extremities within three months through targeted therapeutic interventions to enhance participation in sports, work, and social activities.

5. Improve FPT scores by 20% within three months to enable safe and effective participation in competitive running again.
6. Reduce stress and anxiety levels by 30% within three months through targeted psychosocial interventions to improve overall mental health, impacting work, social activities, and athletic performance.

Interventions:

1. **Nutrition Management**: Collaborate with a dietitian to develop a nutrition plan that supports bone health and hormonal balance. The OTP will help the client integrate these dietary recommendations into her daily routine by:
   - **Meal Preparation and Planning**: Assisting the client in preparing and planning healthy, protein-rich meals that include calcium and vitamin D-rich foods. This includes teaching energy-saving techniques for meal prep, using adaptive equipment if necessary, and creating meal plans that minimize reliance on processed foods.
   - **Healthy Eating Strategies**: Educating the client on the importance of balanced nutrition, including how to read food labels, choose nutrient-dense foods, and create balanced meals. The OTP will also provide strategies for maintaining a healthy diet while managing a busy training schedule.
   - **Routine Integration**: Developing strategies to seamlessly integrate healthy eating habits into the client's daily routine. This includes establishing regular meal times, creating a structured grocery shopping list, and utilizing meal prep techniques to ensure consistent adherence to the nutrition plan.
2. **Weight-Bearing Exercises**: Implement a tailored exercise program focusing on weight-bearing activities such as resistance training and low-impact aerobic exercises to improve bone density and overall strength.
3. **Hormonal Regulation Techniques**: Introduce stress management techniques such as mindfulness, yoga, and adequate sleep hygiene to help regulate hormonal balance and improve menstrual regularity. Additionally, support the client in medication management for hormones prescribed by her endocrinologist, and promote healthier eating patterns and regular physical activity to support hormonal health.
4. **Pain Management**: Utilize modalities such as heat therapy, TENS units, and gentle stretching exercises to manage pain in the lower extremities. Introduce strengthening exercises to improve muscular support around affected areas.
5. **Sport-Specific Training**: Develop a progressive training program that includes sport-specific drills and exercises to improve running mechanics, endurance, and strength, facilitating a safe return to competitive running.
6. **Functional Performance Training**: Target specific areas identified in the FPT:
   - **Strength and Power**: Resistance training to build lower extremity and core strength.
   - **Speed and Endurance**: Interval training and cardiovascular conditioning to improve running performance.
   - **ROM and Flexibility**: Stretching and flexibility exercises to enhance range of motion.
   - **Balance and Proprioception**: Balance drills and proprioceptive training to improve running form and prevent injuries.
   - **Agility**: Agility drills to enhance quickness and responsiveness.
   - **Functional and Safe Movement Patterns**: Corrective exercises to address compensatory movement patterns.

7. **Bone Density Scan Collaboration**: While OTPs do not perform or interpret bone density scans, they can utilize the results provided by a radiologist or physician to tailor the intervention plan. Specifically:
    - **Incorporate Recommendations**: Integrate recommendations from the client's physician regarding bone health into the therapy plan, ensuring exercises and activities are safe and beneficial.
    - **Monitor Progress**: Work with the client to track improvements in bone health as indicated by follow-up scans, adjusting interventions as needed based on the physician's feedback.
8. **Psychosocial Interventions**: Address the client's mental health and stress levels through targeted interventions:
    - **Cognitive-Behavioural Therapy (CBT)**: Implement CBT techniques to help the client manage anxiety and stress by identifying and reframing negative thought patterns.
    - **Relaxation Techniques**: Teach and practice relaxation techniques such as deep breathing exercises, progressive muscle relaxation, and guided imagery to reduce stress levels.
    - **Mindfulness Training**: Incorporate mindfulness practices to help the client stay present and manage stress effectively.
    - **Social Support Enhancement**: Encourage participation in support groups or peer networks to provide emotional support and reduce feelings of isolation.
9. **Education and Support**: Provide education on the importance of bone health, nutrition, and self-care strategies. Encourage participation in support groups for athletes dealing with similar health issues to enhance social support and motivation.

Outcomes:

- **Post Treatment**: Showed significant improvement in managing osteoporosis, with a 10% increase in bone density and regular menstrual cycles. Enhanced functional independence with COPM scores of 7/10.
- **Functional Independence**: Improved ability to perform daily activities and training with reduced pain and fatigue, maintaining competitive edge in her sport.
- **Pain Reduction**: Reported a 50% reduction in pain levels in the lower extremities, significantly improving her ability to train and compete.
- **Return to Sport**: Achieved a 25% improvement in FPT scores, enabling safe and effective participation in competitive running again.
- **Mental Health Improvement**: Demonstrated a 30% reduction in stress and anxiety levels, enhancing overall well-being and performance.
- **Overall Well-being**: Demonstrated improved nutritional status, hormonal balance, and overall health, contributing to better athletic performance and quality of life.

At the conclusion of therapy, the client demonstrated marked improvements in bone health, hormonal balance, functional independence, pain management, athletic performance, and mental health. These outcomes highlight the effectiveness of a comprehensive, client-centered approach in addressing the unique health challenges faced by female athletes. The client's commitment to therapy and collaboration with the occupational therapy team resulted in sustainable improvements, showcasing resilience and adaptive skills in managing her health and athletic career.

416   Occupational Therapy and Women's Health

CASE B: Alternative Medicine and Holistic Nutrition

Background and Medical History: The client is a 48-year-old woman experiencing chronic migraines and digestive issues. She has a history of anxiety and insomnia, which she believes exacerbate her symptoms. Her medical history includes irritable bowel syndrome (IBS) and a previous diagnosis of generalized anxiety disorder. She has consulted with various healthcare providers and has recently shown interest in exploring alternative medicine and holistic nutrition as part of her treatment plan. Her physician has conducted a comprehensive assessment, including blood tests to check for nutrient deficiencies and an evaluation of her gastrointestinal health.

Prior Level of Function:

- **Work**: Full-time dentist, managing a busy practice and multiple patients daily.
- **Social**: Actively involved in community events and social gatherings.
- **Hobbies**: Enjoyed visiting art museums, which require a lot of walking, camping, and swimming.
- **ADLs**: Independent in all activities of daily living, including personal care, meal preparation, and household chores.
- **IADLs**: Efficiently managed her dental practice, financial responsibilities, and transportation needs.

Household Living Arrangements and Social History:

- **Living Situation**: Resides with her spouse and two adult children in a suburban home.
- **Family and Social Support**: Strong support system with family and close friends, though her participation has been limited recently due to health issues.

Change in Functional Status and Challenges:

The client reports significant disruptions in her daily activities due to chronic migraines, digestive issues, and associated symptoms. Specific areas affected include:

ADLs:

- Difficulty with personal self-care tasks such as grooming, bathing, lower body dressing due to migraine-related pain and fatigue.
- Challenges with meal preparation due to nausea and dietary restrictions related to IBS.
- Reduced frequency of engaging in hobbies like visiting art museums, camping, and swimming due to fatigue and pain.

IADLs:

- Struggles with managing household chores such as cleaning and grocery shopping due to decreased energy levels.
- Difficulty coordinating her dental practice, including patient scheduling and administrative tasks, due to frequent absences and decreased concentration.

Work:

- Increased absenteeism due to severe migraines and digestive issues.
- Difficulty maintaining productivity and concentration during patient appointments, impacting the quality of care.

- Increased anxiety and stress related to managing her practice while coping with health issues.

Social Activities:

- Reduced participation in community events and social gatherings due to fatigue and pain.
- Difficulty maintaining relationships and engaging in social interactions.

Emotional and Psychological:

- Increased anxiety and insomnia exacerbating her physical symptoms.
- Feelings of isolation and frustration due to her health conditions.

Occupational Therapy Assessments:

- **Canadian Occupational Performance Measure (COPM):** Identified significant difficulties in managing self-care, productivity, and leisure activities, with a performance satisfaction score averaging 3/10.
- **Beck Anxiety Inventory (BAI):** Scores reflecting moderate to severe anxiety symptoms, with a total score of 25.
- **Gastrointestinal Symptom Rating Scale (GSRS):** Assessed the severity of digestive issues, indicating significant discomfort and impact on daily life with a total score of 45.
- **Migraine Disability Assessment (MIDAS):** Evaluated the impact of migraines on occupational performance and daily activities, revealing a score of 20, indicating severe disability.
- **Role Checklist:** Assessed the client's roles and satisfaction with these roles, identifying areas of role transition stress, particularly in her professional and social roles.
- **Occupational Balance Questionnaire (OBQ):** Evaluated the client's balance between work, leisure, and self-care activities, indicating significant imbalance with a score of 30/100.

Occupational Therapy Plan of Care and Goals:

The client will receive skilled occupational therapy services twice a week for 12 weeks to improve her independence in ADLs, manage her symptoms, and enhance her ability to balance her roles as a dentist and mother.

Goals:

1. Client will achieve a 50% reduction in the severity and frequency of migraines using alternative medicine techniques within 12 weeks, enabling her to attend work regularly and perform her duties as a dentist without disruption.
2. Client will independently manage personal care tasks with minimal fatigue, using energy conservation techniques, achieving a 30% improvement in COPM scores within 12 weeks, thereby maintaining her grooming and hygiene to support professional appearance and self-esteem.
3. Client will establish a consistent meal preparation routine using holistic nutrition principles, improving adherence to a healthy diet within 12 weeks, ensuring she has the energy and nutritional support needed to manage her dental practice and family responsibilities effectively.

4. Client will manage household chores efficiently, using time management and energy conservation techniques, achieving a 40% improvement in IADL performance as measured by self-report within 12 weeks, maintaining a clean and organized home environment to support her and her family's well-being.
5. Client will improve work performance and attendance, reducing absenteeism and enhancing focus, as measured by MIDAS scores and employer feedback within 12 weeks, ensuring she can meet the demands of her dental practice and provide quality care to her patients.
6. Client will reduce anxiety symptoms, with BAI scores decreasing to below 15 within 12 weeks through targeted psychosocial interventions, enhancing her emotional stability and ability to engage in work and social activities.
7. Client will increase participation in social activities, re-engaging in at least one community event or social gathering per week, as measured by self-reported participation and satisfaction within 12 weeks, promoting a sense of community and support to improve her overall well-being.

Occupational Therapy Interventions:

The following interventions will be tailored to meet the client's specific needs and address the outlined goals:

1. **Alternative Medicine Techniques**

   - **Acupuncture**: Implement acupuncture sessions to reduce migraine frequency and severity.
   - **Herbal Supplements**: Educate on the use of herbal supplements to manage digestive issues and anxiety.
   - **Biofeedback**: Use biofeedback techniques to help the client manage stress and pain.

2. **Holistic Nutrition Education**

   - **Dietary Planning**: Develop a nutrition plan that supports digestive health and reduces migraine triggers.
   - **Meal Preparation**: Teach meal preparation techniques that are quick, nutritious, and tailored to her dietary needs.

3. **Activity Modification and Energy Conservation**

   - **Energy Conservation**: Educate the client on energy conservation techniques, such as pacing activities and incorporating frequent rest breaks.
   - **Activity Modification**: Advise on modifying activities to reduce fatigue, such as breaking tasks into smaller, manageable steps.

4. **ADL and IADL Training**

   - **Adaptive Equipment**: Provide training on the use of adaptive equipment designed for individuals with limited energy, such as ergonomic tools for personal care tasks.
   - **Household Management**: Develop strategies for efficient household management, including time-saving techniques and organizational tools.

5. **Work-Life Balance**

   - **Structured Schedule**: Develop a structured schedule that balances work, parenting, and self-care activities.

- **Organizational Tools**: Provide advanced organizational tools and strategies to help the client keep track of work tasks, deadlines, and personal responsibilities.

6. **Social and Emotional Support**

    - **Peer Support**: Facilitate connections with peer support groups and community resources to provide emotional support and reduce feelings of isolation.
    - **Stress Management**: Implement stress management strategies to help stabilize mood and enhance overall mental well-being.
    - **Cognitive-Behavioural Therapy (CBT) Techniques**: Integrate CBT techniques to address negative thought patterns and develop healthier coping mechanisms.
    - **Motivational Interviewing**: Use motivational interviewing to enhance motivation and commitment to treatment plans.

Outcomes:

Post Treatment:

- **Symptom Management**: Significant reduction in migraine frequency and severity, enabling the client to attend work regularly and perform her duties as a dentist without disruption.
- **ADL and IADL Independence**: Improved engagement in personal care and household tasks, maintaining a clean and organized home environment and supporting professional appearance and self-esteem.
- **Nutritional Adherence**: Established a consistent meal preparation routine, ensuring the client has the energy and nutritional support needed to manage her dental practice and family responsibilities effectively.
- **Work Performance**: Improved work performance and attendance, reducing absenteeism and enhancing focus, ensuring the client can meet the demands of her dental practice and provide quality care to her patients.
- **Emotional Stability**: Reduced anxiety symptoms, enhancing the client's emotional stability and ability to engage in work and social activities.
- **Social Engagement**: Increased participation in social activities, promoting a sense of community and support to improve the client's overall well-being.

Follow-Up Visits:

- **Continuous Reinforcement**: Continuously reinforce stress management techniques and activity modifications to ensure the sustainability of the client's improvements in daily activities and work tasks.
- **Ongoing Support**: Provide ongoing support and adjust the client's treatment plan based on her feedback, changes in her symptoms, and any new challenges that arise in managing her role as a dentist and parent.
- **Holistic Practices Integration**: Ensure the client continues to integrate holistic practices into her routine, such as maintaining her nutrition plan and using alternative medicine techniques for symptom management.

The client demonstrated significant improvement in managing her migraines, digestive issues, and stress, enhancing her overall functionality and independence. She is now capable of performing daily tasks and work activities with greater efficiency and less anxiety. The tailored occupational therapy interventions enabled her to balance her roles as a dentist and a parent effectively. Through the collaborative and holistic approach of occupational therapy, the client has regained a better quality of life and improved her capacity to engage in meaningful activities.

Further Reading

Ardern, C. L., Hooper, N., O'Halloran, P., Webster, K. E., & Kvist, J. (2022). A psychological support intervention to help injured athletes "get back in the game": Design and development study. *JMIR Formative Research*, *6*(8), e28851. https://doi.org/10.2196/28851

de Borja, C., Chang, C. J., Watkins, R., & Senter, C. (2022). Optimizing health and athletic performance for women. *Current Reviews in Musculoskeletal Medicine*, *15*(1), 10–20. https://doi.org/10.1007/s12178-021-09735-2

Dixon, S., Keating, S., McNiven, A., Edwards, G., Turner, P., Knox-Peebles, C., Taghinejadi, N., Vincent, K., James, O., & Hayward, G. (2023). What are important areas where better technology would support women's health? Findings from a priority setting partnership. *BMC Women's Health*, *23*(1), 667. https://doi.org/10.1186/s12905-023-02778-2

Haraldsdottir, K., & Watson, A. M. (2021). Psychosocial impacts of sports-related injuries in adolescent athletes. *Current Sports Medicine Reports*, *20*(2), 104–108. https://doi.org/10.1249/JSR.0000000000000809

Heeb, R., Putnam, M., Keglovits, M., Weber, C., Campbell, M., Stark, S., & Morgan, K. (2022). Factors influencing participation among adults aging with long-term physical disability. *Disability and Health Journal*, *15*(1), 101169. https://doi.org/10.1016/j.dhjo.2021.101169

Hosseini, S. A., & Padhy, R. K. (2023). Body image distortion (Archived). In *StatPearls*. StatPearls Publishing.

Liberty, A., Rubin, E. S., Bullard, K. A., & Au, K. (2022). Human milk-expression technologies: A primer for obstetricians. *Obstetrics and Gynecology*, *139*(6), 1180–1188. https://doi.org/10.1097/AOG.0000000000004804

Lyzwinski, L., Elgendi, M., & Menon, C. (2024). Innovative approaches to menstruation and fertility tracking using wearable reproductive health technology: Systematic review. *Journal of Medical Internet Research*, *26*, e45139. https://doi.org/10.2196/45139

Munguba, M. C., Valdés, M. T., & da Silva, C. A. (2008). The application of an occupational therapy nutrition education programme for children who are obese. *Occupational Therapy International*, *15*(1), 56–70. https://doi.org/10.1002/oti.244

Plapler, P. G., Cecatto, R. B., Socolowski, M. D., & Martins, F. (2023). Disability prevalent conditions in women. *Revista da Associacao Medica Brasileira (1992)*, *69*(suppl 1), e2023S115. https://doi.org/10.1590/1806-9282.2023S115

Reitz, S. M., Scaffa, M. E., Commission on Practice, & Dorsey, J. (2020). Occupational therapy in the promotion of health and well-being. *The American Journal of Occupational Therapy: Official Publication of the American Occupational Therapy Association*, *74*(3), 7403420010p1–7403420010p14. https://doi.org/10.5014/ajot.2020.743003

Rogers, D. L., Tanaka, M. J., Cosgarea, A. J., Ginsburg, R. D., & Dreher, G. M. (2024). How mental health affects injury risk and outcomes in athletes. *Sports Health*, *16*(2), 222–229. https://doi.org/10.1177/19417381231179678

Index

Pages in *italics* refer to figures and pages in **bold** refer to tables.

abdominal hysterectomy *see* hysterectomy
abortion: spontaneous (miscarriage) 139–140, *139*; rights and access 7, 411
Acceptance and Commitment Therapy (ACT) **216**
acupuncture 406, **408**, 418
across lifespan 339–368; case studies 359–364, 365–368; early adulthood 347–350; later life 354–357; middle years 350–354; pediatric and adolescent girls 339–347, 359–364
adolescents *see* pediatric and adolescent girls' health
adrenal insufficiency **158**, 162–163
advocacy 409–412; aims, needs 409; birth control, reproductive health and rights 7, 8, 411; chronic conditions 411; gender equity and professional development 5, 15–16, **16**, 17, 27; gender-based violence 383, 412; holistic health care 7; maternal health 411; medical choice 125; menstrual care access 341; mental health 411; non-cisgender health needs, gender diversity 208–209, **214**, 218; strategies 410; *see also* women's health movements
alternative medicine techniques 406–409, 418, **408**; acupuncture 406, **408**, 418; aromatherapy 406,**408**; chiropractic therapy 406–407; client preferences and values 408–409; common practices 406, **408**; contraindications 407–408, **408**; case study 416–420; herbal medicine 406, **408**; massage therapy **124**, 406, **408**; physical exercise, sport 63, 99, **100**, 169–170, 396, 406, **408**; reflexology 407, **408**; reiki 407, **408**; safety and efficacy considerations 407
American Cancer Society (ACS) 290–291, 298, 301, 303
American Joint Commission on Cancer 293
anorexia nervosa 269, **270**, 282–285

assessment 29–33; assistive technology fit 254–255; cardiovascular health 251–253; client-centered **23**; cognitive and emotional 32–34; culturally competent and sensitive 25, **26**; disabilities 398; eating-related disorders, obesity, nutrition 273, **273**, 400–401, 403; ergonomic **18**; gynecological conditions 64; inter-partner violence impact 373–375; pain 57–60, **60**, 104–106; pelvic health 52, 57–60, **60**, 65, 111, **112**; physical and functional 31–32; physical activity levels and barriers 276, **276**; *see also* pregnant patient evaluation and assessments; sleep health 267, **267**; substance use disorder 280–281, **280**; trauma-informed 380, **381–382**
Assessment of Motor and Process Skills (AMPS) **110**
assigned female at birth (AFAB), occupational function and OT interventions 203; community and social participation 207–208; competent-provider lack 209; discrimination and bias, health care 208–209; financial/healthcare cost barriers 210; gender-affirming care/surgeries 204–206, 209–210; healthcare disparities, access barriers 208–212; health care needs knowledge lack 209; identity and role transitions 207; mental health challenges and interventions 206, 215–217, **216–217**; *see also* non-cisgender health; pelvic floor muscle functions 48–49, **48**; self-care and health management 207; social support needs 206–207; specific occupational needs 207
assigned male at birth (AMAB) 48–49, **48**; *see also* non-cisgender health
assistive technology *see* technology, supportive devices
athletes 393–397; case study 412–415; holistic health approach 396; injury prevention,

rehabilitation 394–395; nutritional needs 401; performance enhancement 395–396; physiological challenges 345–346, 393–394; psychosocial well-being 396
autoimmune conditions 177–201; case studies 194–201; celiac disease 190–193, 198–201; Hashimoto's thyroiditis 185–190, 178–182; SLE (systemic lupus erythematosus) 182–185, 194–197
avoidant/restrictive food intake disorder (ARFID) 269, **270**

Barthel Index (BI) for activities of daily living (ADL) Score **110**
beauty standards 20–21
Beck Depression Inventory (BDI) 375
billing in occupational therapy 29–31, **30**, 36–37, **37**
binge-eating disorder 269, **270**, 273, 274, 278, 347
biofeedback 54–55, **60**, 61, 129, **130**, 169, 418
biopsychosocial perspectives and approaches: Biopsychosocial Model, OT framework 69; infertility support 226; menopause 226; sexual health 224–226
bipotential neonatal brain 92, *94*
body image 20–21, 33, 269–270, 271, 291, 296, **297**, 302, 305, **307**
bottle feeding 131, 132, 237–238; education, counseling 132; ergonomic positioning **101**, 129, 130; supportive devices 131; techniques 131; transition from breastfeeding 131, 237
breast cancer 290–298, 313–315; awareness campaigns 7; body image concerns 291; case study 313–315; diagnosis, examination 290–291, 293; impact 291; incidence, survival rates 290; lymphedema 298, 308; medical management 294–295, 298; occupational performance barriers 295–296; OT interventions 296–298, **297**; pathology 292, *292*–293; rehabilitation 9–10; stages 293–294, *293*, *294*; symptoms 295
breast health: anatomy, breast 292, *292*; assistive technology 389–390; breast self-examination (BSE) 290–291, 389; hormonal influence 88, **88**, **157**
breastfeeding 235–237; assistive technology and devices 131,237, 389–390, 391; bottle feeding transition 237–238; and contraceptive planning 167; education 132, 236–237, **236**, 236; emotional support 237; environment 237; ergonomic positioning **101**, 129, 236; latching techniques 131, 236; OT support and interventions **101**, 129–130, 131, 132, 235–237; prolactin **157**; pumps 131, 389; routine, structure 237
bulimia nervosa 269, **270**

Canadian Model of Occupational Performance and Engagement (CMOP-E) 69
Canadian Occupational Performance Measure (COPM) **110**, 375
cardiovascular health 246–262; *see also* heart disease
case studies: alternative medicine, holistic nutrition 416–420; anorexia nervosa 282–285; athlete, injuries, hormonal imbalance 412–415; autoimmune diseases 194–201; celiac disease 198–201; endocrine health 172–176; gynecological health 77–81, 81–85; health across lifespan (adolescent dysmenorrhea) 359–361; health across lifespan (middle adulthood role transition, divorce, stress) 365–368; health across lifespan (teen pregnancy) 361–364; heart disease (CAD) 259–262; infertility 240–244; neurological health (early-stage Alzheimer's) 335–337; neurological health (ischemic stroke) 333–335; non-cisgender health 219–222; obstetric health (postpartum) 145–149; obstetric health (pregnancy) 149–152; oncology 313–315; polycystic ovary syndrome (PCOS) 81–85; SLE (systemic lupus erythematosus 194–197; trauma-informed care (substance abuse, sleep) 285–288
celiac disease 190–193, 198–201
Centers for Disease Control and Prevention (CDC) 342, 347, 352, 354, 355, 370, 372, 377, 397
cerebrovascular accident (CVA) *see* stroke, cerebrovascular accident (CVA)
cervical cancer 4, 301, 303, **304**
cervical dysplasia **70**
Cesarean section (C-section): breastfeeding adaptation, bottle-feeding support 129, 131; pelvic floor rehabilitation 129, **130**; post-cesarean scar management and activity modifications 127–130; postoperative rehabilitation 75, 126; preparation 127
chemotherapy 294, 296, **297**, 300, **302**, 304, **307**
childbearing, empowering agency 230–232, **231**
cholesterol 247, *247*, 252, *252*, 257
chronic conditions 136–137; across lifespan 10; cerebral palsy **135**, 137; cystic fibrosis **135**, 137; diabetes (type 1 and type 2) **158**, 161–162, 352; hypertensive disorders 136; later life 354–355, 358; lymphedema 43, **68**, 295, 296, 298, 308–312, 313, 314, 315;

middle years 350, 351, 352; multiple sclerosis (MS) 135, 136, 325–329; nutritional needs 403; and pregnancy 136–137; prevalence 350, 351; rheumatoid arthritis (RA) 178–182, *179*, **180–182**; SLE (systemic lupus erythematosus 136–137, 182–185, 194–197; spinal cord injury **135**, 136; sport performance impact **394**; women's health advocacy and policy 411
clinical breast exam (CBE) 290–291
coeliac disease *see* celiac disease
cognitive-behavioral therapy (CBT) 169, **181**, 190, **216**, 268, 274, 281, 352–353, 377, 399
compression therapy 310–311, *311*
coronary artery disease (CAD) 247, 259–262
cultural competency: addressing cultural factors **24**; aspects/actionable steps 383–385, **384**; building, OTP strategies 22, **23**; community engagement 380–382; defining 383; cultural awareness, knowledge and skills 25, 383–384, **384**; cultural and societal norms 2, 3, 11, 18, 20–22, 23–25, **24**, 280, 291, 371

diabetes: gestational mellitus (GDM) 122, 135, **135**; type 1 and 2 **158**, 161–162, 352
dialectical behavior therapy (DBT) **216**
dysmenorrhea **58**; adolescent, prevalence 339, 341; case studies 77–81, 359–361
dyspareunia **58**, **226**

early adulthood women's health 347–350; mental health and emotional well-being 349–350; preventive health and lifestyle choices 350; reproductive health and family planning 348–349; role transitions (work, personal) 347–348; work-life balance and career development 349
eating disorder inventory (EDI) **273**
eating disorders 269–272; age group-related frequency 269–270; anorexia nervosa 269, **270**, 282–285; binge-eating disorder 269, **270**, 273, 274, 278, 347; bulimia nervosa 269, **270**; causes, contributing factors 270; healthy eating education 403, 414; mental health correlation 10, 269; *see also* nutrition, nutrition management; occupational performance impact 272–273; OT framework, assessment and interventions 270–271, 273–275, **273**, 402, 405; other specified feeding or eating disorder (OSFED) 269, **270**; prevalence 269; rumination disorder **270**
Ecological Model of Human Performance (EMHP) 69
embryological and fetal development stages **90–91**, *92*

emotional well-being *see* mental health and emotional well-being
endocrine health 155–176; adrenal insufficiency 162–163; case studies 172–176; contraception, family planning 165–166; diabetes, type 1 and 2 **158**, 161–162, 352; hyperthyroidism 159–160; hypothyroidism 158–159; perimenopause and menopause 163–165, 167–172; polycystic ovary syndrome (PCOS) 160–161; reproductive hormones 49–50
endometrial (uterine) cancer 301, 303, **304**
endometriosis, endometriosis excision **58**, 69, **70**, 72–73, **75**, 77–81
estrogen 50; cardiovascular system protection 250; menopause, perimenopause **158**, 163, 164, 168, 189, 351; migraines 317; neuroprotective effects 329; ovaries 45; pregnancy 88, **88**; puberty 50, 339; sleep pattern effect 265; type, function 50, **157**, 340
evaluation 29–33; cognitive and emotional 32–34; complexity levels 30–31, **30–31**; cultural sensitivity 25; physical and functional 31–32; pregnant patient 103–112, **104**, **107–108**, **110–112**
expressive arts therapy **216**

fecal incontinence 50, 51–52, 56, 111
feeding, newborn 235–238, **236**; bottle **101**, 131, 132, 237–238; breastfeeding 131–132, **157**, 235–238, 390–391; ergonomic positioning **101**, 129, 236; prolactin **157**; supportive devices and technology 131, 237, 389, 391
FemTech *see* technology and women health
Fertility Quality of Life Questionnaire (FertiQoL) 229
fibroid embolization 74, 76
Five F trauma responses (fight, flight, freeze, fawn, flop) 372–373, *373*

gender diversity terminology **204**
gender equity/disparities: contraceptive access 4; digital health interventions (DHIs), telemedicine 253; economic productivity, workforce participation 4; gender bias and medical outcome 12, 249, 353; gender role expectations 17, 21, **24**, 371; global causes and significance 1–2, 3, 4–5; health advocacy 411; health outcome, mortality 4; healthcare access/outcome 5, 11–17, 208–212; infertility treatment 3–4; intersectionality 26–27; maternal and child health 4; medical research 11–14, **15**; OT intervention, role and potential 5; racial 290; rehabilitation outcomes 12–14, **15**;

workplace, professional development 15–16, **16**, 18–20, **19**, 249
gender-affirming care 204–206, 209–210; *see also* non-cisgender health
gestational diabetes mellitus (GDM) 122, 135, **135**
global perspective 1–5; conflict zones 2–3; developed nations 5; Eastern Europa 3–4; health disparities, significance 4–5; Latin America, Caribbean 3; Middle East and North Africa (MENA) region 2; Oceania, Pacific Islands 4; South Asia 2; Southeast Asia 3; Sub-Saharan Africa 2
goal setting 34–35, 112
gonadotropins 50, 88
gynecological cancers 301–307; anatomy, pathology 303; cervical 4, 301, 303, **304**; clinical presentation **70**; incidence and mortality rate 301; medical management 304–305; occupational performance symptoms and barriers 305–306; OTP interventions **70**, 306–307, **306–307**; ovarian 301, 303, **304**; screening and screening access 4, 303; stages 304, **304**; uterine (endometrial) 301, 303, **304**; vaginal 301, **304**; vulvar 303, **304**
gynecological conditions 64–71; assessments, signs and symptoms 64–66, **65**, **66**; ADL, IADL adaptation strategies 66–**67**; case study, endometriosis 77–81; cancers 301–307; cervical dysplasia **70**; emotional and psychological support 66; endometriosis, endometriosis excision 58, 69, **70**, 72–73, **75**; infertility 3–4, 69, **71**, 226–228, 229, 241–244; menopause-related symptoms **71**, 156, 164, **168**; menstrual disorders **70**; OT theory frameworks and interventions 66, **67**–68, 68–69; ovarian cysts **70**, 73; pain management 66; pelvic floor rehabilitation 66, **107**, **112**; pelvic organ prolapse **59**, **60**, 66, 69, **71**, 73, **112**; polycystic ovary syndrome (PCOS) 50, **70**, 81–85, **158**, 160–161; premenstrual syndrome (PMS) **71**, 341; uterine fibroids / uterine fibroid embolization (UFE) 45, 69, **70**, 74
gynecological health management 39–85; case studies, endometriosis 77–81; case studies, polycystic ovary syndrome (PCOS) 81–85; gynecological conditions 64–71; gynecological surgery, rehabilitative strategies 71–77; pelvis and perineum 39–64; *see also each under own heading*
gynecological surgery 71–77; Caesarian section (C-section) **75**, 127–130; collaboration, OTP-surgical teams 76–77; endometriosis excision 73, **75**; fibroid embolization 74, 76; hysterectomy 72–73, **75**, 204; ovarian cystectomy 73; patient preparation and education 72–74; pelvic organ prolapse repair 13–14, 73, **75**, 76, 129; postoperative rehabilitation, recovery support 74–76, **75**; uterine fibroids / uterine fibroid embolization (UFE) 45, 69, **70**, 74

Hashimoto's thyroiditis 185–190; exercise interventions 188–189; as hypothyroidism cause 185–186; and menopause 189–190; OT interventions 187–188, **187–188**, 189–190; symptoms *186*
heart disease 246–262; arrhythmias 248; case study, CAD 259–262; cholesterol as cause 247, *247*, 252, *252*, 257; coronary artery disease (CAD) 247, 259–262; heart failure 247–248; high risk populations 255–259, **256**; impact daily functioning 248; OT in cardiac rehabilitation 248–253; prevalence, mortality cause 246–247; prevention strategies 257–258; types 247–248; valvular heart disease 248
heart health, technology and innovation 253–255; advanced imaging and diagnostic tools 254; assessment, client's technology fit 254–255; mobile apps 254; OT impact potential 253; OT interventions example 254–255; telehealth, remote monitoring 254; wearable devices 253–254
herbal medicine 406, **408**
hemorrhagic stroke 319, **320**
high-risk pregnancies 134–137, **135**, **138**, 139
history of women's health care 6–10; current trends, future directions 8–10; OT emergence and development 8–10; women health movements 7–8
holistic health approach **214**, 396; case study: holistic nutrition 416–420; 21st century/current 10–11; holistic assessment methods 116–118; holistic wellness programs 169–170, **233**, 235; WHO health definition 6; Women's Health Movement (1970s–1980) 7
hormonal imbalances/disorders *see* endocrine health
hormonal therapies in cancer treatment 204, 294, 305
hormone replacement therapy (HRT) 49, 204, 207, 211–212, **211**, **218**, **219**
human papillomavirus (HPV) 4, **70**, 301, 303, 304, 344
hypertensive disorders 136
hyperthyroidism 159–160
hypothyroidism 158–159
hysterectomy 72–73, **75**, 204

immune system-related diseases *see* autoimmune diseases
immunotherapy 295, 300, 305
incontinence 13–14, 49, 51–52, 56, 111, **112**
infertility **71**; case study 241–244; emotional coping 226, 227; Fertility Quality of Life Questionnaire (FertiQoL) 229; OT support 69, 226–228, 229; treatment access 3–4
insomnia 266, **266**; cognitive behavioral therapy for insomnia (CBT-I) 268; insomnia severity index (ISI) **267**
inter-partner violence (IPV) 370–387; case study 385–387; community engagement 382; *see also* cultural competency; economic dependency and 371; health consequences and economic costs 370, 372; impact assessment 373–375; non-verbal indicators 374, **374**; occupational performance impact factors 371–372; OT settings **381–382**; power dynamics, control relationships 371; prevalence 370; reproductive coercion, sexual violence 371; sensitive questioning techniques 374; social norms, gender roles and 371; trauma response, types 372–373, *373*; trauma-healing 374; *see also* trauma-informed care (TIC); violence, nature and severity 371
intersectionality 26–27
ischemic stroke 319, 333–335

Katz Index of independence in activities of daily living **110**
Kawa Model 69, 215
Kegel exercises 52–54, *54*, 63

labor and delivery 123–125, **124**; Cesarean section (C-section) **75**, 126, 127–130, **130**; labor positions, strategies and adaptations 123–124, **125**
later life women's health 354–357; chronic conditions 354–355; cognitive decline 355; loss experience (death) 356–357; mental health and social isolation 356; mobility issues 355; physical changes and exercise recommendations 357–358; retirement transition 356
Lawton Instrumental Activities of Daily Living Scale (IADL) **110**
Life Events Checklist (LEC) 375, **381**
lifespan 339–368; case studies 359–364, 365–368; early adulthood 347–350; later life 354–357; middle years 350–354; pediatric and adolescent girls 339–347, 359–364; *see also each under own heading*
lifestyle choices 276–279; adolescent obesity 342; OT assessment and interventions 52, 276–278, **276**; preventive health and 350; promotion 279; substance use 343; unhealthy, impact and examples 278–279
lung cancer 298–301, **302**; anatomy, pathology 298–299; incidence rate, prevalence 298; medical management 299–300; occupational performance, symptoms and barriers 300–301; OT interventions (pre-/post-surgery) **302**; OTP interventions 301, 303; screening 298; stages 299, **299**
lupus *see* SLE (systemic lupus erythematosus)
lymphedema 43, **68**, 296, 308–312; care training, certification 309; case study 313, 314, 315; management, breast cancer 295; management: breast cancer 298; management methods *310*; OTP interventions, management methods 309–312, *310*; primary, secondary 308; stages 308–309; symptoms, effects/impact 308

mammogram 291, 294
manual lymphatic drainage (MLD) 310, *310*
manual muscle testing (MMT) 64, **66**
massage therapy **124**, 406, **408**
maternal mental health 141–145, 235–237; conditions 142–143; long-term support 145; multidisciplinary collaboration 145; OT interventions 143–145; prevalence 141
menopause 168, 350; body changes *239*; eating disorders, weight gain 270; and Hashimoto's thyroiditis 189–190; hormonal changes 155–156, **156**, **157**, **158**, 328; impact daily life and management **158**, 168–170, **168**; incidence, onset age 164, 238, 350; menopause-related symptoms, gynecological conditions **71**; mental health, biopsychosocial approach 238; OT interventions 163–164, 238–241, 351–352; OTP transition report 28; *see also* perimenopause; post-menopause 156, **156**; sexual health changes, addressing 171–172, **226**; sleep disturbances 265; symptoms and impact **71**, 156, 164, **168**; technology integration, tracking 170–171
menstrual cycle: athlete's training adaptation 345, 394, 395; menstrual migraine 317–318, *317*; multiple sclerosis (MS) 329; puberty 339–340; regulation (estrogen, progesterone) 50, **156**, **157**
menstrual disorders **70**
menstrual hygiene: assistive technology 392–393; multiple sclerosis (MS) 329; post-stroke 324; product access, adolescents 341
menstruation: assistive technology, tracking 166, 392; case study 81–85; cessation, perimenopausal and menopausal transition

164, 168–169, **168**, 211, 238, 351; menstrual cramps *see* dysmenorrhea; menstrual disorders **70**; onset, adolescent 156; premenstrual syndrome **71**; stages 339–340, *340*

mental health and emotional well-being: breastfeeding 235–237; case study: infertility 241–244; case study: non-cisgender health 219–222; childbearing, empowering agency 230–232, **231**; children and adolescent girls 342–343; early adulthood 349–350; emotional and cognitive assessments 32–34; *see also* infertility; later life 356; gender disparity in research and treatment 11, 12; maternal mental health 141–145, 235–237; *see also* menopause; middle life 352–353; mental health stigma 21; non-cisgender health 206–208, 215–217; OT history 10; postpartum 132; pregnancy, psychiatric symptom management 102, 110–111, **111**, 232, **232–233**, 232–235; roles variety 16, 17; sexual health 224–226, **226**; women's health advocacy and policy 411; workplace, work-life balance 15, 16, **19**, 34, 231–232, **231**, 347, 349

middle life women's health 350–354; caregiving responsibilities 353; case study role transition, divorce, stress 365–368; chronic conditions 352; mental health, emotional well-being 352–353; *see also* perimenopause, menopause; physiological changes 350–351; work-life balance and career development 353–354

migraines 317–319; causes, trigger 317; menstrual migraine 317–318; occupational functioning, impact 318, **318**; OT approach and interventions 319, **320**; phases 318, **318**; prevalence 317; types **317**

miscarriage (spontaneous abortion) 139–140, *139*

Model of Human Occupation (MOHO) 68–69

Modified Barthel Index **110**

multiple sclerosis (MS) 325–329; fatigue management 326, 327, 329; high-risk pregnancies **135**, 136; menstruation/pregnancy hormonal effects **325**, 329; mobility management 329; occupational functioning impact 325–326; phases, symptoms **326**; phases: occupational performance changes **326**; phases: OT approaches 327; types **325**

musculoskeletal health and disorder (MSDs): evaluation 31; pregnancy 87, 89, **93**, **94**, 102–103, 106–109, **107–108**, 112, **113–114**; workplace 16

National Institute on Aging 238

neuroanatomical changes in pregnancy: amygdala 92, *93*, 96; bonding preparation 96–97; emotional and cognitive adaptations 96; frontal lobe 93, 95; occipital lobe 96; parietal lobe 95; prefrontal cortex 93, 96; temporal lobe 95–96; white matter 92–93, 95, 96

neuroanatomical diversity 92, *94*

neuroanatomy 92–97; bipotential neonatal brain 92, *94*; lobes 92–96, *95*; male vs female brain 92, *94*

neurological health 317–337; Alzheimer's disease (AD) 329–333, 335–337; case studies 333–337; migraines 317–319; multiple sclerosis (MS) 325–329; stroke 319–324, 333–335; *see also each under own heading*

neuropathy, peripheral 196, 197, 200, 201, 296, **297**, **307**

non-cisgender health needs 203–222; advocacy 28; community and social participation 207–208; competent-provider lack 209; discrimination and bias, health care 208–209; financial/healthcare cost barriers 210; gender diversity terminology **204**; healthcare disparities, access barriers 208–212; inclusive healthcare environment creation 210–215, **213–214**; legal and administrative education and support 218; mental health challenges and interventions 215–217, **216–217**; OT interventions 204–208, 217–218; self-care and health management 207; social support needs 206–207; specific occupational needs 207; unique health needs (AFAB) 203–204

non-cisgender gender-affirming care 204–206, 209–210, **218**; access limitations 209–210; hormone replacement therapy (HRT) 49, 204, 207, 211–212, **211**, **218**, **219**; OT interventions 205–206, 217–219, **217**; puberty blockers **218**; surgical interventions 204–206, 217, **218**

non-cisgender mental health and wellbeing: case study 219–222; challenges 206; community and social participation 207–208; health promotion 215–217, **216–217**; identity and role transitions 207

nutrition, nutrition management 400–405; adaptive equipment, techniques 405; behavioral OT interventions 405; case study, holistic nutrition 416–420; celiac disease 191–192, **192**; cultural factors **24**; diabetes, type 1 and 2 163; eating-related disorders 269–272; education, healthy eating 403; Hashimoto's thyroiditis, hypothyroidism

118, 189; meal planning, preparation 403–405; menopause 163; nutritional needs assessment 403, **404**; obesity and weight management 272–275, 342; OTP role, support 400–402; perimenopause, menopause 170, 351; pregnancy **101**, 118, 235

obesity 272–275; adolescent 342; and anxiety disorder correlation 273; associated health issues 272; body mass index (BMI) 272, **273**; causes, contributing factors 272; emotional, psychological distress 273; lifestyle 278; occupational challenges 273; OT assessment and interventions 273–275, **273**; physical health issues 272; prevalence 269; as public health concern 272

obstetric health management 87–152; case study: postpartum care 145–149; case study: pregnancy care 149–152; childhood disability 140; labor and delivery 123–125; maternal mental health 141–145, 235–237; miscarriage, stillbirth 139–140; postpartum care 125–134; pregnancy 87–97, 134–139; prenatal care 97–123

occupation-centered practice 27–29

Occupational Adaptation (OA) model 69

occupational balance 231–232, **231**, 347, 349, 366

occupational therapy: billing 29–31, **30**, 36–37, **37**; emergence and development 8–10; evaluation, assessment 29–34, **30**; goal setting, treatment planning 34–36; intersectionality 26–27; practitioner roles **18**; women and occupation 25–29

oncology 290–315; breast cancer 290–298, 313–315; case studies 313–315; gynecological cancers **70**, 301–307; lung cancer 298–301, **302**; lymphedema 308–312; *see also* each under own heading

osteoporosis: perimenopausal and menopausal transition 168; pregnancy changes **108**, **114**; physical exercise, sport **394**

ovarian cancer 301, 303, **304**

ovarian cystectomy 73

ovarian cysts **70**, 73

pediatric and adolescent girls' health 339–346; adolescent obesity 342; athletics as meaningful occupation 345–346; case study, adolescent dysmenorrhea 359–361; case study, teen pregnancy 361–364; hygiene product, access 341; obstetric and gynecologic issues 344–345; psychological development and depression 342–343; puberty and menstrual cycle 339–341; sexual abuse, teen pregnancy 343–344; sexually transmitted diseases (STDs) 344; substance use 343

pelvic floor muscles 45–46, *45*, **46**, *48*; assessment 111, **112**; biofeedback 54–*55*; floor health 48–49, 59, 225; exercises 52–54, *54*, *55*, 63; functions / dysfunction 13–14, 45, 48–49, **48**, 51–52, **107**, 111, **112**; pelvic diaphragm 45; sports 345

pelvic health: in OT history 10; rehabilitation research 13–14, 49

pelvic organ prolapses **59**, **60**, 66, 69, **71**, 73, **112**

pelvic organ prolapses repair / pelvic rehabilitation 13–14, 66, 73, **75**, 76, **107**, **112**, 129, **130**

pelvic pain 56–64; assessment, evaluation 57, 59, **60**; characterization 56; related conditions and disorder 56; impact 56–57, **107**; OT strategies **58**–59, 60–64; types **58**–**59**

pelvis and perineum 39–64; anatomy 39–43, *40*; blood vessels and nerves 42–43; bony pelvis anatomy 39–41, *40–41*; health, dysfunction 50–56; joints and ligaments 42; male vs female 41, *41*; *see also* pelvic floor muscles; perineum *48*, 49; pelvic organs 42; reproductive system (internal, external genitalia) 43–45, *44–45*

perimenopause 163–164, 168, 351; hormonal changes **158**; impact daily life and management 163–164, 168–169, **168**; OT interventions 351–352; sexual health changes 171, 172; symptoms, daily 168, **168**

perineum *48*, 49

Person-Environment-Occupation (PEO) model 68

physical activity 275–279; barriers 276, **276**; daily functioning, occupational performance impact 276; hyperthyroidism 159, 161, 162; obesity and 272, **273**, 274, 275; OT assessment and interventions 276–278, **276**; pregnancy, postpartum 121–122, 136, 138; sleep quality 268; WHO recommendation 275

physical activity log 273

Pittsburgh sleep quality index (PSQI) 118, **267**

polycystic ovary syndrome (PCOS) 50, **70**, 81–85, **158**, 160–161

postpartum health and care 125–134, **126**; C-section, postoperative rehabilitation **75**, 126, 127–130, **130**; feeding (breast, bottle) 131–132, 235–238, **236**; infant care training 132–133; mental health, emotional well-being 132; postpartum depression, anxiety, psychosis 142–143; return to work and daily activities 133–134 pregnancy 87–97, 134–139; cardiovascular changes 89; child disabilities 140–141; embryological and fetal development stages **90–91**, *92*; gastrointestinal changes 89; high-risk pregnancies 134–139; hormonal changes 87–88, **88**, 89; *see also* labor and delivery support; miscarriage (spontaneous abortion) 139–140, *139*; *see also* maternal mental health; musculoskeletal changes 87, 89–**90**, 93, *94*, 102–103, 106–109, **107–108**, 112, **113–114**; neuroanatomical differences and changes 92–97, *94*; *see also* neuroanatomy; physiological and anatomical changes 87, **93**; *see also* postpartum care, prenatal care; psychiatric symptoms **232–233**, 232–235; stillbirth 140

pregnant patient evaluation and assessments 103–118; ADLs and IADLs 109–110, **110**; environmental and ergonomic 110; functional mobility 106, 108–109; holistic 116–118; mental health and psychosocial well-being 110–111, **111**; pain 104–106; patient interview and history 103–104, **104**; pelvic floor 111, **112**; physical examination 106, **107–108**; TIC 115–116, **117**

Pregnancy Mobility Index (PMI) 106

Pregnancy-Related Pelvic Girdle Pain Questionnaire (PGQ) **110**

premenstrual syndrome (PMS) **71**, 341

prenatal care 97–123; comprehensive care interventions 97, **98**; emotional, psychological support **98**, 102; environmental modification 102; key areas, holistic approach 100–102, **101**; mental health and psychosocial assessment 110–111, **111**; musculoskeletal issues and dysfunction 102–103, **107–108**, **113–113**; patient evaluation, treatment planning 103–123; physical support/exercises by trimesters 97, 99–100, **99–101**

prenatal care, patient evaluation and treatment planning 103–123; ADLs, IADLs 109–110, **110**; environmental and ergonomic assessment 110; goal setting, treatment planning 112–115, **113–114**; holistic assessment methods 116–118; mobility assessment 106, 108–109; Motivational Interviewing (MI) 121–122; pain assessment 104–106; parenthood, adaptation and compensation strategies 118–121, *119*, *120*; patient interview and history 103–104, **104**; pelvic floor assessment 111, **112**; physical examination 106; trauma-informed care (TIC) 115–116, **117**; unhealthy performance patterns addressing 122–123

professional development empowerment 15–16, **16**, 18–20, **19**

progesterone 50; menopause, perimenopause **158**, 163, 164, 168; menstruation cycle **157**, 340; ovaries 45; pregnancy 50, 88, **88**, **157**; puberty 339; sleep pattern effect 265

PTSD Checklist (PCL) 375

pubic symphysis 40, *40*, 41, 42, **107**, **113**

radiation therapy 294, 300, 304, 308

range of movement (ROM) 64, **65**, 109

reiki 407, **408**

reflexology 407, **408**

reproductive coercion 371

reproductive health, women's health advocacy and policy 411

reproductive system: genitalia (internal, external) 43–45, *44–45*; hormones 49–50; *see also* estrogen; gonadotropins; progesterone

restless legs syndrome (RLS) **266**

rheumatoid arthritis (RA) 178–182; gender specific differences 179–180; OT interventions **180–182**, 182–182; stages 178–179, *179*

rumination disorder **270**

safety assessment 375, **381**

SAMHSA (Substance Abuse and Mental Health Services Administration) 376

sciatica 56, 105, **107**, **113**

self-esteem 20–21, 82, 225, 237, 296, **297**, **302**, 305, **307**

sensitive questioning techniques 25, 374

sexual counseling **226**

sexual health 224, **224–226**; biopsychosocial perspective 224–226; body image concerns 291, 301; dyspareunia **58**, **226**; education, counseling 225; emotional support 225; gynecological cancers **307**; intercourse, pleasure 43–44; OT interventions **226**; pelvic floor health 48–49, 59, 225; perimenopause, menopause 169, 171–172, **226**; physical interventions 225; physical limitations, adaptive strategies 225; relationship and communication skills 225; Sexual Health Inventory for Women (SHIW) 195; sexually transmitted diseases (STDs) 344; stigma 2; systemic lupus erythematosus (SLE) 182–183

sexual violence and coercion 371; adolescent girls 343; inter-partner violence (IPV) 370, 371, 372; political and military conflict zones 2–3

shift work 17, **18**, 266

SLE (systemic lupus erythematosus) 182–185, 194–197; case study 194–197; late onset 185; occupational therapy 136–137, 182, 183–185, **184**; sexual functioning 182; symptoms 182, 183, *183*

sleep and sleep disturbances: apnea **266**; perimenopause, menopause 163–165, 168, **168**, 190, 240, 263–269; Alzheimer's disease (AD) **331**; assessment, interventions 118, 266–269, **266**; case study 285–288; circadian rhythm, melatonin and cortisol fluctuations 264–265, *265*; duration, requirements and lack 264–265, 279; Hashimoto's and hyperthyroidism 160, 190; insomnia 266, **266**, **267**, 268; multiple sclerosis (MS) **326**; non-rapid eye movement (NREM) 263–264; pelvic pain impact 57; pregnancy **88**; rapid eye movement (REM) 264; restless legs syndrome (RLS) **266**; shift work impact 17, **18**; sleep apnea **266**; sleep disorders 266–267, **266**; sleep disturbances impact 265–266; sleep hygiene **98**, 278, 279; sleep-disordered breathing **266**; stroke **321**

SMART (specific, measurable, achievable, relevant, and time-bound) goals 34

sociocultural perspectives of women's health 20; cultural competency **23**, **24**, 380–282, 383–385, **384**; cultural/societal norms 2, 3, 11, 18, 20–22, 23–25, **24**, 280, 291, 371

spinal cord injury **135**, 136

spontaneous abortion (miscarriage) 139–140, *139*

sport: athletes 393–397, 412–415; gender-specific physiological performance impact **394**; holistic health approach 396; injury prevention, rehabilitation 394–395; as meaningful adolescent occupation 345–346; nutritional needs 401; performance enhancement 395–396; physiological challenges 345–346, 393–394, **394**; and psychosocial well-being 396; tai chi 406, **408**; yoga 63, 99, **100**, 169–170, 406, **408**

State-Trait Anxiety Inventory (STAI) 371, 375

stigma: non-cisgender individuals 215; mental health conditions 21, 206; obesity 273; sexual and reproductive health 2

stillbirth 140

Stress Urinary Incontinence (SUI) 51

stroke, cerebrovascular accident (CVA) 319–324; adaptive equipment 324; case study 333–335; cause 333–335; hemorrhagic 319, **320**; ischemic 319, **320**; phases, occupational performance impact and OT approaches 321–324, **321**, **322–324**; sexual health **321**, 324; transient ischemic attack (TIA) / mini stroke **320**; unique post-stroke challenges 324

substance use, addiction 279–282; case study 285–288; contributing factors, causes 279, 280; daily functioning, occupational performance impact 280; and inter-partner violence (IPV) risk 343, 372; OT assessment and interventions 280–282, **280**; and pain management 279; teenage 343

surgical site infection (SSI) 127

systemic lupus erythematosus *see* SLE (systemic lupus erythematosus)

tai chi 406, **408**

technology support 388–393; breast health 388–390; feeding, newborn (breastfeeding, bottle) 131, 237, 389, 391; dressing devices 391–392; heart health 253–255; menstrual management assistance 166, 392–393; reproductive health 388–391; sports, female athletes 393–394

telehealth 11, 170–171, 209, 254

testosterone, testosterone therapy 49, 204, **211**, 358, **394**

thyroid: Hashimoto's thyroiditis 185–190; hyperthyroidism, hypothyroidism 158–160

TNM (Tumor, Nodes, Metastasis) classification system: breast cancer 293; lung cancer 299, **299**

trauma responses: Five F responses (fight, flight, freeze, fawn, flop) 372–373, *373*; inter-partner violence (IPV) 372

Trauma Symptom Inventory (TSI) 375, **381**, 385

trauma-informed care (TIC) 370–378; assessment, evaluation 116, 380, **381–382**; case study IPV and TIC 385–387; community engagement 383–383; cultural competence 383–385, **384**; *see also* inter-partner violence (IPV); non-cisgender clients **217**; OTP integration 375, 380; pregnancy 115–116, **117**; principles 115–116, 376, 379–380; sexual abuse and teen pregnancy 343–344

treatment planning, occupational therapy 34, 35–36

U.S. Transgender Survey (2015) 208

urinary incontinence 13–14, 49, 50–51, 52, 56, 111

urge incontinence 51

uterine (endometrial) cancer 301, 303, **304**

uterine fibroids / uterine fibroid embolization (UFE) 45, 69, **70**, 74

vaginal cancer 301, **304**

valvular heart disease 248

violence against women: advocacy against 412; *see also* inter-partner violence (IPV); political conflict zones 2–3; workplace 17

vulvar cancer 301, 303, **304**

women's health advocacy and policy 409–412; chronic conditions 411; focus, key areas

411–412; mental health 411; reproductive and maternal health 411; strategies 410–411; violence against women 412

women's health movements: 1830s–1900s: early stirrings 7; 1900s–1960s: reproductive rights fight 7; 1970s–1980s: Women's Health Movement, holistic health care 7; 1990s–2000s: advances, challenges 7–8; 2020–Present: global challenges respond 8

work-life balance/integration 15, **16**, **19**, 34, 231–232, **231**, 347, 349

workplace: gender inequities 15–16, **16**; health issues related to 16–17; intersectionality 27; occupational balance 231–232, **231**, 347, 349, 366; OTP role and interventions 18–20, **18–19**; professional development 15–16, **16**, 18–20, **19**; violence 17

World Health Organization (WHO) 6, 230, 235, 301

yoga 63, 99, **100**, 169–170, 406, **408**

Made in the USA
Monee, IL
03 May 2026